Fever of Unknown Origin

Wenhong Zhang • Xinhua Weng
Editors

Fever of Unknown Origin

Integration of Clinical Practice

SSTP

Springer

Editors
Wenhong Zhang
Huashan Hospital
Fudan University
Shanghai, China

Xinhua Weng
Huashan Hospital
Fudan University
Shanghai, China

ISBN 978-981-95-1400-7 ISBN 978-981-95-1401-4 (eBook)
https://doi.org/10.1007/978-981-95-1401-4

The printed edition is not for sale in Mainland of China. Customers from Mainland of China please order the print book from Shanghai Scientific & Technical Publishers.

This Springer imprint is published by the registered company Springer Nature Singapore Pte Ltd.
The registered company address is: 152 Beach Road, #21-01/04 Gateway East, Singapore 189721, Singapore

Preface

For infectious disease physicians, fever of unknown origin (FUO) has always been one of the most challenging syndromes that tests clinical skills. In 1961, Dr. Petersdorf and Dr. Beeson, who were renowned in the field of infectious diseases and rheumatology, first proposed the concept of FUO, which refers to a group of diseases characterized by fever persisting for more than three weeks, with a temperature exceeding 38.3 °C at least three times, and despite at least one week of systematic and comprehensive examination in outpatient or inpatient settings, a definitive diagnosis cannot be reached. With the development of clinical medicine, in 1991, Dr. Durack and Dr. Street proposed that the definition of FUO should be revised for inpatients and specific populations such as the immunocompromised.

FUO can stem from over 200 etiologies, but ultimately, all the causes of FUO can be classified into five categories: neoplastic diseases, infectious diseases, non-infectious inflammatory diseases, other causes, and unknown causes. With the changing times, the spectrum of diseases is also changing. More and more non-infectious disease patients appear in front of us. Among these, there is a particularly unique group of patients who have persistent fever with an elusive cause.

With the improvement of diagnostic technologies, especially in the past two decades with the rapid advancement of molecular biology and imaging technology, our understanding of FUO has taken a step further. Understanding FUO serves as a way for both general practitioners and specialists to quickly improve their clinical reasoning and broaden their medical perspectives.

Fudan University Affiliated Huashan Hospital, originally founded as the general hospital of Red Cross Society in 1907, stands as one of the most esteemed hospitals in China and even internationally, boasting an excellent reputation. Infectious diseases are one of its nationally renowned disciplines, ranking first in China since 2010. The founder of the Department of Infectious Diseases was Professor Dai Ziying who obtained his doctoral degree from Oxford University in 1950, under the mentorship of Howard Walter Florey, who was credited with the successful isolation and purification of penicillin for clinical use. Florey shared the Nobel Prize in Physiology or Medicine in 1945 with Sir Alexander Fleming and Ernst Boris Chain. Professor Dai Ziying is also celebrated as the founder of clinical antibiotic science in China. In 2021, the Huashan Hospital Infection Department was designated as the National Infectious Disease Medical Center because of its tirelessly exploring precise diagnosis and treatment of challenging infectious diseases. Currently, it has become the national referral center for infectious diseases and FUO cases in China.

Since 2012, we have been annually publishing a series of books featuring difficult cases solved in our department, with the 12th volume released in 2023. These series of books have garnered admiration from Chinese clinical doctors. In the present book, we introduced a diagnostic and management algorithm for FUO based on the experiences of our center. Through the selected cases from the previous book series, we hope to systematically demonstrate the basic rules and techniques of managing FUO cases, and to help clinicians improving clinical reasoning. All these cases are divided into four chapters, covering various causes of FUO: infection (such as tuberculosis, endocarditis, HIV infection, malaria, amoebiasis, and histoplasmosis), malignant neoplastic diseases, autoimmune and autoinflammatory diseases, and other causes. Many new diagnostic tools, such as PET/CT (positron emission tomography/computed tomography), mNGS (metagenomics and next-generation sequencing), and whole genome sequencing, also play a great role in diagnosing FUO. We hope this book can provide a practical, clinically oriented, and trainee-friendly resource for the diagnosis and treatment of FUO.

I would like to thank all those who contributed to the preparation of this book. A special thanks goes to the dedicated young staff, especially Ruan Qiaoling, Hu Yuekai, Zhao Huazhen, Zhou Xian, Zhang Bingyan, and Liu Qihui.

Shanghai, China
March 11, 2024

Zhang Wenhong

Editor's List

Editor-in-Chief

Zhang Wenhong, Department of Infectious Diseases, Huashan Hospital, Fudan University, Shanghai, China
Weng Xinhua, Department of Infectious Diseases, Huashan Hospital, Fudan University, Shanghai, China

Editors

Ruan Qiaoling, Department of Infectious Diseases, Huashan Hospital, Fudan University, Shanghai, China
Hu Yuekai, Department of Infectious Diseases, Huashan Hospital, Fudan University, Shanghai, China
Liu Qihui, Department of Infectious Diseases, Huashan Hospital, Fudan University, Shanghai, China
Zhao Huazhen, Department of Infectious Diseases, Huashan Hospital, Fudan University, Shanghai, China
Zhang Bingyan, Department of Infectious Diseases, Huashan Hospital, Fudan University, Shanghai, China
Zhou Xian, Department of Infectious Diseases, Huashan Hospital, Fudan University, Shanghai, China

Other Members of the Editors

Chen Chen, Department of Infectious Diseases, Huashan Hospital, Fudan University, Shanghai, China
Chen Mingquan, Department of Infectious Diseases, Huashan Hospital, Fudan University, Shanghai, China
Chen Peidong, Department of Infectious Diseases, Huashan Hospital, Fudan University, Shanghai, China
Chen Shu, Department of Infectious Diseases, Huashan Hospital, Fudan University, Shanghai, China

Fan Qingqi, Department of Infectious Diseases, Jing'an District Central Hospital of Shanghai, China
Hu Yuekai, Department of Infectious Diseases, Huashan Hospital, Fudan University, Shanghai, China
Huang Yuxian, Department of Infectious Diseases, Huashan Hospital, Fudan University, Shanghai, China
Jin Jialin, Department of Infectious Diseases, Huashan Hospital, Fudan University, Shanghai, China
Jiang Weimin, Department of Infectious Diseases, Huashan Hospital, Fudan University, Shanghai, China
Li Ning, Department of Infectious Diseases, Huashan Hospital, Fudan University, Shanghai, China
Li Qian, Department of Infectious Diseases, Huashan Hospital, Fudan University, Shanghai, China
Li Tao, Department of Infectious Diseases, Huashan Hospital, Fudan University, Shanghai, China
Liu Qihui, Department of Infectious Diseases, Huashan Hospital, Fudan University, Shanghai, China
Liu Yuanyuan, Department of Infectious Diseases, Huashan Hospital, Fudan University, Shanghai, China
Mao Richeng, Department of Infectious Diseases, Huashan Hospital, Fudan University, Shanghai, China
Qin Yanli, Department of Infectious Diseases, Huashan Hospital, Fudan University, Shanghai, China
Ruan Qiaoling, Department of Infectious Diseases, Huashan Hospital, Fudan University, Shanghai, China
Shao Lingyun, Department of Infectious Diseases, Huashan Hospital, Fudan University, Shanghai, China
Sun Feng, Department of Infectious Diseases, Huashan Hospital, Fudan University, Shanghai, China
Wang Ting, Department of Infectious Diseases, Jing'an District Central Hospital of Shanghai, China
Wang Xuan, Department of Infectious Diseases, Huashan Hospital, Fudan University, Shanghai, China
Wang Xinyu, Department of Infectious Diseases, Huashan Hospital, Fudan University, Shanghai, China
Wen Xiao, Department of Infectious Diseases, Jing'an District Central Hospital of Shanghai, China
Xu Bin, Department of Infectious Diseases, Huashan Hospital, Fudan University, Shanghai, China
Yang Feifie, Department of Infectious Diseases, Huashan Hospital, Fudan University, Shanghai, China
Yu Shenglei, Department of Infectious Diseases, Huashan Hospital, Fudan University, Shanghai, China

Zhang Bingyan, Department of Infectious Diseases, Huashan Hospital, Fudan University, Shanghai, China
Zhang Jiming, Department of Infectious Diseases, Huashan Hospital, Fudan University, Shanghai, China
Zhang Shu, Department of Infectious Diseases, Huashan Hospital, Fudan University, Shanghai, China
Zhao Huazhen, Department of Infectious Diseases, Huashan Hospital, Fudan University, Shanghai, China
Zheng Jianming, Department of Infectious Diseases, Huashan Hospital, Fudan University, Shanghai, China
Zhu Haoxiang, Department of Infectious Diseases, Huashan Hospital, Fudan University, Shanghai, China
Zhu Liping, Department of Infectious Diseases, Huashan Hospital, Fudan University, Shanghai, China

Translators

Chen Jingwen, Department of Infectious Diseases, Huashan Hospital, Fudan University, Shanghai, China
Cheng Jiahui, Department of Infectious Diseases, Huashan Hospital, Fudan University, Shanghai, China
Fu Zhangfan, Department of Infectious Diseases, Huashan Hospital, Fudan University, Shanghai, China
Ge Shijia, Department of Infectious Diseases, Huashan Hospital, Fudan University, Shanghai, China
Guo Xiaoxiao, Department of Infectious Diseases, Huashan Hospital, Fudan University, Shanghai, China
Han Jiajia, Department of Infectious Diseases, Huashan Hospital, Fudan University, Shanghai, China
He Jingjing, Department of Infectious Diseases, Huashan Hospital, Fudan University, Shanghai, China
He Zhangyufan, Department of Infectious Diseases, Huashan Hospital, Fudan University, Shanghai, China
Hua Wenya, Department of Infectious Diseases, Huashan Hospital, Fudan University, Shanghai, China
Huo Meisi, Department of Infectious Diseases, Huashan Hospital, Fudan University, Shanghai, China
Li Rong, Department of Infectious Diseases, Huashan Hospital, Fudan University, Shanghai, China
Lin Ke, Department of Infectious Diseases, Huashan Hospital, Fudan University, Shanghai, China
Lin Siran, Department of Infectious Diseases, Huashan Hospital, Fudan University, Shanghai, China

Liu Wanling, Department of Infectious Diseases, Huashan Hospital, Fudan University, Shanghai, China
Luo Yu, Department of Infectious Diseases, Huashan Hospital, Fudan University, Shanghai, China
Qi Xiao, Department of Infectious Diseases, Huashan Hospital, Fudan University, Shanghai, China
Qin Xiangyu, Department of Infectious Diseases, Huashan Hospital, Fudan University, Shanghai, China
Wang Hongyu, Department of Infectious Diseases, Huashan Hospital, Fudan University, Shanghai, China
Wang Xuyang, Department of Infectious Diseases, Huashan Hospital, Fudan University, Shanghai, China
Weng Taoping, Department of Infectious Diseases, Huashan Hospital, Fudan University, Shanghai, China
Yang Jingshu, Department of Infectious Diseases, Huashan Hospital, Fudan University, Shanghai, China
Yang Qingluan, Department of Infectious Diseases, Huashan Hospital, Fudan University, Shanghai, China
You Ruirui, Department of Infectious Diseases, Huashan Hospital, Fudan University, Shanghai, China
Zhang Chubin, Department of Infectious Diseases, Huashan Hospital, Fudan University, Shanghai, China
Zhang Haocheng, Department of Infectious Diseases, Huashan Hospital, Fudan University, Shanghai, China
Zhang Lu, Department of Infectious Diseases, Huashan Hospital, Fudan University, Shanghai, China
Zhang Miaoqu, Department of Infectious Diseases, Huashan Hospital, Fudan University, Shanghai, China
Zhang Qiran, Department of Infectious Diseases, Huashan Hospital, Fudan University, Shanghai, China
Zhang Wei, Department of Infectious Diseases, Huashan Hospital, Fudan University, Shanghai, China
Zhang Yi, Department of Infectious Diseases, Huashan Hospital, Fudan University, Shanghai, China
Zhang Yu, Department of Infectious Diseases, Huashan Hospital, Fudan University, Shanghai, China
Zhou Jingyu, Department of Infectious Diseases, Huashan Hospital, Fudan University, Shanghai, China
Zhou Linghong, Department of Infectious Diseases, Huashan Hospital, Fudan University, Shanghai, China

Contents

1 **Fever of Unknown Origin** 1
Zhang Wenhong, Ruan Qiaoling, Liu Qihui, Zhao Huazhen, Zhang Bingyan, and Zhou Xian

2 **Fever of Unknown Origin in Infectious Diseases** 15
Zhang Wenhong, Zhu Liping, Wang Ruiying, Jiang Weimin, Hu Yuekai, Huang Yuxian, Wang Ting, Jin Jialin, Zhang Jiming, Li Qian, Shao Lingyun, Yu Shenglei, Liu Yuanyuan, Xu Bin, Mao Richeng, Zhu Haoxiang, Wang Xuan, Lin Jie, Dong Minhui, Zhu Beidi, Wang Xinyu, Yang Yuling, Zhang Shu, Li Tao, Zhu Zuiyun, Li Ning, Li Yuxin, Wang Chao, Chen Mingquan, Jia Wen, Weng Shanshan, Zhu Xiaoxue, Liang Daobin, Yang Feifie, Zhou Xian, Chen Shu, Zheng Jianming, Lin Siran, Liang Jun, Li Li, Liu Hong, and Zhong Wen

3 **Fever of Unknown Origin in Malignant Diseases** 157
Li Ning, Chen Shu, Mao Richeng, Zou Mingde, He Fanrong, Wu Ping, Chen Mingquan, Zhang Jiming, Shao Lingyun, Huang Yuxian, Zhang Wenhong, Chen Peidong, Jia Wen, Zheng Jianming, Du Zunguo, Zhang Bingyan, and Jin Jialin

4 **Fever of Unknown Origin in Noninfectious Inflammatory Diseases** 211
Jin Jialin, Chen Mingquan, Yang Feifie, Chen Shu, Huang Yuxian, Bao Suxia, Zheng Jianming, Li Ning, Zhang Jiming, Fan Qingqi, Jia Wen, Shao Lingyun, Zhang Wenhong, Liu Yuanyuan, Qin Yanli, Zhang Shu, Hu Yuekai, Zhang Yanliang, Ruan Qiaoling, Wu Jing, and Wang Xinyu

5 **Fever of Unknown Origin Other Disease** 277
Chen Chen, Chen Shu, Yu Shenglei, Zhu Chong, Li Ning, Zhang Jiming, Zhu Haoxiang, Sun Feng, Wang Ting, Yang Feifie, Huang Yuxian, and Liu Qihui

Fever of Unknown Origin

1

Zhang Wenhong, Ruan Qiaoling, Liu Qihui, Zhao Huazhen, Zhang Bingyan, and Zhou Xian

1.1 Clinical Overview and Perspective

The diagnosis of prolonged fevers has posed a clinical challenge for centuries. In 1907, the related concepts of "fever of unknown origin," "fever of undetermined origin," and "unexplained fever" appeared. The original diagnostic criteria for fever of unknown origin (FUO), established by Petersdorf and Beeson in 1961, required a fever ≥38.3 °C (101 °F) persisting for over 3 weeks, remaining undiagnosed after one week of inpatient evaluation. Evaluation of fever of unknown origin (FUO) can be conducted in the outpatient setting. Petersdorf further categorized FUO into four major groups: infectious, malignant (neoplastic), rheumatic or non-infectious inflammatory, and miscellaneous disorders. In 1991, D. T. Durack and A. C. Street refined the FUO definition initially outlined by R. B. Petersdorf in 1961. They suggested differentiating classical FUO from three specific subtypes: nosocomial FUO, neutropenic FUO, and HIV-associated FUO (Table 1.1). This refined classification reflects significant differences in disease patterns, with the latter groups more frequently associated with infections, malignancies, and drug-induced cases. Additionally, the diagnostic and management approaches for these subtypes require distinct clinical considerations. In this book, we will focus on the classical FUO.

In China, "fever of unknown origin" first appeared in literature in 1962. In 1981, Xin-hua Weng and Zhao-yue Xu published the first article that described the epidemiology of fevers of unknown origin and the categories of causes.

Z. Wenhong (✉) · R. Qiaoling · L. Qihui · Z. Huazhen · Z. Bingyan · Z. Xian
Department of Infectious Diseases, Huashan Hospital, Fudan University, Shanghai, China
e-mail: zhangwenhong@fudan.edu.cn

W. Zhang, X. Weng (eds.), *Fever of Unknown Origin*,
https://doi.org/10.1007/978-981-95-1401-4_1

Table 1.1 Definitions of fever of unknown origin (FUO)

Type	Definition
Classical FUO	Repeated fever episodes of ≥38.3 °C Duration lasting at least 3 weeks Diagnosis remains unclear after 3 days of thorough in-hospital evaluation or following three outpatient visits
Nosocomial FUO	Occurs in hospitalized patients Repeated fever episodes of ≥38.3 °C No infection present or incubating at admission Diagnosis remains unclear after 3 days of comprehensive investigations, including microbiological cultures incubated for at least 48 h
Neutropenic FUO	Neutrophil count below $500/mm^3$ Repeated fever episodes of ≥38.3 °C Diagnosis remains unclear after 3 days despite detailed investigations, with a minimum 48-h incubation of cultures
HIV-associated FUO	Confirmed HIV infection Repeated fever episodes of ≥38.3 °C Duration of fever ≥4 weeks for outpatients or ≥3 days for hospitalized patients Diagnosis remains unclear after 3 days of appropriate investigations, including at least 48 h of incubation of microbiological cultures

Fevers of unknown origin remain a difficult diagnostic challenge because over 200 disorders are in the differential diagnosis. The courses of fevers of unknown origin can be classified into four categories: infectious, malignant/neoplastic, rheumatic/noninfectious inflammatory, and miscellaneous disorders. The causes of fever of unknown origin (FUO) can vary depending on patient age, geographic location, time period, and the level of available medical resources. Here, we list several causes of FUO by category and prevalence (Table 1.2).

Usually, FUO patients have a long course of the disease, and abuse of antibiotics, glucocorticoids, and antipyretics is common in clinical practice. This not only wastes a lot of medical resources but also delays and interferes with the correct diagnosis and treatment of the disease. Therefore, when dealing with similar patients, it is crucial to emphasize finding the causes of FUO. Currently, there is no generally accepted diagnostic protocol for fever of unknown origin (FUO). Effective evaluation relies on an FUO-relevant history, detailed physical examination, and critical use of nonspecific laboratory investigations, rather than excessive testing.

Table 1.2 Classification and prevalence of etiologies of fever of unknown origin

Category	Common diseases	Uncommon diseases	Rare diseases
Infectious disease			
Bacterial	Bacterial abscess (abdominal cavity, pelvic cavity, central nervous system (CNS)), infective endocarditis, odontogenic infection, pyelonephritis, extrapulmonary tuberculosis (kidney, bone, and CNS), nontuberculous mycobacterial infection, listeriosis, Bruce mycosis, Legionnaires' disease, typhoid fever, nocardiasis, chronic sinusitis, infectious aneurysm, etc.	Pylephlebitis, implant infections, Yersinia infection, chronic meningococcalemia, gonorrhea, actinomycosis, spinal osteomyelitis, etc.	Suppurative thrombophlebitis of the internal jugular vein, mediastinitis, aortoenteric fistula, rat-bite fever (*Streptobacillus moniliformis* infection), xanthogranulomatous pyelonephritis, etc.
Fungal	Aspergillosis, candidiasis, cryptococcosis, *Pneumocystis jiroveci* pneumonia, etc.	Histoplasmosis, blastomycosis, sporotrichosis, coccidioidomycosis, malassezia infection, etc.	Zygomycosis, paracoccidioidomycosis, etc.
Parasitic	Amoebiasis, toxoplasmosis, malaria, echinococcosis, etc.	*Babesia*, leishmaniasis, fascioliasis, liver fluke, schistosomiasis, etc.	Trichinosis, strongyloidosis, trypanosomiasis, etc.
Other	Lyme disease, Epstein-Barr virus infection, cytomegalovirus infection, rickettsial disease, etc.	Psittacosis (*Chlamydia psittaci* infection), leptospirosis, ehrlichiosis, syphilis, cat scratch disease (*Bartonella henselae* infection), etc.	Venereal lymphogranuloma (*Chlamydia trachomatis* infection), Whipple disease (*Tropheryma whipplei* infection), louse-borne relapsing fever (*Borrelia recurrentis* infection), tick-borne relapsing fever (*Borrelia duttonii* infection), microspirillum infection, Rocky Mountain spotted fever, etc.
Non-infectious inflammatory disease			

(continued)

Table 1.2 (continued)

Category	Common diseases	Uncommon diseases	Rare diseases
Autoimmune disease	Systemic lupus erythematosus, temporal arteritis/polymyalgia rheumatica, dermatomyositis/polymyositis, Behçet's disease, ankylosing spondylitis, autoimmune hepatitis, mixed connective tissue disease, reactive arthritis, rheumatic fever, etc.	Polyarteritis nodosa, Takayasu arteritis, relapsing polychondritis, Sjogren's syndrome, sarcoidosis, urticarial vasculitis, allergic vasculitis, Churg–Strauss syndrome (eosinophilic granulomatosis with polyangiitis), antiphospholipid syndrome, cryoglobulinemia, Felty syndrome (rheumatoid arthritis, splenomegaly, and neutropenia syndrome), etc.	Vogt–Koyanagi–Harada syndrome (uveomeningoencephalitis syndrome), etc.
Autoinflammatory disease	Adult Still's disease, Crohn's disease, ulcerative colitis, hemophagocytic lymphohistiocytosis, gout, etc.	Pseudogout, Sweet's syndrome, recurrent idiopathic pericarditis, etc.	Blau syndrome (early onset granulomatous arthritis, uveitis, and skin rash), cryopyrin-associated periodic syndromes, deficiency of the interleukin-1 receptor antagonist (DIRA), familial Mediterranean fever, PAPA syndrome (pyogenic arthritis, pyoderma gangrenosum, and acne), PFAPA syndrome (periodic fevers with aphthous stomatitis, pharyngitis, and adenitis), SAPHO syndrome (synovitis, acne, pustulosis, hyperostosis, and osteitis), Schnitzler syndrome (chronic urticaria, recurrent fever, bone pain, arthralgia or arthritis, and lymphadenopathy), tumor necrosis factor receptor-associated periodic syndrome (TRAPS), hyperimmunoglobulin D syndrome (HIDS), etc.

Category	Common diseases	Uncommon diseases	Rare diseases
Neoplastic disease			
Hematological malignancies	Lymphoma, preleukemia /acute myeloid leukemia, myelodysplastic disease, multiple myeloma, myelodysplastic syndrome, plasmacytoma, etc.	Castleman disease, bone marrow fibrosis, amyloidosis, etc.	Systemic mastocytosis, etc.
Solid malignant tumor	Liver and CNS metastases, renal cell carcinoma, liver cancer, colon cancer, pancreatic cancer, breast cancer, CNS tumors, etc.		
Benign tumor		Cavernous liver hemangioma, atrial myxoma, angiomyoma, etc.	
Others	Acute disseminated encephalomyelitis, drug fever, subacute thyroiditis, factitious fever, subacute necrotizing lymphadenitis, etc.	Adrenal insufficiency, aneurysm, Mollaret's meningitis, Caroli disease (congenital dilatation of the intrahepatic bile ducts), complex partial status epilepticus, extrinsic allergic alveolitis, pulmonary embolism, nonbacterial osteitis, pyoderma gangrenosum, tubulointerstitial nephritis and uveitis syndrome (TINU), etc.	POEMS syndrome (Polyneuropathy, Organomegaly, Endocrinopathy, Monoclonal protein, and Skin changes), cyclic neutropenia, primary hyperparathyroidism, retroperitoneal fibrosis, anhidrotic ectodermal dysplasia, Erdheim-Chester disease, Fabry disease (angiokeratoma corporis diffusum), Gaucher disease (glucocerebrosidosis), Hamman-Rich syndrome (acute interstitial pneumonia), Rosai-Dorfman disease (sinus histiocytosis with massive lymphadenopathy), thrombosis, inflammatory pseudotumor, linear immunoglobulin-A bullous dermatosis, myotonic dystrophy, post-cardiac injury syndromes, sclerosing mesenteritis, etc.

1.2 Clinical Diagnostic Approaches

The etiology of FUO is complex, and the clinical manifestations are diverse. However, if clinicians could collect a comprehensive medical history, perform a detailed physical examination, and take necessary laboratory examinations, most of the causes of fever can be identified.

For clinical management of classical FUO, we suggest a stepwise diagnostic approach as follows (Fig. 1.1). The diagnosis and treatment process includes four steps: 1. Determine whether the patient belongs to classical FUO; 2. Stage 1st: initial screening; 3. Stage 2nd: specific examination; 4. Treatment (including symptomatic treatment and diagnostic treatment).

When we are making a diagnosis, we should obey the role of clinical thinking. First of all, the accuracy of diagnosis can be significantly improved by carrying out

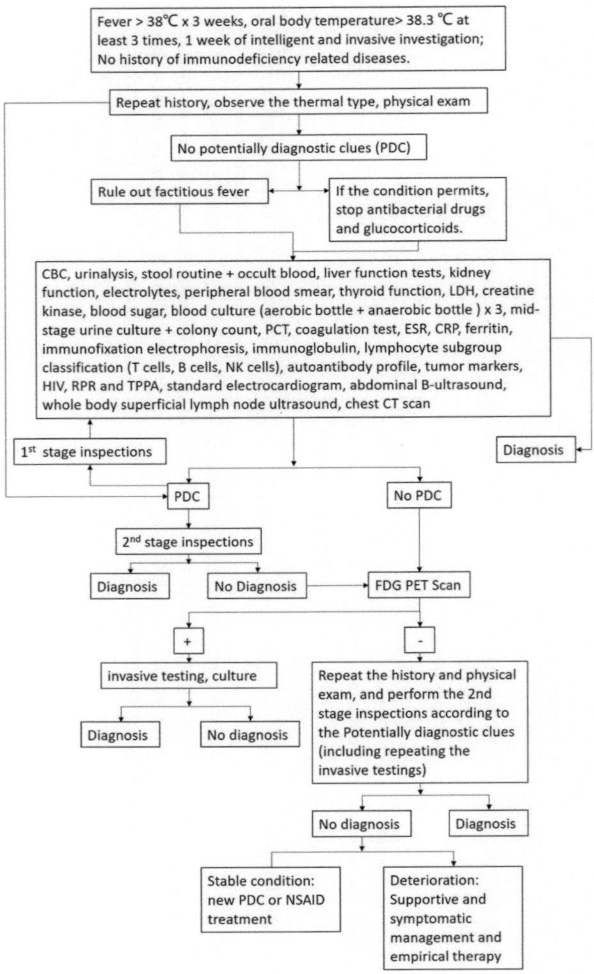

Fig. 1.1 Suggested diagnostic and management algorithm for fever of unknown origin (FUO). The approach should be individualized on the basis of the specific clinical scenario. *CBC* complete blood count, *CRP* C-reactive protein, *CT* computed tomography, *ESR* erythrocyte sedimentation rate, *FDG PET-CT* ^{18}F-fluorodeoxyglucose positron-emission tomography with CT, *HIV* human immunodeficiency virus, *LDH* lactate dehydrogenase, *NSAID* nonsteroidal anti-inflammatory drug, *PCR* polymerase chain reaction, *PCT* procalcitonin, *RF* rheumatoid factor, *RPR* rapid plasma reagin test, *TPPA Treponema pallidum* antibody, *TSH* thyrotropin

etiological diagnosis and differential diagnosis according to the following sequence of thinking: First, the common clinical manifestations of common diseases are considered; second, consider the rare clinical manifestations of common diseases; third, the common clinical manifestations of rare diseases were considered; and finally, the clinical manifestations of rare diseases should be carefully identified.

1.3 History

A comprehensive history is a cornerstone of the evaluation of FUO. Special attention should be paid to patients with FUO:

1. Verification of Fever and Fever Pattern

   The first step in evaluating a patient with FUO is to verify the presence of fever. If necessary, record the oral and rectal temperatures at the same time. In fact, a series of patients who complain of fever have been proven to have disguised fever or no significant fever at all.

   Many febrile diseases have a special fever pattern, which can sometimes play a role in prompting diagnosis. For example, sustained fever is more common in typhoid fever, typhus, lobar pneumonia, etc.; remittent fever is more common in rheumatic fever, sepsis, and systemic inflammation reaction symptoms, as well as in liver abscess, severe tuberculosis, etc.; intermittent fever can be found in malaria, pyelonephritis, lymphoma, etc.; irregular fever can be seen in influenza, amebic liver abscess, tuberculosis, etc.; and undulant fever is common in brucellosis.

   It should be noted that during the course of the disease, two or more fever patterns may present at the same time and interact with each other, such as lobar pneumonia complicated by empyema and lung abscess. The fever pattern can change from a typical sustained fever to a remittent fever. On the other hand, due to the widespread application of antibacterial drugs, the infection could be controlled in time. The fever pattern can also become atypical due to the application of antipyretic drugs and adrenal cortex hormones. In addition, the fever pattern is also related to individual reactions. For example, in shock-type pneumonia in the elderly, the fever may not be high or may not even be present. Therefore, a specific analysis should be made for patients with fever in order to make a correct diagnosis of the disease.
2. Fever Course and Accompanying Syndrome

   The duration of the fever is of great reference value for FUO diagnosis. Generally speaking, a patient with a short fever duration and obvious toxic symptoms (such as fatigue and chills) is likely to have a diagnosis of infectious diseases. And they may show a good treatment response to interventions like antibiotics, lesion resection, or abscess drainage. Tumors are more common in those with moderate fever duration and gradual exhaustion. A long fever duration, absence of toxic symptoms, and alternating episodes and remissions are conducive to the diagnosis of connective tissue diseases. A study showed that only 6% of FUO patients with a fever duration of more than 6 months were finally diagnosed with infectious diseases.

Accompanying syndromes, such as fever with chills, conjunctival congestion, skin rash, respiratory symptoms, neurological symptoms, cardiovascular system symptoms, gastrointestinal symptoms, jaundice, hepatomegaly, splenomegaly, lymphadenopathy, and bleeding phenomena, have important reference value. The corresponding diagnosis can be made according to the characteristics of symptoms and signs.

3. Medical History

A comprehensive medical history is an important part of correct diagnosis, especially in patients with a long-standing fever who lack objective physical signs. Routine medical history interviews could miss some vital information due to the patient's unclear memory. Retracing the medical history can sometimes provide new clues for the final diagnosis. Special attention should be paid to the history of fever, medication, surgery, blood transfusion, animal contact, occupation, hobbies, and travel. For example, brucellosis is more common in people engaged in animal husbandry (especially animal delivery); homosexuals and intravenous drug addicts are more likely to be diagnosed with AIDS or combined opportunistic infections.

1.4 Physical Examinations

Clinicians need to observe the general condition of the patient daily, including the skin, nail beds, lymph nodes, facial features, heart, lungs, liver, gallbladder, spleen, vulva, anus, spine, limbs, and nervous system, among others. It is necessary to pay attention to the newly appearing symptoms and signs, especially transient symptoms and signs, and to perform relevant examinations accordingly, as this can be of great significance for the diagnosis.

1.5 Laboratory Investigations

Laboratory tests are of great significance in diagnosis, but they should be selectively and purposefully carried out based on specific cases. If necessary, they should be repeated to increase the positive rate. Clinical diagnosis should be based neither on an overreliance on test results nor on a neglect of them. It is unrealistic to screen all patients with FUO for all causes. It not only increases the economic burden on society and patients but also complicates some cases that can be easily diagnosed.

The nonspecific auxiliary examinations that are suitable for FUO are mostly cheap, common, noninvasive, or minimally traumatic. Recommended examinations include the following: a. Basic Blood & Urine Tests (blood routine, urine routine, stool routine + occult blood; liver function, kidney function, electrolytes; DIC complete set; blood sugar, lactate dehydrogenase, creatine kinase; erythrocyte sedimentation rate, C-reactive protein, procalcitonin, ferritin). b. Infectious Disease Workup (lood culture [aerobic + anaerobic bottles]; mid-stream urine culture + colony count; HIV, TPPA, RPR) c. Hematologic & Immunologic Studies (peripheral blood smear; immunofixation, immunoglobulin levels; lymphocyte subset analysis [T-cells, B-cells, NK cells]; autoantibody profile). d. Other Specialized Tests (thyroid function; tumor markers). e. Imaging & Procedures (electrocardiogram; abdominal ultrasound; superficial lymph nodes ultrasound; chest CT). After the first stage of routine screening, some patients will have a clear diagnosis. Others may have diagnostic clues that require specific examinations such as tumor markers, autoimmune antibodies, CT, MRI, radionuclide, PET/CT, etc. Histopathologic examination of tissues obtained by excisional biopsy, needle biopsy, or laparotomy can provide a definitive diagnosis in some cases. An etiological diagnosis is always the most important evidence in the diagnosis of infectious diseases. Traditional pathogenic diagnosis depends on blood culture, sputum culture, or culture from any other sterile body fluid. Recently, with the development of molecular diagnostic technologies like *metagenomics, next-generation sequencing*, *GeneXpert MTB/RIF, and FilmArray*, clinicians have been able to identify a series of rare and complicated infectious diseases.

1.6 Treatment Principles for FUO

1.6.1 Control of the Body Temperature

If a patient has a fever with body temperature ≤39 °C, he should maintain the balance of water and electrolytes without antipyretic treatment. Antipyretic treatment can interfere with the type of fever, cover the relationship between body temperature and pulse (for example, making the pulse become relatively slower), etc. It can not only affect the diagnosis and prognosis but also affect the evaluation of the treatment effect. Fever is considered to be an important defense mechanism of the body. Whether it is physical cooling or antipyretic drugs, it will reduce or even eliminate the synthesis of inflammatory mediators and weaken the body's defenses. In addition, there are adverse reactions to antipyretic treatment. Physical cooling accelerates heat loss through skin heat transfer, resulting in convulsion and evaporation, which can cause chills, blood vessel contractions, coronary spasms, and reflexive hypothermia. The use of antipyretic drugs can cause a sudden drop in body temperature accompanied by a large amount of sweating, which can easily lead to shock. These drugs also carry risks of liver and kidney toxicity and gastrointestinal bleeding.

1.6.2 High Temperature >39 °C or Hyperpyrexia Lasting for a Long Time

Hyperthermia not only increases the metabolic rate but also triggers an excessive immune response, causing acid-base balance disorders, cell protein degeneration, tissue hypoxia, and multiple system damage. It can even cause changes in consciousness, such as confusion, disorientation, and epilepsy. At this time, physical cooling and antipyretic drugs should be used to lower the core body temperature below 39 °C. Water and electrolyte balance should be maintained. Sedation and anti-epileptic treatment should be given. It is not recommended to use physical cooling alone when the body temperature regulation mechanism is normal. The reason is that it will increase thermogenesis, metabolic rate, and oxygen consumption. It is recommended to only use it in combination with antipyretic drugs to lower the set point of body temperature. For patients with hyperthermia >40 °C or who may be at risk of brain damage or septic shock, the skin should be wiped with cold or ice water or a fan, an ice blanket, and an ice pack should be used to increase water evaporation to quickly control the core body temperature and protect the organ functions while using antipyretics.

1.6.3 Diagnostic Therapy

When some specific diseases are suspected clinically, but there is no evidence, diagnostic treatment can be carried out without further examination to make a clinical diagnosis based on the obtained curative effect. For example, for patients with epidemiological history and suspected malaria, if the malaria parasite is not found in multiple blood smears or bone marrow smears, they can try antimalarial drugs for treatment. After successful treatment, clinical diagnosis of malaria can be achieved. For patients suspected of tuberculosis infection, diagnostic anti-tuberculosis treatment can also be administered. However, it needs to be pointed out that the observation time should be long enough for the diagnosis and treatment of suspected tuberculosis patients, generally more than 3 to 4 weeks, during which attention should be paid to the adverse reactions of antituberculosis drugs and changes in the condition. Other diseases, such as amoebic liver abscess, are also common diseases that can be diagnosed and treated. It must be pointed out that the diagnostic treatment should use specific, effective, and safe therapeutic drugs; the dosage should be sufficient and the entire course of treatment should be completed; and the therapeutic drugs should not be changed without special reasons. Only in this way can the diagnostic treatment be effective before it can be used as a basis for clinical diagnosis.

1.6.4 Empirical Use of Antimicrobial Agents

In classic FUO, the use of antimicrobial drugs should be strictly based on clinical etiological evidence. In the case where pathogenic evidence is not available but clinically suspected of infection, clinicians need to analyze possible infection sites, make empirical pathogenic judgments, and strictly follow the indications for the use of antimicrobial drugs. After necessary laboratory examinations and various culture specimens are taken, empirical anti-infection treatment can be given based on the preliminary clinical diagnosis. Currently, there is a phenomenon of abuse of antimicrobial drugs in the clinical practice of FUO. Not only does it cause a huge economic waste and a decrease in the positive rate of pathogenic examinations, but it can also cause adverse drug reactions, drug fever, double infection, and the production of drug-resistant bacteria, which interfere with the correct diagnosis of the primary disease. Therefore, in clinical practice of FUO, the application of antimicrobial drugs should not be used as a means of routine diagnostic treatment. For patients who are clinically suspected of infectious fever, they should actively retain specimens to search for pathogenic evidence.

1.6.5 The Use of Glucocorticoids

Glucocorticoids have inhibitory effects on both infectious and non-infectious inflammations, so they have a good antipyretic effect on fever due to most causes, including infection, connective tissue disease, and tumors. In addition, glucocorticoids can also dilate blood vessels, improve microcirculation, enhance myocardial contraction, and improve the body's tolerance to bacterial endotoxins. It can be used for the treatment of shock, multiple organ failure, and severe inflammatory response syndrome. However, due to the remarkable curative effect, the abuse of steroids in fever patients in primary hospitals has become increasingly serious. The abuse of steroids not only changes the original fever type and clinical manifestations and makes diagnosis more difficult, but long-term use can also spread potentially infectious diseases or induce double infections, delaying necessary treatment. Therefore, in principle, it is not recommended to use steroids in patients with FUO, especially not as antipyretic drugs.

1.6.6 Long-Term Follow-Up

About 4.7% to 19.2% of patients still cannot be diagnosed after a comprehensive assessment. For some patients with mild symptoms whose cause is still unclear after detailed examination, long-term follow-up can be carried out in specialist clinics to observe changes. Some patients need nonsteroidal anti-inflammatory drugs to control their symptoms. If there are new clues, they need to be readmitted to the hospital and evaluated according to the FUO diagnostic process. Some patients do not experience any disease progression during long-term follow-up, and usually have favourable prognosis.

1.7 17 Recommendations Based on Expert Consensus on Clinical Management of Fever of Unknown Origin

Recommendation 1: "Fever of unknown origin (FUO)" was suggested as the unified name.

Recommendation 2: FUO can be divided into four categories: classical FUO, FUO in hospitalized patients, FUO in patients with agranulocytosis, and FUO in HIV-infected patients.

Recommendation 3: The diagnosis of classical FUO should be combined with the course of disease, temperature, and previous disease history. It should be noted that the patients should be those who cannot be diagnosed after a comprehensive examination.

Recommendation 4: Systematic and comprehensive examination should include blood routine test, urine routine test, fecal routine test and occult blood, liver function, renal function, electrolytes, blood culture (from 3 different parts at different times), chest X-ray, and abdominal ultrasound (liver, gallbladder, pancreas, spleen, and kidney).

Recommendation 5: A complete history collection should include a complete thermal record, thermal type analysis, accompanying symptoms, examination results in other hospitals, and a detailed history.

Recommendation 6: Body temperature monitoring should be conducted at least four times a day. When a central system-associated fever is considered, the body temperature of multiple parts can be measured at the same time.

Recommendation 7: The general condition of patients should be observed and evaluated once a day, including skin, nail bed, lymph node, five senses, heart, lung, liver, gallbladder, spleen, vulva and anus, spine, limbs, and nervous system. Special attention should be paid to new symptoms and signs, especially transient ones.

Recommendation 8: It is suggested that the screening items in the first stage should include blood routine test, urine routine test, stool routine test + occult blood, liver function, renal function, electrolyte, peripheral blood smear, thyroid function, lactate dehydrogenase, creatine kinase, blood glucose, blood culture (aerobic and anaerobic bottle), midstream urine culture and colony count, procalcitonin, DIC, erythrocyte sedimentation rate, C-reactive protein, ferritin, immunofixation electrophoresis, immunoglobulin, lymphocyte subsets (T lymphocyte, B lymphocyte, natural killer cell), autoantibody spectrum, tumor markers, HIV, syphilis RPR and TPPA, standard electrocardiogram, ultrasound of abdomen and whole body superficial lymph node, and chest CT scan.

Recommendation 9: Two principles should be paid attention to in the second stage: high specificity and from noninvasive to invasive procedures.

Recommendation 10: In cases difficult to diagnose, invasive examination for clinical clues can be repeated if necessary.

Recommendation 11: PET CT or PET MRI is not recommended as a routine screening method for FUO. The significance of PET CT is to indicate the location of suspicious lesions and to point out the direction for further examination.

Recommendation 12: For fever with body temperature no more than 39 °C, it is recommended to maintain the balance of water and electrolytes without treatment of fever.

Recommendation 13: For fever with body temperature between 39 °C and 40 °C, physical cooling and antipyretic drugs should be actively used to reduce the core body temperature below 39 °C and maintain the balance of water and electrolytes. It is not recommended to use physical cooling alone when the temperature regulation mechanism is normal.

Recommendation 14: For fever patients whose body temperature is more than 40 °C or who may have the risk of brain tissue damage or septic shock, it is suggested to wipe the skin with cold water or ice water or use fans, ice blankets, and ice bags after wiping the skin to increase the evaporation of water, on the basis of antipyretic drugs.

Recommendation 15: Diagnostic treatment should be limited to malaria, tuberculosis infection, and other specific diseases that can be clinically diagnosed by curative effect and should not be used as conventional treatment.

Recommendation 16: Anti-infective drugs should not be used as a routine diagnostic treatment.

Recommendation 17: In principle, hormones are not recommended for patients with fever with unknown etiology, especially as antipyretic drugs.

References

1. Janeway TC, Mosenthal HO. A study of nitrogen metabolism in a case presenting short paroxysms of fever of unknown origin. Proc Soc Exp Biol Med. 1908;5(4):111–2.
2. Ashby H. An address on some cases of unexplained fever in infants and children [J]. Br Med J. 1907;2(2449):1637–9.
3. Durack DT, Street AC. Fever of unknown origin- reexamined and redefined [J]. Curr Clin Top Infect Dis. 1991;11:35–51.

4. Bennett JE, Dolin R, Blaser ML. Mandell, Douglas, and Bennett's principles and practice of infectious diseases [M]. 8th ed. Philadelphia: Elsevier Saunders; 2014. p. 2583–9.
5. Goldman L, Schafer AL. Goldman's Cecil medicine [M]. 24th ed. Philadelphia: Saunders; 2012. p. 1768–74.
6. Kasper DL, Fauci AS. Harrison's infectious diseases [M]. 2nd ed. New York: McGraw-Hill; 2013. p. 135–41.
7. Schlossberg D. Clinical infectious diseases [M]. 2nd ed. Cambridge: Cambridge University Press; 2015. p. 1–12.
8. ter Haar NM, Oswald M, Jeyaratnam J, et al. Recommendations for the management of auto inflammatory diseases [J]. Ann Rheum Dis. 2015;74(9):1636–44.
9. Brown M. Pyrexia of unknown origin 90 years on: a paradigm of modern clinical medicine [J]. Postgrad Med J. 2015;91(1082):665–9.
10. Shi XC, Liu XQ, Zhou BT, et al. Major causes of fever of unknown origin at Peking Union Medical College Hospital in the past 26 years [J]. Chin Med (Engl). 2013;126(5):808812.
11. Baicus C, Bolosiu HD, Tanasescu C, et al. Fever of unknown origin-predictors of outcome. A prospective multicenter study on 164 patients. Eur Intern Med. 2003;14(4):249–54.
12. Efstathiou SP, Pefanis AV, Tsiakou AG, et al. Fever of unknown origin: discrimination between infectious and noninfectious causes [J]. Eur Intern Med. 2010;21(2):137–43.
13. Johnston V, Stockley IM, Dockrell D, et al. Fever in returned travellers presenting in the United Kingdom: recommendations for investigation and initial management [J]. J Infect. 2009;59(1):1–18.
14. Bleeker-Rovers CP, Vos FJ, de Kleijn EM, et al. A prospective multicenter study on fever of unknown origin: the yield of a structured diagnostic protocol [J]. Medicine (Baltimore). 2007;86(1):26–38.
15. Dittrich S, Tadesse BT, Moussy F, et al. Target product profile for a diagnostic assay to differentiate between bacterial and non-bacterial infections and reduce antimicrobial overuse in resource-limited settings: an expert consensus [J/OL]. PLoS One. 2016;11(8):e0161721.
16. Knockaert DC, Dujardin KS, Bobbaers HJ. Long-term follow-up of patients with undiagnosed fever of unknown origin [J]. Arch Intern Med. 1996;156(6):618–20.
17. Mackowiak PA, Bartlett JG, Borden EC, et al. Concepts off ever: recent advances and lingering dogma[J]. Clin Infect Dis. 1997;25(1):119–38.
18. Knockaert DC, Vanderschueren S, Blockmans D. Fever of unknown origin in adults: 40 years on [J]. Intem Med. 2003;253(3):263–75.
19. Blockmans D, Knockaert D, Maes A, et al. Clinical value of [(18)F] fluoro-deoxyglucose positron emission tomography for patients with fever of unknown origin [J]. Clin Infect Dis. 2001;32(2):191–6.
20. Dong MJ, Zhao K, Liu ZF, et al. A meta-analysis of the value of fluorodeoxyglucose PET/PET-CT in the evaluation of fever of unknown origin [J]. Eur J Radiol. 2011;80(3):834–44.
21. Balink H, Veeger NJ, Bennink RJ, et al. The predictive value of C-reactive protein and erythrocyte sedimentation rate for18F-FDG PET/CT outcome in patients with fever and inflammation of unknown origin [J]. Nucl Med Commun. 2015;36(6):604–9.
22. Robine A, Hot A, Maucort-Boulch D, et al. Fever of unknown origin in the 2000s: evaluation of 103 cases over eleven years [J]. Presse Med. 2014;43(9):e233–40.
23. Cunha BA, Lortholary O, Cunha CB. Fever of unknown origin: a clinical approach [J]. Am J Med. 2015;128(10):1138.e1–15.
24. Gerfaud-Valentin M, Maucort-Boulch D, Hot A, et al. Adult-onset still disease: manifestations, treatment, outcome, and prognostic factors in 57 patients [J]. Medicine (Baltimore). 2014;93(2):91–9.
25. Bryan CS, Ahuja D. Fever of unknown origin: is there a role for empiric therapy? [J]. Infect Dis Clin North Am. 2007;21(4):1213–20.
26. Haidar G, Singh N. Fever of unknown origin. N Engl J Med. 2022;386:463–77.

2 Fever of Unknown Origin in Infectious Diseases

Zhang Wenhong, Zhu Liping, Wang Ruiying, Jiang Weimin, Hu Yuekai, Huang Yuxian, Wang Ting, Jin Jialin, Zhang Jiming, Li Qian, Shao Lingyun, Yu Shenglei, Liu Yuanyuan, Xu Bin, Mao Richeng, Zhu Haoxiang, Wang Xuan, Lin Jie, Dong Minhui, Zhu Beidi, Wang Xinyu, Yang Yuling, Zhang Shu, Li Tao, Zhu Zuiyun, Li Ning, Li Yuxin, Wang Chao, Chen Mingquan, Jia Wen, Weng Shanshan, Zhu Xiaoxue, Liang Daobin, Yang Feifie, Zhou Xian, Chen Shu, Zheng Jianming, Lin Siran, Liang Jun, Li Li, Liu Hong, and Zhong Wen

Infectious diseases have been the main cause of fever of unknown origin (FUO) for a long time. In recent years, this kind of disease has declined, especially in the economically developed areas, and its proportion has dropped to about 30%. However, in developing countries, including China, about 40%–50% of FUO is caused by infectious diseases, which is still the most common cause.

The infectious diseases causing FUO are mainly bacterial infections, which can be divided into systemic and local infections. It is generally believed that systemic infection is the main cause of infectious fever. However, in recent years, foreign literature has reported that focal bacterial infection may be more common. Local abscess, urinary tract infection, and biliary tract infection are common local infections, which are often neglected because of no obvious localized lesions or local

Z. Wenhong (✉) · Z. Liping · W. Ruiying · J. Weimin · H. Yuekai · H. Yuxian · J. Jialin · Z. Jiming · L. Qian · S. Lingyun · Y. Shenglei · L. Yuanyuan · X. Bin · M. Richeng · Z. Haoxiang · W. Xuan · L. Jie · D. Minhui · Z. Beidi · W. Xinyu · Y. Yuling · Z. Shu · L. Tao · Z. Zuiyun · L. Ning · L. Yuxin · W. Chao · C. Mingquan · J. Wen · W. Shanshan · Z. Xiaoxue · L. Daobin · Y. Feifie · Z. Xian · C. Shu · Z. Jianming · L. Siran · L. Jun · L. Li · L. Hong · Z. Wen
Department of Infectious Diseases, Huashan Hospital, Fudan University, Shanghai, China
e-mail: zhangwenhong@fudan.edu.cn

W. Ting
Department of Infectious Diseases, Jing'an District Central Hospital of Shanghai, Shanghai, China

W. Zhang, X. Weng (eds.), *Fever of Unknown Origin*,
https://doi.org/10.1007/978-981-95-1401-4_2

symptoms. Viral infection of the upper respiratory tract may be the cause of fever only in children, but it is rare in adults.

The etiological distribution of infectious diseases in FUO is shown in the general table, among which the classic ones are briefly introduced as follows:

Tuberculosis (TB) In some countries of the third world and some poor areas of our country, as well as among the elderly in industrially developed countries, tuberculosis has risen to the first place in the etiology of infectious long-term fever. Extrapulmonary tuberculosis is far more than intrapulmonary tuberculosis, which can affect the liver, spleen, bone, kidney, meninges, peritoneum, pericardium, etc. In some cases, fever may be the only initial clinical manifestation. Fever occurs in 80%–98% of the patients with liver tuberculosis, but it is often misdiagnosed because the disease has no specific symptoms and signs or is covered by the symptoms of tuberculosis in other parts, or there is no tuberculosis focus outside the liver (about 1/4~1/3 of the cases have normal chest film). The diagnosis of renal tuberculosis is also difficult. Only 20% of the autopsy patients were diagnosed with renal tuberculosis. Therefore, clinicians should pay more attention to this disease. Interferon-gamma (IFN-γ) release test is widely used in clinics, and its sensitivity and specificity can reach more than 90%, but it is still difficult to identify active and latent tuberculosis infection. In recent years, the progress of tuberculosis molecular diagnosis, including Xpert MTB/RIF and second-generation sequencing, has greatly helped the diagnosis of tuberculosis.

Typhoid and Paratyphoid: Typhoid and paratyphoid are still the most important causes of fever in China. Typhoid fever has changed significantly in clinical practice. Atypical manifestations are more common than bradycardia and typical roseola. The patients with drug-resistant strains have severe conditions, a long course of disease (the longest fever course is 101 days, with an average of 33.58 days), many complications, a high recurrence rate, and multiple-drug resistance. Combined with irregular drug use in the early stage, the positive rate of bacterial culture is low, which makes the diagnosis difficult. However, the onset of the disease is still seasonal and should be paid attention to in the diagnosis. It must be pointed out that the diagnostic value of the Widal test—used for over 90 years—has been challenged. A key concern is its high false positive rate: conditions such as tumor diseases (lymphoma, various solid tumors), connective tissue diseases (systemic lupus erythematosus, Behcet's disease), non-typhoidal acute infectious diseases (viral hepatitis, pneumonia, tuberculosis, liver abscess), ulcerative colitis, and enteritis may all lead to high-titer positive results in the Widal test. The mechanism of the Feida test's false positive has not been fully elucidated.

Infective Endocarditis: Infective endocarditis (IE) is a common cause of long-term fever, with complex manifestations and a high misdiagnosis rate. In the past 20 years, great changes have taken place in the clinical characteristics of IE: Euclidean nodule, Janeway nodule, and Roth point are rare, and there are more and more patients without a heart murmur and negative blood culture, which makes the diagnosis more difficult. The endocarditis without a heart murmur and negative blood culture may be caused by the application of antibiotics in advance, involvement of the right side of the heart, and improper culture of special infectious factors such as *Rickettsia* and fungi. Persistent fever of unknown origin and recurrent embolism suggest the possibility of the disease. In recent years, it has been considered that microaerobic, anaerobic, or L-form bacteria can cause infective endocarditis. Therefore, anaerobic culture and L-form bacteria culture should be performed in some cases. Echocardiography can detect the location, size, number, and shape of vegetations, which is of great diagnostic value.

Intraperitoneal Infection or Abscess in Other Parts: In foreign countries, it is believed that intraperitoneal infection is the most common cause of fever, especially liver abscess and subphrenic abscess, followed by pelvic abscess. If there are clinical manifestations such as fever, hepatomegaly and tenderness, limited right diaphragm activity, and jaundice, the diagnosis of liver abscess is not difficult. However, the above common symptoms can only appear in the late stage of the disease. In the early stage of the disease, fever can be the only symptom. Liver pain can be absent or appear as late as 3 months after fever. However, the serum alkaline phosphatase (AKP) of most patients is increased, and the proportion of serum albumin is decreased or even decreased. Inversion, hepatic computed tomography (CT) and MRI, and hepatic arteriography are helpful for early diagnosis. The clinical symptoms of subphrenic abscess depend on the course of the disease and the location of the lesion. In the early stage, there are only chills, fever, and elevated white blood cells but no local symptoms. With the progress of the disease, subcostal pain and tenderness, pleural effusion, atelectasis of the lower lobe, and limited or disappeared diaphragmatic activity of the diseased side appear. Combined lung and liver scanning is a good method for the diagnosis of subphrenic abscess. A pelvic abscess may have no abdominal pain, only fever as the main manifestation. It should be emphasized that the effect of anti-infective drugs alone is very little, and early diagnosis and surgical drainage should be made. In addition to abdominal abscess, sometimes a gingival abscess and brain abscess may also be the cause of fever of unknown origin. In the literature, it is called odontogenic fever, chronic alveolar fistula, and gingival abscess, and the thermal process can be as long as several months.

Detailed medical history is an important part of correct diagnosis, including body temperature, heat type, heat course, and accompanying symptoms. In particular, some epidemiological history is of great significance for infectious diseases; pay attention to comprehensive and repeated physical examination (P.E.), such as rash characteristics and location, lymphadenopathy, hepatosplenomegaly, and cardiac murmur; at the same time, pay attention to new symptoms and signs, and make relevant examination accordingly. Laboratory examination is of great significance in the diagnosis, but it should be carried out selectively and purposefully according to the specific cases. When necessary, the specimens for such examinations should be submitted repeatedly to improve the positive rate. Make full use of all kinds of noninvasive examinations and new detection technology, shorten the diagnosis time, and reduce the pain of patients, but most patients often need one or more invasive examinations to be clear. When patients lack specific clinical symptoms and signs, a comprehensive laboratory examination should be carried out. Once abnormal findings are found, they should be followed up.

In this book, we include not only the classic infectious diseases of fever, including tuberculosis infection, *Nontuberculous mycobacteria* (NTM) infection, *Brucella* infection, Epstein–Barr virus (EBV) infection, infective endocarditis, liver abscess, and implant-related infection, but also some rare infectious diseases, such as *Scedosporium acuminatum* meningitis, *Babesia*, psittacosis, Lyme disease, and *Fasciola hepatica*. For the patients with fever and unknown infectious diseases, we should pay attention not only to repeatedly inquiring about the epidemiological history and life contact history of the patients to obtain suspicious clues, such as the history of living at home and abroad, the history of animal contact, the history of mosquito bites, eating habits, drowning, and so on, but also to exploring the host factors behind the spread of infection, such as tumor, autoimmune disease, organ transplantation, and idiopathic CD4. In recent years, the number of immunodeficient patients with IFN-γ autoantibodies has been reduced. These patients may be infected with a variety of pathogens. Compared with patients with normal immunity, their condition is more complex and changeable.

2.1 Fever with Progressive Enlargement of the Liver and Spleen Due to Disseminated *Mycobacterium avium* Infection Simulating Malignancy

Zhang Wenhong

The patient, a 52-year-old female, was admitted to the hospital on March 12 due to "recurrent fever for 2 months." The patient's right purlicue was punctured by a wood thorn two months ago, and the lymph nodes under her arm were enlarged. On January 9, the patient underwent "right underarm lymph node abscess resection" at the local hospital. She had recurrent fever after the operation, about two or three times a day, mainly in the afternoon and night. The patient first experienced chills, followed by profuse sweating once the fever developed. This profuse sweating was sufficient to soak the patient's clothes and quilts, and the body temperature fluctuated between 36 and 39°X. Fever was sometimes accompanied by nausea and vomiting of stomach contents but no headache, chest tightness, palpitations, abdominal pain, or diarrhea. Blood routine on February 17 revealed the following: white blood cell (WBC) count: 24.5×10^9/L, neutrophils: 91%, and hemoglobin (Hb): 77 g/L. On February 18, due to cough and sputum, she had a chest CT examination, showing "possible infection in the upper lobe of the left lung, small nodules in the upper and lower lobes of the right lung and the upper lobe of the left lung," but the symptoms did not improve after oral administration of cefuroxime. On March 3, the patient was given piperacillin and sulbactam 5 g IVGTT q8h combined with levofloxacin

0.2 IVGTT bid for anti-infective treatment. After 3 days, the treatment was changed to vancomycin 1 g IVGTT bid and piperacillin and sulbactam 5 g IVGTT q8h treatment, but the fever still persisted. The patient underwent bone marrow aspiration on March 9, and her bone marrow cytology showed that leukocytosis was closely related to the inflammation caused by the infection, and hematological tumors were basically excluded. The patient was then admitted to our department. Since the onset of the illness, the patient had dry mouth, polydipsia, hyperhidrosis, anorexia, fatigue, and a weight loss of about 10 kg within 2 months.

2.1.1 Past History

The patient had hypertension for 6 or 7 years, and her blood pressure was well-controlled by taking antihypertensive drugs.

2.1.2 Physical Examination

T: 37 °C, HR 88 bpm, R 20 breaths/min, and BP 110/80 mmHg. Physical examination revealed consciousness, lethargy, no yellowing of the skin and mucous membranes, dry and desquamated skin, and no swelling of superficial lymph nodes all over the body. The sclera was not yellowish, the pupils were equal to the same circle, and there was normal light reflection. The neck was soft, the trachea was in the middle, and the thyroid gland was not enlarged. A surgical incision of about 7 cm in length was seen in the right armpit, with a wound of about 1 × 2cm^2, with a built-in gauze drainage strip, with pale bloody exudate. On physical examination, a 3 cm × 4 cm mass was palpated in her right breast. The left lung breath sounded clear, the right lower lung breath sounded low, and there were no dry or wet rales. The heart rate was 88 bpm, the rhythm was uniform, and murmurs were not heard in each valve area. The abdomen was soft, and there was light tenderness under the xiphoid process and no rebound pain. The liver edge and splenic edge were palpable >2 cm below the right and left costal margins, respectively. There was pitting edema in the lower back, tenderness in the posterior superior iliac spine, and edema in the right forearm. The range of motion of the limbs was normal. There was no edema in the lower extremities. The neurological examination was normal.

2.1.3 Workup After Admission

Blood routine after admission revealed the following: WBC: 6.77 × 10^9/L, neutrophils: 90.5%, hemoglobin: 62 g/L, mean corpuscular hemoglobin: ↓21.9 pg, mean corpuscular hemoglobin concentration: ↓297 g/L, and mean corpuscular volume: ↓73.9fl. Stool routine, urine routine, and liver and kidney function test results were normal, albumin was ↓20 g/L, and autoimmune antibody sets were all normal. The full set of viral hepatitis, HIV antibody, and rapid plasma reagin test (RPR) was all negative. The tumor markers (alpha fetoprotein (AFP), carcinoembryonic antigen (CEA), cyfra 21-1 (CY21-1), and neuron-specific enolase (NSE)) were all negative. Erythrocyte sedimentation rate (ESR) was ↑107 mm/h, C-reactive protein (CRP) was ↑158 mg/L, and *Brucella* antibody titer was <1:25(−); CD4/CD8 quantity and ratio were in the normal range. Ultrasound showed that "several enlarged lymph nodes were seen in bilateral neck, left supraclavicular, left axilla, and bilateral groin, which may be reactive hyperplasia; hepatosplenomegaly, with multiple solid masses in the spleen. The gallbladder wall was edematous; there was a solid mass in the right breast, which might be a fibroadenoma"; chest CT showed "possible pneumonia in left upper lung and right lower lung, right pleural effusion"; abdominal CT showed "hepatosplenomegaly, uneven enhancement of the splenic in vein phase, multiple lymph nodes in the posterior peritoneum." The right axillary lymph node section showed "(right axillary) lymph node acute suppurative inflammation." The patient was given doxycycline, ceftriaxone, levofloxacin, compound trimethoprim, and other antibiotics, but the effect was not obvious, with progressive liver, spleen, and lymph node enlargement. The liver was enlarged to 3 cm below the costal margin, and the spleen was enlarged to 4 cm below the costal margin. Bone marrow biopsy showed "solid tumor (including lymphoma) bone marrow invasion," and PET-CT showed "multiple bone marrow infiltration by lymphoma." A biopsy of the lymph node in front of the right ear was performed on April 8. It showed "(in front of the right ear) lymph node granulomatous inflammation with coagulative necrosis." After discussion, it was considered that it was probably an inflammation of infection. As a result, the patient was actively treated with anti-infective medicine (cefepime, isepamicin, fluconazole, vancomycin, micafungin, linezolid, etc.) and supportive treatment. Although her body temperature still fluctuated, it decreased, and purulent secretions still exuded from the wound gauze drainage. Later, three blood cultures and one pleural fluid culture all reported the growth of mycobacteria, and the acid-fast staining was positive. The colloidal gold method and 16sRNA sequencing method identified *Mycobacterium avium*. Therefore, the patient was given rifampicin + ethambutol + clarithromycin and levofloxacin. At last, the patient's body temperature returned to normal, and the wound gradually healed. After 1 year of treatment, the patient presented with decreased vision, which might be an adverse reaction to ethambutol, as her vision gradually recovered after stopping ethambutol. She was asked to continue the remaining triple therapy for six months and then stop the drug. So far, the patient is generally well and has no recurrence.

2.1.4 Discussion

Nontuberculous mycobacteria (NTM) refers to *Mycobacterium*, which does not include *Mycobacterium tuberculosis complex* (human, bovine, African, and *Mycobacterium microti*) or *Mycobacterium leprae*, both of which are conditional pathogens. Nontuberculous mycobacterial disease refers to infection with NTM, which causes corresponding organ or tissue pathological changes, the most common of which is chronic lung disease. In addition, NTM can also cause skin and lymph node lesions and systemic disseminated lesions. More than 150 types of NTM have been discovered so far, 37 of which have been reported to cause diseases. In 1993, the Huangshan Conference officially named NTM as *nontuberculous mycobacteria*. According to bacterial colony morphology, color, light, culture temperature, and growth rate, NTM is divided into four groups. Currently, the Runyon classification method is the most used. In addition, the NTM complex classification is proposed based on the similarity of pathogenicity to humans and animals and biological characteristics, including *Mycobacterium avium-intracellulare* complex (MAC), *Mycobacterium gordonae* complex, *Mycobacterium kansasii* complex, *Mycolicibacter terrae* complex, and *Mycobacterium fortuitum* complex. Among them, MAC is the most common conditional pathogen.

At the beginning, the patient's right hand was punctured by a wooden thorn. Subsequently, high fever, pulmonary infection, systemic lymph nodes, and hepatosplenomegaly occurred, and multiple solid masses were seen in the spleen. The leukocyte count and percentage of neutrophils were significantly increased, suggesting infectious diseases. However, the anti-infective treatment for common bacteria was not effective, and she even developed wasting symptoms such as anemia, hypoproteinemia, and thrombocytopenia. Purulent discharge could be seen in the wound. Lymph node biopsy revealed granulomatous inflammation and coagulative necrosis, suggesting a special infection. After culture and acid-fast staining, it was confirmed that it was an infection by *Mycobacterium avium*, so the diagnosis was clear. *Mycobacterium avium* infections, especially systemic disseminated infections, mostly occur in people with severe immunodeficiency, including acquired immunodeficiency syndrome (AIDS) patients and HIV patients who have been treated with corticosteroids or immunosuppressants for a long time. This patient had neither immunodeficiency nor underlying disease, so it is relatively rare. The patient's clinical manifestations included fever, hepatosplenomegaly, and lymphadenopathy throughout the body. PET-CT showed multiple bone marrow infiltrations of lymphoma, so it was seriously misunderstood during the diagnosis process, but no lymphoma was found on multiple biopsies. Therefore, this was a false positive of PET-CT in the diagnosis of lymphoma. Since F^{18}-FDG (18F - Fluorodeoxyglucose) is a nonspecific tumor imaging agent, it needs to be combined with other clinical manifestations to make a comprehensive judgment.

References

1. Juweid ME. FDG-PET/CT in lymphoma. Methods Mol Biol. 2011;727:1–19.
2. Claudio Piersimoni, Claudio Scarparo. Extrapulmonary infections associated with nontuberculous mycobacteria in immunocompetent persons. Emerg Infect Dis. 2009,15(9):1351–8.
3. Cook JL. Nontuberculous mycobacteria: opportunistic environmental pathogens for predisposed hosts. British Medical Bulletin, 2010,96: 45–9.

2.2 A 31-Year-Old Man with Recurrent Fever, Myalgia, Headache, and Projectile Vomiting

Zhu Liping and Wang Ruiying

2.2.1 Lyme Disease with a 5-Month History of Chronic Meningitis

A 31-year-old man was admitted to the hospital on November 17, 2003, for a 5-month history of recurrent fever. He had traveled to a primeval forest in Nujiang, Yunnan Province, China, 5 months ago and camped there for one night. He found himself bitten by an unknown bug and had a focal red bump. Three days later, he developed a fever at a maximum temperature of 39.5 °C, with no obvious cold or chills. He also had a paroxysmal dry cough. At the local hospital, cephalosporins, ciprofloxacin, azithromycin, and ampicillin were successively administered. The body temperature decreased to the normal level after 2 weeks, but he developed myalgia and fatigue and was unable to take things or walk. The pain relieved spontaneously 4 days later. One month later, he had a fever again, with headache and projectile vomiting of stomach contents. Lumbar puncture examination at the local hospital revealed the following findings in cerebral spinal fluids (CSFs): WBC: 655×10^6/L, multinuclear cells that accounted for 90%, protein: 522 mg/L, and glucose: 2.4 mmol/L. Cranial CT scan revealed a low-density patchy area on the right frontal lobe. Empiric antituberculosis treatment (isoniazid, rifampicin, and ethambutol) and dexamethasone 20 mg per day were administered, and the fever disappeared the next day. CSF examinations every week for six times were all normal. When glucocorticoids were decreased to prednisone 5 mg per day, this patient had a fever again with a maximum temperature of 38.5 °C, then he was transferred to our hospital for further diagnosis and treatment.

2.2.2 Physical Examination

This patient was afebrile. There were no skin rashes, no palpable lymph nodes, no abnormal findings in cranial nerve examination, no nuchal rigidity, and no abnormal findings in cardiopulmonary auscultation. The abdomen was soft, with no tenderness or rebound tenderness. The liver and spleen were not palpable. Movement of the upper and lower limbs was normal. There was no focal redness or swollen lower limbs. Kernig sign was negative, and pathologic reflexes were not present.

2.2.3 Diagnosis and Treatment

Laboratory examinations after hospitalization yielded the following findings: white blood cells: 7.5 × 10^9/L, neutrocytes that accounted for 80%, hemoglobin: 101 g/L, and platelets: 283 × 10^9/L. Urine routine test, liver and kidney function tests, and blood glucose were normal. C-reactive protein (CRP) was 151 mg/L, and antinuclear antibodies (ANA), extractable nuclear antigen (ENA), and dsDNA were negative. HIV antibody was negative. Ultrasound revealed a mild splenomegaly, with normal liver, gallbladder, pancreas, and kidney. There were no abnormal findings on the electrocardiogram (ECG) and lung CT scan. Lumbar puncture yielded normal CSF pressure, routine test, and biochemical test. Bacterial, fungal, and tuberculosis cultures of CSF were negative. There were no abnormal findings in bone marrow examination. Blood antibody for *Borrelia burgdorferi* was positive, with a titer of 1:1000.

After administration of ceftriaxone 4 g per day and penicillin 19,200,000 units per day, divided into two times for 3 weeks, the body temperature decreased to the normal level, and generalized myalgia and fatigue were relieved. This therapy continued for 5 weeks.

2.2.4 Key Points

Lyme disease, also known as Lyme borreliosis, is a zoonotic disease first found in the town of Lyme, United States, in 1975. It is a systemic infectious disease caused by *Borrelia burgdorferi.* Humans and animals can be infected when bitten by ticks and develop serial clinical symptoms. Besides erythema chronicum migrans (ECM) and arthritis, cardiac impairment and nervous system involvement are also common, which can lead to permanent disability or even death. This disease is widely spread, with approximately 300,000 cases every year around the world, and has become one of the most important emerging infectious diseases.

This patient had a 5-month history of recurrent fever, with subsequent generalized myalgia, failure to catch things or walk on the ground, headache, and abnormal CSF examination. He had a clear history of traveling to a primeval forest and a focal red bump from a bug bite. Blood anti-*Borrelia burgdorferi* antibody was a strong positive. Symptoms were relieved after effective anti-spirochetal treatment. Above all, Lyme disease was clearly diagnosed.

However, this patient did not have typical symptoms, like ECM, the characteristic skin damage of Lyme disease, while studies reported that ECM could be missing in 15–40% patients. Cardiac impairment could be found in some cases, like myocarditis or arrhythmia, while this patient had no palpitation or chest tightness or abnormal ECG findings. Besides, this patient first presented with fever and generalized myalgia 2 weeks after the tick bite but without common arthralgia. As for the change of nervous system, related symptoms appeared 2 months after the tick bite, which was rare because it happened between the acute and chronic phases and presented as meningitis. Therefore, epidemiological history and serology tests are very important for atypical cases.

References

1. Wormser GP, Nadelman RB, Dattwyler RJ, et al. Practice guidelines for the treatment of Lyme disease. Clin Infect Dis. 2000;31:S1–14.
2. Hengge UR, Tannapfel A, Tyring SK, et al. Lyme borreliosis. Lancet Infect Dis. 2003;3:489–500.
3. Singh SK, Girschick HJ. Molecular survival strategies of the Lyme disease spirochete *Borrelia burgdorferi*. Lancet Infect Dis. 2004;4:575–83.
4. Embers ME, Ramamoorthy R, Philipp M. Survival strategies of *Borrelia burgdorferi*, the etiologic agent of Lyme disease. Microbes Infect. 2004;6:312–8.
5. XJ Yu, MF Liang, SY Zhang, et al. Fever with thrombocytopenia associated with a novel Bunyavirus in China. N Eng J Med. 2011;364:1523–32.

2.3 A 50-Year-Old Woman Was Admitted with the Chief Complaint of Fever for Eight Weeks

Jiang Weimin

The patient developed a fever eight weeks ago, and her body temperature fluctuated between 37.6 °C and 38.7 °C. She denied experiencing shivers, chills, cough, expectoration, abdominal pain, diarrhea, urinary urgency, frequency, dysuria, fatigue, night sweats, chest pain, hemoptysis, etc. Blood and urine test and chest radiograph results were unremarkable. She had been given "ceftriaxone, levofloxacin, azithromycin, ribavirin, ganciclovir" for treatment, but her symptoms remained the same. A month ago, the patient began having a dry cough with no sputum, and her body temperature remained at about 38.0 °C. No obvious abnormalities were found in lung CT or cardiac ultrasound. No pathogens were found in the blood culture or sputum culture. The erythrocyte sedimentation rate was 104 mm/h. Then, she was successively given fluconazole, azithromycin, and cephalosporin for treatment. However, her temperature did not drop, and her symptoms still remained the same. Then the patient came to our hospital for further diagnosis and treatment. Besides, the patient had a 2-year history of keeping parrots and had close contact with her parrots.

2.3.1 Physical Examination

The patient was clear in consciousness and was in a generally good condition. She had conjunctival congestion. Her superficial lymph nodes were not swollen all over the body. Breath sounds in both lungs were clear, with no dry or wet rales. No pathological murmurs were heard in the heart valve area. Her abdomen was soft, with no tenderness or rebound pain. No positive signs were found during the other physical examinations.

2.3.2 Diagnosis and Treatment

2.3.2.1 Complete Examination After Admission

Blood routine results showed the following: white blood cell: 4.34×10^9/L, neutrophils: 65.6%, hemoglobin: 110 g/dl, and platelet count (PLT): 297×10^9/L. There was no abnormality in liver and kidney function results. ESR was 104 mm/h, and the absolute count of eosin was 22×10^6/L. Tumor markers (AFP, CEA, CA125, CA199, PSA, CY211, NSE, and CA50) and ANA, ENA, dsDNA, ANCA, C3, C4, and rheumatoid factor (RF) were all within the normal range.

After admission, the patient was found to have a cough, obviously with small amounts of sputum. So, considering the possibility of "endobronchial tuberculosis," fiberoptic bronchoscopy was performed. But the result was negative.

According to the patient's past history of raising parrots and being in close contact with parrots, doctors considered whether the patient had *Chlamydia psittaci* infection. Then the psittacosis complement fixation test came out positive. According to the results of the psittacosis complement fixation test, the patient was given doxycycline 100 mg bid orally. After two days, the patient's body temperature returned to normal. The patient was discharged from the hospital after taking doxycycline for another 2 weeks. During the half a year of follow-up, the patient did not have fever again.

2.3.3 Case Comments

Parrot fever is caused by *Chlamydia psittaci* and is also known as bird fever. It is an infectious disease of birds and poultry, including chickens and ducks. It can also be transmitted to humans. So it is a kind of zoonosis. In 1879, the Swiss doctor Girit stated that a family of seven had suffered from pneumonia after contact with tropical birds. In 1890, Moranche identified parrots as the source of infection and named this disease psittaci. There are about 130 species of birds that can be infected with *Chlamydia psittaci*. When infected, they can develop symptoms or only become pathogen carriers. But all of them can excrete the pathogen.

Humans usually become infected through close contact with the pathogens. In most cases, humans become infected while inhaling dry feces, feathers, and dust of sick birds through the respiratory tract; humans can also be infected through damaged skin and mucous membranes. Occasionally, the disease can be transmitted orally through contaminated hands or food. Laboratory infection is also an important route of transmission. The population is generally susceptible, and poultry farm workers, bird farmers, zoo managers, and laboratory workers studying *Chlamydia psittaci* are more susceptible.

The incubation period of this disease is 7–15 days or longer. The main clinical manifestations are fever and pneumonia. The disease has an acute onset, usually with chills, high fever, rapid rise of body temperature, headache, fatigue, muscle pain, relatively slow pulse (body temperature rises, but pulse does not accelerate accordingly), etc. Severe cases may have neuropsychiatric symptoms, such as lethargy, delirium, irritability, and even coma. Symptoms of pneumonia may also appear, including dry cough, coughing a small amount of sticky sputum, bloody sputum, chest pain, shortness of breath, and cyanosis in severe patients. On chest X-ray examination, single or multiple flaky inflammatory shadows can be seen. The shadows can be diffuse, large-leaf, nodular, or miliary. Pleurisy, splenomegaly, and mild liver enlargement may also occur. It can also be complicated by myocarditis, pericarditis, endocarditis, encephalitis, acute renal failure, jaundice, etc. White blood count is usually normal or slightly lower.

The course of the disease is generally 7–10 days and 12–21 days for severe patients.

The diagnosis depends on laboratory tests, such as the following:

1. Complement Fixation Test

   The complement fixation test usually starts to be positive 2–3 weeks after the infection. The antibody titer reaches the peak at 4–6 weeks. It is of diagnostic importance that the antibody titer of double serum in the acute and recovery phases increases by four times.
2. Isolation of *Chlamydia*

   At the early stage, taking the serum or sputum of patients and inoculating it in chicken embryo yolk sac or tissue culture medium may isolate *Chlamydia psittaci*.
3. Fluorescent Quantitative PCR

   It is faster and more sensitive than ordinary PCR methods, which overcomes the deficiencies of the ordinary PCR quantitative method. It is also an important method.

As for drug therapy, tetracycline, oxytetracycline, and chlortetracycline have good therapeutic effects, and doxycycline is now widely used. The treatment duration must be at least 10 days after fever regression to prevent recurrence. Adrenal cortex hormones can be used in severe cases. The case fatality rate is about 20% before the emergence of effective treatment drugs. Now it has fallen below 1%. The majority of deaths were of elderly and young children.

In this case, the patient had a fever for eight weeks, accompanied by an irritating dry cough. Various antibiotics (including drugs against gram-positive cocci, negative bacilli, anaerobic bacteria, and viruses) did not work. The results of chest radiograph, chest CT, fiberoptic bronchoscopy, blood culture, and sputum culture were all negative. Analysis of the therapeutic effect of doxycycline associated with the history of close contact with parrots and the result of the psittacosis complement fixation test suggested a clinical diagnosis of "psittacosis." The symptoms of *Chlamydia psittaci* are often severe. Common symptoms are fever, cough, chest pain, and chills. Severe cases may develop respiratory failure. This patient only had mild symptoms, including fever and a dry cough. Signs on pulmonary physical examination and imaging findings were negative. So patients like this are often missed. The key to diagnosing psittacosis is a careful investigation of medical history. The most reliable method to help with diagnosis is to do a *Chlamydia psittaci* culture. Any of the nasopharyngeal or posterior pharynx swabs, tracheal and bronchial aspirates, alveolar lavage fluid, and other specimens can be used for bacterial culture. The application of *Chlamydia psittaci* species–specific monoclonal antibodies and PCR test is helpful for diagnosis. But at the same time, it is necessary to pay attention to quality control to prevent false positive results.

References

1. Feng Yue, Zhang Zhonghua, Gong Fuming, Liu Chenjian. Establishment and application of a TaqMan-MGB probe-based fluorescent quantitative PCR detection method for Chlamydia psittaci. J Zoonoses. 2010;26(11):1041–4.
2. Zhang Jun, Tang Guangjian, Wang Shulan, et al. Imaging features of Psittacosis Pneumonia. Chin J Radiol. 2005;39(11):1134–7. https://doi.org/10.3760/j.issn:1005-1201.2005.11.004.
3. Yang J, Ling Y, Yuan J, Isolation and characterization of peacock Chlamydophila psittaci infection in China Avian Dis. 2011;55(1):76–81.
4. Becker Y. Chapter 39: Chlamydia. In: Baron S, editor. Medical microbiology. 4th ed. Galveston (TX): University of Texas Medical Branch at Galveston; 1996.
5. Dickx V, Vanrompay D. Zoonotic transmission of Chlamydia psittaci in a chicken and turkey hatchery. J Med Microbiol. 2011;60(Pt 6):775–9. Epub 2011 Mar 10.

2.4 EBV Infection-Related Hemophagocytic Lymphohistiocytosis

Hu Yuekai and Huang Yuxian

A 26-year-old man, who is a building worker, was admitted to the hospital with a month of fever.

The patient developed nasal congestion, a runny nose, and a sore throat without an obvious cause and felt no fever at the end of March 2012. The symptoms were relieved after taking oral cold medicine. A few days later (April 4), he developed chills and rigors after catching a cold, followed by the body temperature rising to 40 °C. On April 5, he received a 6-day anti-infective treatment (details unclear), but the fever was not alleviated. Then, he presented to a provincial hospital with fever of unknown origin (FUO) and was given levofloxacin tablets 0.5 qd (from Apr 26 to May 13), ganciclovir 0.3 bid (from May 2 to May 9), imipenem and cilastatin sodium 0.5 q8h (from May 7 to May 9), Solu-Medrol 40 mg IVGTT (from May 11 to May 13), dexamethasone 10 mg (from May 11 to May 13), and dexamethasone 3 mg (from May 13 to May 16) and was intermittently given symptomatic treatment, such as Celebrex and indomethacin, and the decrease in body temperature was not obvious. On May 17, 2013, he was admitted with a fever for further investigation. During the course of the disease, the patient's highest body temperature was 40.9 °C, which was an irregular heat type. After using antipyretics, the body temperature would drop to normal. There was no dizziness, no headache, no cough and sputum, no chest tightness, no shortness of breath, no abdominal pain, no diarrhea, no urgent and frequent urination, no pain with urination, no rash, no bleeding points, no joint pain, no oral ulcers, and no history of skin ulceration and trauma before the onset. Two days before admission, vision loss occurred without visual rotation. On the day before admission, there was intermittent dull pain and discomfort in the left upper abdomen without an obvious cause, which was alleviated when lying supine. Since the illness, the patient had been in good mental state, with normal appetite and sleep and normal bowel movements, and had suffered a weight loss of about 10 kg. He denied any history of surgery or trauma. He denied the history of infectious diseases such as hepatitis, tuberculosis, typhoid fever, and schistosomiasis. The patient denied any history of allergy to penicillin and sulfa drugs or of basic diseases, such as high blood pressure and diabetes. The history of vaccination was unknown.

2.4.1 Physical Examination (P. E.)

Conscious, fair spirit, normal development, active position, stepped into the ward, able to cooperate in physical examinations, and answered relevant questions. Slightly yellowish skin and sclera, no skin rash and bleeding spots, palpable swollen rice-sized lymph nodes on both sides of the neck and left groin, soft and movable. The head was not deformed, the facial features were regular, the neck was soft, the trachea was in the middle, and the thyroid gland was not enlarged. Breathing movements on both sides were normal and symmetrical, breathing sounds in both lungs were clear, and no obvious dry or wet rales were heard. The HR was 80 beats per min. The heart rhythm was uniform, and pathological murmurs in each valve area were not heard. The abdomen was flat and soft, with no tenderness or rebound pain; the liver was three fingers below the ribs; the spleen was three fingers below the ribs; there was normal movement of the limbs, no edema of the lower limbs, and symmetrical knee reflexes (++) and NS (-).

2.4.2 Hospital Course (Table 2.1)

Table 2.1 The laboratory test indicators on April 11 and April 26

	Leukocyte (10^9/L)	Hemoglobin (g/L)	Monocyte (%)	Platelets (10^9/L)	Alanine aminotransferase (ALT) (U/L)
April 11	3.4	97	12.1	140	47
April 26	3.0	97	12.8	107	55
	Total bilirubin (μmol/L)	Albumin (/L)	TG (mg/L)	LDH (IU/L)	ESR (mm/h)
April 11	<12	31.2	3.22	338	27
April 26	<12	24.5	3.35	407	

Ferritin: 17870.9↑ng/mL and blood β2 microglobulin: 5100 mg/L↑

Lymphocyte subset: CD3+: 80.12%, Th cells (CD3+/CD4+): 44.76%, T cells (CD3+/CD8+): 23.6%, B cells (CD19+): 5.4%, and NK cells (CD3−/CD16+56+): 5.84% Pathogenic examination: HIV antibody, RPR, tuberculosis T-SPOT, *Toxoplasma* antibody immunoglobulin G (IgG)/IgM, *Enterovirus* RNA, Coxsackievirus B antibody IgM, herpes simplex virus I-IgG/IgM, herpes simplex virus II-IgG/IgM, cytomegalovirus (CMV) IgM/IgG, rubella virus IgG, *Mycoplasma pneumoniae*/*Chlamydia pneumoniae* antibody, *Mycobacterium tuberculosis* antibody, blood and bone marrow cultures, bacterial endotoxin, heterophilic agglutination test, peripheral blood smear for *Plasmodium*, and viral hepatitis indicators were all negative. EB virus IgG was negative on April 11 and positive on April 26.

Cardiac ultrasound and chest CT showed no abnormalities, and abdominal CT showed splenomegaly and a small amount of pelvic effusion. Head CT showed no abnormalities. B-scan showed multiple gallbladder polyps and splenomegaly and multiple lymph nodes in the neck, axilla, and groin on both sides.

Inguinal lymph node puncture: scattered lymphocytes, mature cells (chronic inflammation of lymph nodes)

Bone marrow puncture: The smear showed that the bone marrow hematopoietic tissue was actively proliferating and G/E was normal. Erythrocytes of all stages were visible. Granulocytes were mostly band neutrophil and partial left shift, and megakaryocytes were scattered. AML-ETO, BCR/ABL, and PML-RARA were all negative. CD3 (+), CD20 (-), CD45 (+), MPO (+).

May 17

Blood test: leukocyte: 5.5×10^9/L, hemoglobin: 98 g/L, erythrocyte: 3.13×10^{12}/L, platelets: 68×10^9/L, and monocytes: 13.8%

Peripheral blood smear: monocytes: 11%↑, abnormal lymphocytes: 2%, myelocytes: 1%, metamyelocytes: 1%, and metarubricytes: 2%

ALT: 433↑U/L, total protein: 43↓g/L, albumin: 20↓g/L, total bilirubin <32.1umol/L, CHO: 1.76 mmol/L, TG: 5.49 mmol/L, and ferritin >646.00 ug/L

Rheumatism immunology indicators: ANA, ENA, ANCA, AMA, dsDNA, RF, ASO, urine Bence-Jones protein, immunoglobulin, and serum immunofixation electrophoresis Coombs test: No abnormal findings were revealed. CRP was 13.40↑mg/L, and total IgE was 544.80 ng/ml.

Pathogen test: Multiple blood cultures and urine cultures were negative, *Plasmodium* was not found, and the *Cryptococcus* latex agglutination test, G test, and CMV-DNA were negative.

The tumor markers were normal.

No obvious abnormalities were found in the cardiac ultrasound.

According to the symptom of fever, hepatomegaly, splenomegaly, abnormal items of blood cell reduction (involving peripheral blood ≥2/3 blood cells lines, Hb <90 g/L, and PLT<100 × 10^9/L), high triglycerides (triglycerides ≥3 mmol/L after vegetarian diet), and ferritin ≥500 μg/L, the diagnosis of hemophagocytic lymphohistiocytosis (HLH) was established. However, HLH is a syndrome after all, so what we need to do is to find the cause of HLH as much as possible. The patient received many antibiotics in the other hospital, which were ineffective. In the course of the disease, the EB virus IgG turned from negative to positive, and the peripheral blood smear showed the following: monocytes: 11%↑, abnormal lymphocytes: 2%, myelocytes: 1%, metamyelocytes: 1%, and metarubricytes: 2%. Therefore, EBV infection and hematological tumors needed to be excluded. On May 21, the patient's serum EBV-DNA reached 2.9 × 10^6 copics/mL. Whole-body PET-CT showed enlarged liver, with a mild diffuse increase in FDG metabolism (indicating benign lesions), laryngitis, mild left pleural thickening, splenomegaly, suspected gallbladder stones, and pelvic effusion. At the same time, reexamined bone marrow smears on admission showed (Fig. 2.1) a proliferative bone marrow, with granulocytes and megakaryocytes all showing maturation disorder; some granulocytes exhibited degeneration. Erythrocyte hyperplasia was active, some with hemoglobin insufficient filling; iron staining showed iron utilization disorder. Mononuclear phagocyte system proliferation was active, hematopoietic cells were easy to see (2.5%), and a small amount of abnormal lymphocytes could be seen.

According to the proliferation of mononuclear phagocyte system on the bone marrow smear, hemophagocytic cells were easy to see (2.5%), which was another diagnostic basis for HLH. So far, six of the eight criteria for diagnosing HLH had been met. Clinical diagnosis of hemophagocytic syndrome (HPS) was doubtless. Moreover, neither previous lymph node biopsy nor PET-CT had shown any evidence of lymphoma or other tumors. The repeated serological tests and pathogenic cultures of the other hospital and our hospital had no evidence of other serious

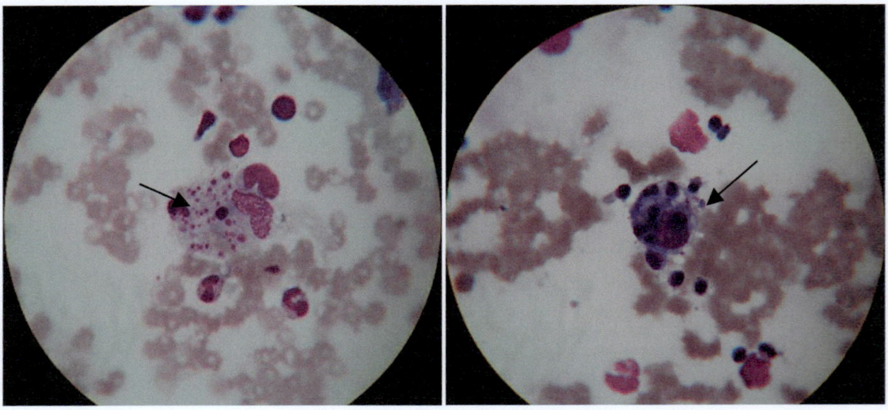

Fig. 2.1 Bone marrow smear: Wright's stain, optical microscopy 100*, arrow pointing to hematopoietic cell

infections, and repeated immunological indicators were also negative, combined with clinical manifestations, and it was difficult to diagnose autoimmune diseases, so a positive result of serum EBV-DNA could indicate that the patient suffered from EBV infection–related HLH.

The patient received treatment with methylprednisolone 40 mg bid IVGTT and ganciclovir 0.25 bid IVGTT from May 21, and the peak body temperature dropped to 37.5 °C. After three days, the body temperature rebounded to a maximum of 39 °C, but the patient's spirit and appetite improved. Platelets and albumin increased. After that, the therapeutic regimen was switched to dexamethasone, combined with VP-16, cyclosporine, and other treatments (see Table 2.2 for detailed laboratory indicators and medications), and strengthened anti-infective and supportive therapy was used. The condition of the patient gradually stabilized, and he was transferred to the Department of Hematology to continue treatment.

2.4.3 Comments

Hemophagocytic syndrome (HPS), also known as hemophagocytic lymphohistiocytosis (HLH), is a group of immune abnormal diseases, whose main pathological features are the CD8+ T lymphocytes and macrophages that proliferate and aggregate in the bone marrow and lymphatic tissues and macrophages that phagocytose blood cells. HLH is divided into two categories: hereditary or primary HLH (familial hemophagocytic lymphohistiocytosis (FHLH)) and secondary HLH.

In the etiology of secondary HLH, infections of multiple pathogens can cause secondary HLH, such as viruses, including *Herpesviridae* virus, HIV, hepatitis virus, adenovirus, influenza virus, and parvovirus; bacteria, including *Typhoid bacilli*, *Escherichia coli*, *Mycobacterium tuberculosis*, *Staphylococcus aureus*, *Mycoplasma*, and *Rickettsia*; fungi, including *Cryptococcus* and *Histoplasma capsularis*; and parasites, including *Leishmania* and *Plasmodium*. In addition, tumors, such as lymphoma, multiple myeloma, leukemia, gastric cancer, and metastatic tumors, and autoimmune diseases, such as systemic lupus erythematosus, rheumatoid arthritis, sarcoidosis, and inflammatory bowel disease, can also cause secondary HLH. Among the causes of viral infection–related HLH, Epstein–Barr virus (EBV) infection takes the first place, especially in children and adolescents, which accounts for up to 74%. It is more common in Asians. However, EBV infection–related HLH is rare in adults.

Table 2.2 Blood test and liver function results after treatment

	Leukocyte (10^9/L)	Hemoglobin (g/L)	Lymphocyte (%)	Platelet (10^9/L)	ALT (U/L)	Total bilirubin (μmol/L)	Direct bilirubin (μmol/L)	Main therapeutic regimen
May 17	5.5	98	13.8	68	433	32.1	23.1	1. Methylprednisolone 40 mg IVGTT bid 2. Ganciclovir 250 mg, IVGTT bid (from May 21 to June 4); ganciclovir 250 mg, IVGTT qd (from June 4 to June 7)
May 20	3.51	89	26.5	45	343	101.8		
May 21	3.66	100	23.8	50	353	110.5	91.3	
May 23	5.15	87	21.9	86	317	63	51	
May 25	5.15	94	23.7	76	226	54.7	42.4	
May 26	5.59	92	26.7	61	191	42.8	32.2	
May 27	4.77	87	31.9	51	157	55.9		1. Dexamethasone 10 mg, IVGTT, qd 2.γ-globulin 20 g IVGTT, qd, × 5d 3.VP-16 150 mg, IVGTT, biw × 2w, then qw 4. Cyclosporin 100 mg q8h po
May 29	3.55	83	34.6	91	104	35.5	27.8	
May 31	3.07	82	37.5	136	94	28.2	21.6	
June 2	2.28	81	35.1	146	77	23.7	18.6	
June 4	2.89	79		207	80	18.8	14.6	
June 6	2.51	82		235	85	19.3	14.4	Dexamethasone 10 mg, IVGTT, bid, combined with VP-16 and cyclosporin

References

1. Evridiki K. Vouloumanou. Current diagnosis and management of infectious mononucleosis. Curr Opin Hematol. 2012;19:14–20.
2. Belyea B, Hinson A, Moran C. Spontaneous resolution of Epstein-Barr virus-associated hemophagocytic lymphohistiocytosis. Pediatr Blood Cancer. 2010,55(4):754–6.
3. Zhang L, Qiu H, Li J. Clinical analysis of 10 cases of secondary hemophagocytic lymphohistiocytosis treated with HLH-2004. Chemother J Exp Hematol. 2010;18(6):1525–30.
4. HLH_2004:diagnostic and therapeutic guidelines for hemophagocytic lymphohistiocytosis. Pediatr Blood Cancer. 2007; 48(2):124–31.
5. Ishi i E, Ohga S, Imashuk US, e t al. Nationwide survey of hemophagocytic lymph o-histiocytosis in Japan [J]. Int J Hematol. 2007; 86(1):58–65.

2.5 A Case of *Brucella* Infection Featured as Lumbar Damage

Wang Ting, Jin Jialin, and Zhang Wenhong

A 59-year-old female farmer, who raised cattle and swine at her farm, was admitted to the hospital for lumbago of 2 months and fever of 20 days on October 14, 2013.

She developed lumbago with no obvious cause in October 2013, which was persistent, presented in the middle of the back, and exacerbated after labor. She had a low fever at first. During several visits to the local outpatient clinics, drugs were orally administered for improving blood circulation and dispersing the stasis, and glucocorticoids were focally injected twice. The back pain was relieved, and the body temperature came down to the normal level. On September 25, 2013, the lower back pain worsened again, which was persistent and exacerbated after labor, with radiating pain in the lower limbs. She was diagnosed with lumbar muscle strain and lumbar disc herniation at the local orthopedic outpatient clinic. Symptoms did not improve after treatment. Blood routine test showed the following: white blood cell (WBC): 3.1 × 10^9/L, neutrocyte: 45.4%, lymphocyte: 46.3%, hemoglobin (Hb): 101 g/L, and platelet count (PLT): 121 × 10^9/L. Three days later, she had hyperpyrexia, with chills sometimes, and was admitted to the infectious disease department at a local grade A tertiary hospital. Blood routine test showed the following: white blood cell (WBC): 2.6 × 10^9/L, neutrocyte: 42.3%, hemoglobin: 103 g/L, and platelet: 136 × 10^9/L. Erythrocyte sedimentation rate (ESR) was 94 mm/h. C-reactive protein (CRP) was 34.8 mg/L. Procalcitonin (PCT) was 0.147 ng/ml. Urine routine test yielded no positive findings. Panipenem 0.5 g q8g IVGTT was administered, along with albumin supplement, supportive treatment, and bed rest. The back pain was partially relieved, while the fever continued and fluctuated around 38–40 °C. Bone marrow puncture was performed, and the bone marrow smear yielded no abnormal findings. She visited our hospital on October 14, 2013, for persistent fever. She was a hepatitis B virus carrier but denied having any other chronic disease.

2.5.1 Physical Examination

Her body temperature was 37 °C on admission, pulse was 82 per minute, respiratory rate was 16 per minute, and blood pressure was 100/60 mmHg. She was clear in consciousness and breathed smoothly and steadily and had no jaundice and no rash or petechia on the skin or mucosa. She had no liver palm. There was no cyanosis on the lips. The breath sound was rough, without dry or wet rales or wheezing. Her heart rate was 78 per minute, without arrhythmia or pathological murmur. The abdomen was soft, without tenderness or rebound tenderness. The upper border of the liver was at the fifth right intercostal space, and neither the liver nor the spleen was palpable under the ribs. There was no percussion pain in the hepatic region and no shifting dullness. There was no deformity of the spine, with mild tenderness at the middle of the L2–4 level and the neighboring soft tissue. There was no edema in the lower limbs. Physiological reflexes existed, and pathological reflexes were not drawn out. Meningeal irritation signs were negative.

2.5.2 Diagnosis and Treatment

The following laboratory tests were completed after hospitalization:

October 15, 2013: Blood routine test: WBC: 3.96×10^9/L, Hb: 90 g/L, PLT: 186×10^9/L, N 40.20%, and L: 49.20%.

October 15, 2013: Ferritin: 467.70 ug/L, high-sensitivity CRP (hs-CRP): 54.10, anti-streptolysin (ASO): 38.30, rheumatoid factor: <20.0 and ESR: 60.00 mm/h.

October 15, 2013: Immunoglobulin G: 13.10 g/L, immunoglobulin A: 1.90 g/L, immunoglobulin M: 1.75 g/L, C3: 1.18 g/L, and C4: 0.34 g/L.

October 15, 2013: Biochemistry test: Total protein: 55.00 g/L, albumin: 28.00 g/L, total bilirubin: 24.10 μmol/L, direct bilirubin: 9.10 μmol/L, indirect bilirubin: 15.00 μmol/L, alanine aminotransferase (ALT): 27.00 IU/L, aspartate aminotransferase (AST): 31.00 IU/L, blood urea nitrogen (BUN): 1.85 mmol/L, serum creatinine (SCr): 51.00 μmol/L, serum potassium (K^+): 3.33 mmol/L, lactate dehydrogenase (LDH): 244.00 U/L, and α-hydroxybutyrate dehydrogenase: 204.00 U/L

October 15, 2013: The coagulation test yielded no abnormal findings.

October 15, 2013: Lung CT scan: There was slight inflammation at the left lower lobe, with pleura thickened on both sides. The spleen was enlarged.

October 16, 2013: Lumbar MRI: There was an abnormal signal at L2–3, which suggested infection according to the history. Subcutaneous soft tissue at the lower back was swollen.

October 17, 2013: Echocardiography: There was slight regurgitation at the mitral and tricuspid valves, with left ventricular diastolic function decreased.

October 18, 2013: Ultrasound yielded no abnormal findings of the liver, gallbladder, pancreas, spleen, and kidneys.

Thyroid function test, tumor indicators, and myocardial enzyme spectrum yielded no abnormal findings.

Blood culture done twice and bone marrow culture done once at the local hospital were positive, and the species identification revealed *Brucella melitensis*.

Further investigation found that the cattle that this patient had raised had gone through a rinderpest. Based on the epidemiological history and culture results, doxycycline 0.1 g bid and rifampicin 0.6 g qd were orally administered the day after admission, the blood sample was sent to the National Institute of Parasitic Disease, China CDC for *Brucella* antibody examination, and 4–5 days after treatment, the peak temperature of the patient gradually dropped to normal. The *Brucella* antibody detected by the CDC was positive with a titer of 1:800. Considering the lumbar impairment, a triple therapy of ceftriaxone, rifampicin, and doxycycline was administered on October 22. This patient was discharged from the hospital on October 25 and continued oral treatment with rifampicin, doxycycline, and levofloxacin. One month later, a lumbar MRI on November 21 yielded an infection damage of the L2–3 vertebrae with a paravertebral small abscess and swollen subcutaneous soft tissue, which had advanced compared with the MRI on October 16. An intensive treatment regimen, including intravenous rifampicin, amikacin, and oral doxycycline (0.1 g bid), was administered from December 9, 2013. Two months later, the lesion was shown to be markedly resolved in a lumbar MRI (Fig. 2.2).

2.5.3 Key Points

Brucellosis is a zoonotic disease caused by the infection–allergy reaction when *Brucella* infects the human body. It has been more than 100 years since *Brucella* was first isolated by Bruce from the spleen of infected soldiers who died of brucellosis in 1887. Brucellosis was first reported in 1905 in China and was well-controlled once. However, this plague has reemerged and spread since 2000. Clinical characteristics of brucellosis include fever, hyperhidrosis, myalgia, arthralgia, fatigue, hepatomegaly, splenomegaly, and swollen lymph nodes. Sometimes, the reproductive system could be involved. Some cases have had cardiac, renal, or neuronal system involvement.

The spondylitis of brucellosis is featured as a persistent pain in the neck, chest, and lower back, along with focal tenderness, percussion pain, muscle spasm, limited spine movement, abscesses of psoas major, radiculalgia of the corresponding nerves, or symptoms of spinal cord compression. It can cause paralysis when the spinal cord is compressed by the epidural abscesses. Spine lesions in brucellosis are mostly located in the lumbar spine, and L4 has the highest incidence. The bone damage is small and multifocal, mostly confined to the edge of the vertebral body. There is obvious hyperplasia and sclerosis around the lesion, with a new destructive lesion in the regenerated bone tissue. Damage to the intravertebral disc is slight, with hyperplasia and sclerosis of the articular surface and increased density of the adjacent bone. Paravertebral abscesses are rare or absent. MRI characteristics

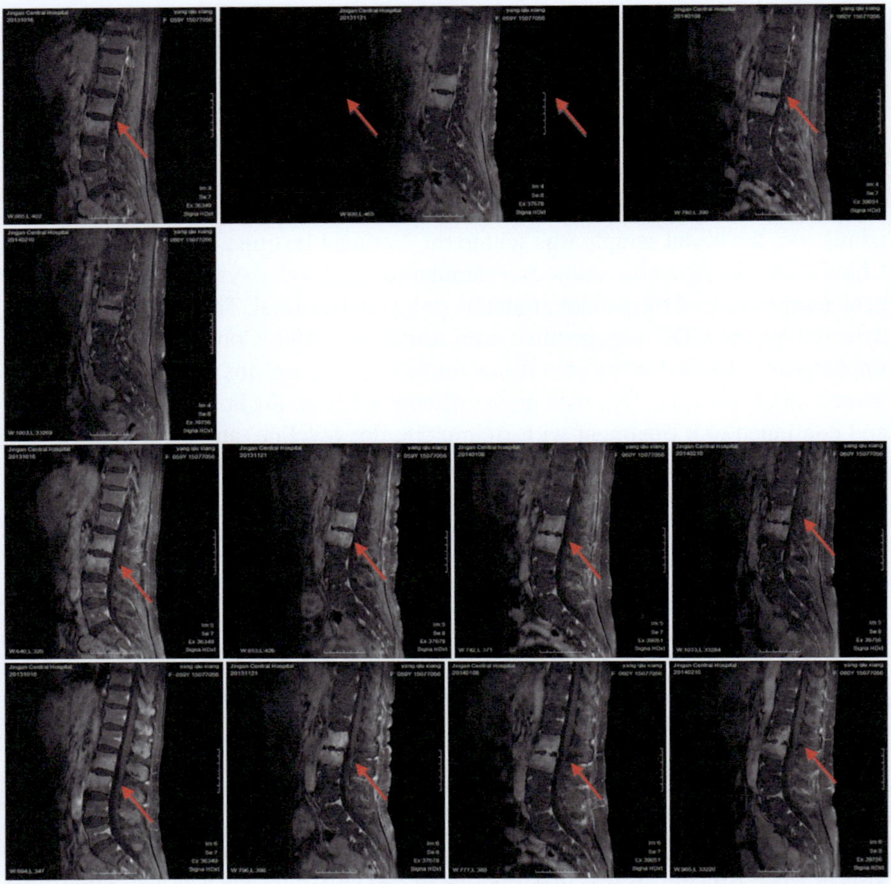

Fig. 2.2 Changes on 2 lumbar MRI cross section of pretreatment (October 16, 2013), 1 month after the two combination oral therapy (November 21, 2013), 2 months after intravenous intensive treatment (January 8, 2014), 1 month after the sequential triple oral therapy (February 10, 2014) from left to right. After a traditional binary therapy of oral rifampicin and doxycycline for 1 month, there is still obvious progress in lumbar lesions, but the range and enhancement degree of vertebral lesions were significantly reduced and weakened after adjustment to intravenous intensive triple therapy.

include the thick and irregularly enhanced abscess wall and paraspinal high signal with an unclear boundary.

This patient was admitted for a fever of unknown origin, with a 2-month history and a 1-month fever. She had a fever with chills and increased inflammation indicators, which suggested a high possibility of an infectious disease. Considering that this patient's history of cattle raising and blood culture yielded *Brucella melitensis*, the diagnosis of brucellosis was clear. The clinical characteristics of brucellosis could vary, but spondylitis is rare (7.5%), which greatly increases the difficulty of treatment and has a high disability rate. This case focused on the clinical characteristics and treatment for brucellosis featured as spondylitis through the real diagnostic and treatment processes.

References

1. Ministry of Culture of the People's Republic of China. Guideline for diagnosis and treatment of Brucellosis. Infect Dis Information. 2012;2(25):323—4, 359.
2. Yang XM, Shi WS, Ya K. Clinical image and pathological characteristics of brucellosis spondylitis. J Prac Radiol. 2008;4(24):522–5.
3. Merdan M, Tian J, Sheng WB. Diagnosis and surgical treatment of brucellosis spondylitis. Chin J Orthop. 2012;4(32):323–30.

2.6 A Case of *Babesia* Infection with Recurrent Fever for More Than 10 Months

Hu Yuekai and Zhang Jiming

A 71-year-old woman, a cartographer from Wuyi Mountain, Fujian, Southeast China, was admitted to the hospital on December 24, 2012, due to "recurrent fever for more than 10 months."

In March 2012, the patient developed intermittent fever, and the highest temperature was 38 °C. The physical examination in May showed a decrease in RBCs, WBCs, and platelets, and the fever recurred several times. In September 2012, a high fever began to appear, accompanied by chills, shivering, and nausea, and the highest temperature was 41 °C. The patient did not respond to antibiotics, and there was no definitive diagnosis. On November 16, 2012, she was transferred to a hospital in Shanghai. Given the decrease in red blood cells (RBCs), white blood cells (WBCs), and platelets, combined with persistent fever and a Widal reaction that revealed O antigen (1:80) and H antigen (1:80), the possibility of typhoid fever could not be ruled out. November 19 to November 30: cefoperazone–sulbactam 3.0 g bid was given for antibacterial treatment, then piperacillin–tazobactam 4.5 g q8h was given in November 30 to December 30, and ornidazole 0.5 g bid in November 30 to December 3. November 28 to December 18, hydroxychloroquine 400 mg bid was given as a diagnostic antimalarial. However, there was no response to the treatment and no improvement in intermittent high fever and chills. After that, doxycycline (0.1 g bid), lincomycin (1.2 g bid 2 days after 0.6 q6h), and azithromycin (0.5 g qd) were given in December 6 to December 13, December 11 to December 18, and December 19, respectively, but no significant decrease in body temperature was observed. She had a history of chronic hepatitis B and had taken entecavir as antiviral therapy.

2.6.1 Physical Examination on Admission

The patient was sane, energetic, and lean. There was no icteric skin or sclera and no swelling in superficial supraclavicular lymph nodes. There was no deformity of the skull, and she presented with a well-featured face and soft neck. The trachea was in the middle, and the thyroid was not enlarged. The respiration movements of both sides were normal and symmetrical. The respiration sounds of both lungs were clear, and no obvious dry or moist rales were heard. HR was 95/min, and there was a regular heart rhythm. No pathological murmur was heard in the auscultatory valve areas. The abdomen was flat and soft, and there was no tenderness or rebound pain in the whole abdomen; no abnormal masses under the liver, spleen, or costal area; no percussion pain in the liver or kidney area; no abdominal shifting dullness; normal bowel sounds; normal limb movement; symmetrical knee reflex; and negative neuropathological signs.

Relevant examinations were completed after admission, as follows:

November 19, 2012: WBC: 1.0 × 10^9/L, N: 47.5%, Hb: 101 g/L, PLT: 73 × 10^{12}/L, reticulocyte (Ret): 3.0, ESR: 53 mm/h, CRP: 20.9 mg/L, ALT: 60 U/L, AST: 134 U/L, and albumin: 33 g/L.

December 20, 2012: WBC: 1.0 × 10^9/L, N: 43%, Hb: 94 g/L, PLT: 43 × 10^{12}/L, ALT: 117 U/L, AST: 184 U/L, and albumin: 31 g/L.

November 30, 2012: Parasite antibodies (*Cysticercus*, *Paragonimus westermani*, *Clonorchis sinensis*, *Schistosoma*, hydatid, *Trichinella*, *Sparganum mansoni*, *Toxoplasma gondii*, *Angiostrongylus cantonensis*, and Filariasis) were negative.

November 30, 2012: Abdominal B-ultrasound: 1. Moderate echo from the left lateral lobe of the liver of size 100 mm × 95 mm; 2. postprandial gallbladder; 3. slight splenomegaly, 0 mm–21 mm below the ribs, with complete capsule and uniform distribution of internal echo; 4. no abnormality was observed in the pancreas; 5. no obvious thrombosis echo was observed in the portal vein; and 6. hypoecho (lymph node) was observed in the retroperitoneum with a size of 10 mm × 7 mm.

November 20, 2012: Enhanced CT: There were abdominal intrahepatic calcification or calculus of bile duct, hepatic cyst, splenomegaly, and multiple enlarged lymph nodes in the hilum hepatis and the retroperitoneal area, and the diameter of the larger ones was about 16 mm. No abnormalities were observed in the kidneys and adrenal glands. Slightly enlarged lymph nodes were observed in the retroperitoneal area. No abnormalities were observed in the pelvic cavity. Chest: chronic bronchitis changes in both lungs, emphysema with multiple inflammatory sequelae, and an old focus in the upper lobe of the left lung. Intracranial: a few lacunar foci in the deep brain on both sides and senile brain atrophy.

December 4, 2012: Plain and enhanced MRI scan of the upper abdomen: cirrhosis, splenomegaly, and multiple microcystic foci in the liver. No obvious abnormalities were observed in the gallbladder and pancreas. There was a slight effusion around the spleen.

Bone marrow puncture indicated that there was active proliferation of bone marrow nucleated cells, active proliferation of both granulocytes and erythrocytes, a normal number of megakaryocytes, and scattered platelets.

Chromosome examination report: Bone marrow cells were cultured for 2 days. Chromosome examination of 20 cells showed no abnormalities in the number or structure of chromosomes associated with tumors.

Bone marrow biopsy pathology: A piece of tissue (posterior superior iliac spine) was 0.3 cm in length. Microscopically, fibrous, adipose, and bone tissue were observed. Two medullary cavities were observed, which were paracortical medullary cavities, most of which were adipose tissue, and a small part comprised hematopoietic components, accounting for 10–20%.

November 29, 2012: Bone marrow smear showed bone marrow mild hyperplasia, granulocyte maturation disorder, and degeneration. A part of the erythroblasts was insufficiently filled with hemoglobin. Plasma cells, monocytes, and macrophages were easy to see, and a part of them was hemophagocytic. Little phagocytized objects were suspected to be unclassified pathogens, and a few atypical lymphocytes were also observed.

After admission, peripheral blood was extracted when the patient was shivering and sent to the Department of Pathogenic Microbiology of the medical college for testing. The sequencing of the pathogenic microorganism gene showed that it was 100% consistent with the *Babesia* gene sequence, so it was considered a *Babesia* infection. After the diagnosis, considering that the patient had been treated with azithromycin and lincomycin with poor results, artesunate was given. However, the body temperature was still fluctuating, and the peripheral blood smear was still positive. Therefore, the medical team advised her family to obtain Malarone and administer it as directed. Afterward, her self-reported symptoms gradually improved, and her body temperature gradually became normal. RBCs, WBCs, and platelets of peripheral blood and liver function also gradually became normal (January 17, 2013: WBC: 4.45×10^9/L, Hb: 101 g/L, PLT: 114×10^{12}/L, CRP: normal, ALT: 26 U/L, AST: 47 U/L, and albumin: 41 g/L). The treatment did not stop until the blood smear was negative for approximately 2 weeks (the first treatment was about 1 month), followed by another 2 weeks of treatment after 1 month. At present, she has been followed up for one year with a stable clinical condition.

2.6.2 Comments

Babesia is a tick-borne protozoan that parasitizes the red blood cells of vertebrates and belongs to the *Babesia* genus of the Babesiidae of Piroplasmida. Babesiosis (piroplasmosis) is a zoonotic parasitic disease caused by the infection of the *Babesia*, which is parasitic in red blood cells, through the bite of ticks. Mammals such as cattle, horses, and sheep are the main sources of babesiosis. It presents as mild influenza-like symptoms in young and healthy people but can develop into malaria-like symptoms after splenectomy or in patients with immunodeficiency and in the elderly. It is characterized by intermittent fever, splenomegaly, jaundice, and hemolysis. *Babesia* parasites reside exclusively within the human red blood cells (Fig. 2.3), exhibiting diverse morphologies, including pear-shaped, round, or oval forms, either singly or in pairs (double pear-shaped, with pointed ends oriented toward each other and blunt ends forming an angle).

In the process of diagnosing FUO, there are sometimes uncommon or rare pathogens, which are difficult to identify. At this time, we should actively search for relevant literature and cooperate with experts in the field to find out the possibility of identifying the pathogen. In this case, babesiosis was a newly emerged parasitic disease, which was not well-known in China. The diagnosis was finally made with the cooperation of the microbiologist and through the gene sequencing of pathogenic microorganisms.

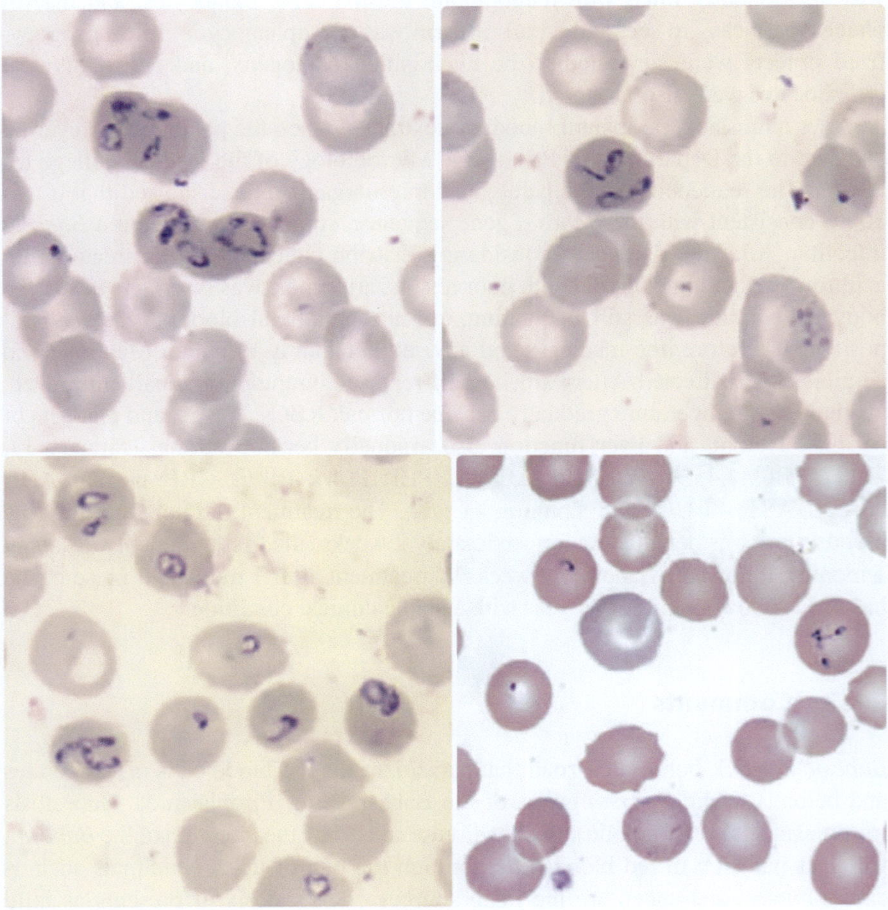

Fig. 2.3 Morphology of *Babesia*-infected red blood cells on a blood smear. (Source: Parasite Image Library, Division of Parasitic Diseases and Malaria (DPDM), Centers for Disease Control and Prevention (CDC), U.S. Department of Health and Human Services.)

Resistance therapy for babesiosis: Symptomatic patients who are negative for *Babesia* on blood smear or in PCR results should not be given resistance therapy. Antigen therapy should be given only to symptomatic patients with *Babesia* detection. Atovaquone + azithromycin for 7–10 days can be a choice for patients with mild infections. Artesunate has also been reported in the treatment for babesiosis. Severe cases may be treated with clindamycin combined with quinine. PCV and parasitemia should be monitored daily during treatment until symptoms are resolved and parasitemia <5%. *Babesia* infection can persist or recur even after satisfactory treatment according to the standard regimen. The DNA positive rate is 36% after 1 month of standard treatment, which is more common in older patients or those with basic immunodeficiency. The treatment of patients like this usually needs more than 6 weeks and should not be stopped until the blood smear is negative for 2 weeks. Patients who are still positive in the blood smear or DNA tests 3 months after the initial treatment should be considered for retreatment.

References

1. Shao LY, Weng XH. Practiced internal medicine. 14th ed. Chapter 13.
2. He DM, Wang YM. Research progress of human babesiosis. Chin J Infect Dis. 2012;10(30):638–40.
3. Vannier E, Gewurz BE, Krause PJ. Human babesiosis. Infect Dis Clin N Am. 2008;22:469–88.
4. Mandell GL, Bennett JE, Dolin R. Principles and practice of infectious diseases. 7th ed. New York: Churchill Livingstone Inc., 2010. p. 3539–45.
5. Lobo CA, Rodriguez M, Cursino-Santos JR. Babesia and red cell invasion[J]. Curr Opin Hematol. 2012;19(3):170–5.

2.7 A Hepatic Fluke Infection Suspected of an Intrahepatic Tumor

Li Qian and Zhang Wenhong

A 54-year-old woman, engaged in the kelp-processing industry, from Ningde, Fujian, in the Southeast of China, was admitted to the hospital for "intermittent fever, progressive emaciation and eosinophilia for more than 2 months."

She had a fever of unknown origin and slight chills since July 2013. Laboratory results of several hospitals revealed eosinophilia, both in the peripheral blood (20–40%) and the bone marrow. The enhanced CT scan of the liver showed "multiple intrahepatic occupying foci." She had received anti-infective and glucocorticoid therapy during hospitalization but still had interrupted irregular fever, with the highest temperature reaching 39.6 °C. Weak positive antibody against *Schistosoma* was found in the blood, and *Blastocystis hominis* was positive in the feces test. On September 17, she was admitted to our department for "eosinophilia." She had been in a poor mental state with poor sleep since the illness, and she had also experienced intermittent diarrhea and abdominal pain in the early stages. She had dry stool two or three times/day in the past 1 month and had a weight loss of 10 kg in the past 3 months. She had a history of diabetes mellitus and duodenal ulcer (S2).

2.7.1 Physical Examination

T:37.8 °C, P:95/min, R: 20/min, BP: 115/75 mmHg, sane, thin, and answering questions. There was no obvious swelling of superficial lymph nodes. Cardiopulmonary auscultation showed no abnormality. Abdomen was flat and soft, and there was no tenderness and rebound pain in the whole abdomen, no abnormal mass, no subcostal reach to the liver and spleen, obvious percussion pain in the liver area, Murphy's sign was negative (−), shifting dullness was negative (−), there was no edema in both lower extremities, and neurological pathological signs were negative (−).

2.7.2 Diagnosis and Treatment

After admission, laboratory studies revealed the following: WBC: 11.43×10^9/L, Hb: 93 g/L, RBC: 3.14×10^{12}/L, platelets: 281×10^9/L, N: 52.8%, and eosinophils: 32.3%. Liver and kidney functions were normal, ESR was 97 mm/h, CRP was 78 mg/L, feces test for parasitic eggs was negative, and T-SPOT.TB was negative (-). Tumor markers were normal, and immune indexes and latex agglutination tests were negative. B-type ultrasound showed no abnormality in the thyroid, and there was a high possibility of diffuse hepatic-occupying foci. There was *biliary sludge* deposition in the gallbladder and no abnormality in the spleen, pancreas, kidney, and the ureter. PET-CT showed a slight increase in liver FDG metabolism inhomogeneity, which was insufficient to consider neoplastic lesions. Magnetic resonance cholangiopancreatography (MRCP) showed "gallstone, cholecystitis, upper common bile duct stone; Multiple abnormal signals in the liver" (Fig. 2.4). Enhanced CT of the liver suggested "multiple intrahepatic occupying foci, considering the

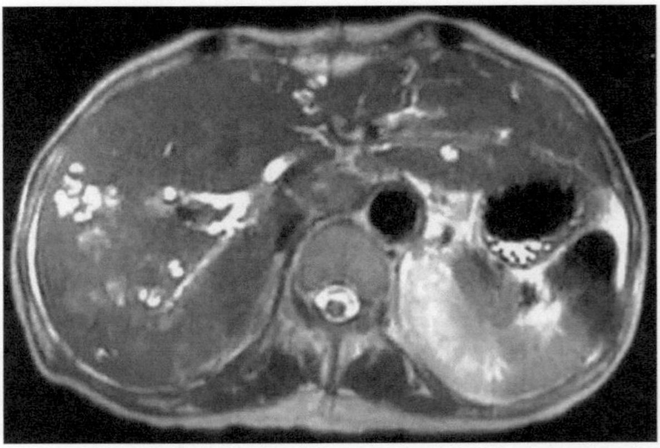

Fig. 2.4 Enhanced hepatic MRCP

possibility of cystic dilatation of intrahepatic bile duct." After admission, she was given supportive treatment. Since intrahepatic infection could not be ruled out, she was given metronidazole with Sulperazon as the anti-infective treatment from September 20. On September 24, medication was switched to vancomycin (1.0 IVGTT q12h) and fosfomycin (8.0 IVGTT q12h) for anti-infective treatment because gram-positive cocci were found in the blood culture. On September 27, she was given Tienam (1.0 IVGTT q12h) for anti-infective treatment, but the body temperature still fluctuated between 39 °C and 40 °C. Due to the obvious eosinophilia in the peripheral blood, the antibacterial effect was not good; considering the possibility of parasitic infection, the antibacterial agents were discontinued, and the treatment was replaced with deworming treatment. Diagnostic albendazole repellent therapy (a total dose of 33 tablets) was initiated on September 30 and ended on October 8. Her body temperature dropped slightly during the treatment, fluctuating between 38.5 °C and 39 °C. Mental state and diet were slightly improved, but the percussion pain in the liver area was not significantly relieved. The patient had the indication of lesion exploration after surgical consultation, which can not only help make a definite diagnosis but also have the effect of treatment. "Partial resection of the right lobe of the liver, cholecystectomy, and common bile duct exploration" were performed under general anesthesia on October 18, during which "No ascites and implant metastasis were observed, and the liver was still soft with slightly blunt edges, and multiple space-occupying lesions were observed in the liver, mainly in the right lobe. The largest lesion was about 5cm in diameter, hard in texture, irregular in shape and clear in boundary." Pathology showed that there was granulomatous inflammation with coagulant necrosis and numerous eosinophils, suggesting parasitic infection (Fig. 2.5). The lesion of the greater omentum was the same as that of the liver. Adult parasites could be seen, and the morphology was consistent with that of hepatic flukes (Fig. 2.6).

The temperature of the patient returned to normal three days after the surgery. Before definitive pathological diagnosis, given the clinical suspicion of parasitic

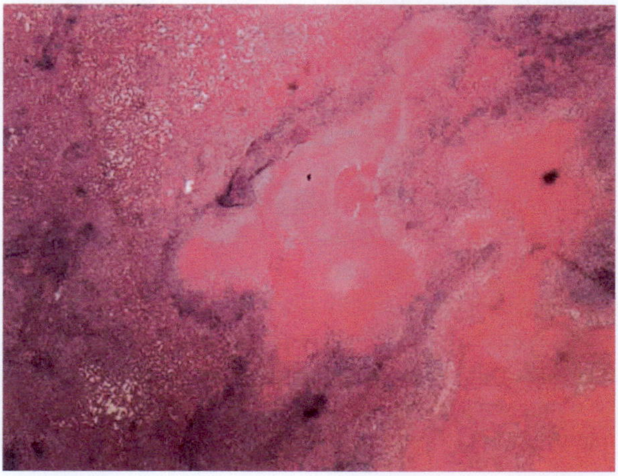

Fig. 2.5 Pathological features of lesions in the right lobe of the liver (Hematoxylin-Eosin staining, HE staining, × 40)

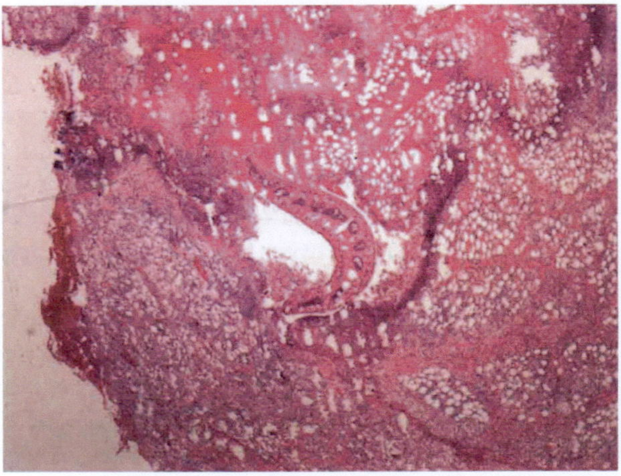

Fig. 2.6 *Fasciola hepatica* seen in nodules of the greater omentum (HE staining, × 100)

infection and and the ineffectiveness of albendazole, praziquantel was prescribed for deworming therapy. The drug specification was 0.2 g per tablet, and the total therapeutic dose was 150 mg/kg body weight. However, the patient's symptoms did not improve significantly, and the proportion of eosinophils also did not decrease, and the T-tube drainage was still turbid. Due to the postoperative pathological findings suggesting hepatic fluidic, she was given triclabendazole (10 mg/kg/d) for two days. After that, the T-tube drainage fluid was cleared, mental state and diet improved, and the eosinophilic cell proportion, erythrocyte sedimentation rate, and C-reactive protein decreased. On November 14, the patient got better and was discharged.

2.7.3 Comments

Fasciola hepatica is a large fluke belonging to the family of Fasciolidae; the adult parasitizes herbivores and other animals in the hepatic bile duct, and the eggs are excreted out of the body in the feces. After the eggs enter the water, they hatch into miracidia, which develop into cercariae in the intermediate host, conidia, and can form metacercariae when the cercariae encounter aquatic plants. Human infection is mainly caused by ingestion of the metacercariae (aquatic plants contaminated with metacercariae or water or cow or sheep viscera containing hepatic flukes). The metacercariae are formed after the excyst penetrates the intestinal wall to invade the liver via the abdominal cavity or enters the biliary tract through the mesenteric vein or lymphatic vessels, and they can live up to 12 years in the human body. Most adults parasitize in the intrahepatic bile duct and present as multiple nodular and cystic lesions in the liver parenchyma. They can also cause ectopic lesions in the subcutaneous tissue, brain, lungs, eyes, and bladder. The hepatic fluke infection can be diagnosed by the discovery of eggs in the fecal or duodenal drainage fluid deposits or by the discovery of adult worms in surgical exploration.

Trematodes and nematodes are the most common worms in the liver. *Clonorchis sinensis* and *Fasciola hepatica* are the most involved in the liver biliary system. Although the lesions in the bile duct system of *Fasciola hepatica* infection are more serious than those of *Clonorchis sinensis* infection, it is difficult to distinguish them clinically, and the identification mainly depends on the eggs or the adults. Due to the clinical rarity of hepatic fluke, albendazole deworming treatment was the first choice on this patient, which only reduced her temperature peak slightly, and the antimicrobial drug treatment was ineffective. In order to clarify the features of liver lesions and treatment, the patient underwent exploratory laparotomy. Tumor or parasitic infection could not be distinguished only from the surgical field of view, and then the worm body was found through pathological sections to confirm the diagnosis. Before the pathology results came back, the patient had been considered to have parasitic infections causing eosinophilia. Although treated with praziquantel and albendazole successively, the patient did not get better. Her symptoms and indexes did not gradually return to normal until the final oral administration of triclabendazole. This brings us to an important point: The treatment for hepatic fluke is distinct from that for parasites and requires special deworming agents, which should be taken seriously in clinical practice.

References

1. Li MD, Wang YM. Practice of infectious diseases. People's Medical Publishing House. p. 1179–83.
2. Aminian K, Rezayat KA, et al. Living Fasciola hepatica in biliary tree: a case report. Ann Hepatol. 2012,11(3):395–8.
3. Giancarlo Albanese and Caterina Venturi. Albendazole: a new drug for human parasitoses. Dermatol Clin. 2003;21:283–90.
4. Dayan AD. Albendazole, mebendazole and praziquantel. Review of non-clinical toxicity and pharmacokinetics. Acta Tropica. 2003;86:141–59.
5. Fairweather I. Triclabendazole: new skills to unravel an old(ish) enigma. J Helminthol. 2005;79:227–34.

2.8 A Case Report of *Plasmodium malariae* Infection with Lymphocyte Hyperplasia

Zhu Liping and Hu Yuekai

A 74-year-old man was admitted with a 3-year history of intermittent shaking chills, severe fever, and sweating on March 10, 2014. He was a retired worker from Shanghai.

His fever had been occurring without any obvious predisposing causes since April 2011. He was experiencing fever of 5–6 hours' duration (temperature as high as 39 °C) every 48–72 h. He had obvious chills preceding the onset of fever but no headache, nausea, or vomiting. The onset of his fever was followed by heavy sweating and severe fatigue. His fever resolved after the sweating. Half a month later, he became febrile every 72 h, with temperature peaking at 41 °C. Besides, he developed dizziness, a sore back, joint pain, and worsening fatigue. Laboratory tests from an outside hospital yielded the following results: white blood cell count: 5.9×10^9/L, of which 54.5% were lymphocytes; hemoglobin: 115 g/L; platelet count: 142×10^9/L; titer of antinuclear antibodies: 1:100; and pANCA: weak positive. His liver and renal functions were normal. The serum tumor markers were within normal limits. Multiple blood smears for malaria and blood culture results were negative. The EBV-DNA assay result was also negative. His bone marrow aspirate smears, biopsy, and immunohistochemistry findings were all unremarkable. Echocardiography found no vegetation in the valves. A mild degree of hepatosplenomegaly was present on abdominal ultrasonography (diameters unspecified). The chest CT detected no abnormalities. A two-week therapy of moxifloxacin and clarithromycin was ineffective, but his fever resolved two months later without further intervention. In January 2013, the patient had another episode of fever with a regular pattern, which abated half a month later without medical intervention. He had a third episode of fever with a pattern similar to the previous two episodes but accompanied by worsened symptoms. Laboratory studies from an outside hospital yielded the following results: white blood cell count: 7.24×10^9/L, of which 73.9% were lymphocytes; hemoglobin: 100 g/L; and platelet count: 76×10^9/L. The results of liver and renal functions were normal. Multiple blood smears for malaria and blood culture results were negative. His bone marrow aspirate smears showed hyperplasia of erythroid, granulocytic, and megakaryocytic lineages, along with immuration of granulocytic and megakaryocytic lineages. The superficial lymph node ultrasound showed a mild enlargement of the bilateral cervical and bilateral inguinal lymph nodes (size peaking at about 5 × 15 mm). The upper abdomen MRI revealed dilation of the main pancreatic duct and the branch duct of the uncinate process and splenomegaly. His PET-CT showed a hypodense lesion in the pancreatic head without remarkable abnormal FDG uptake and splenomegaly with slightly higher FDG uptake. The patient responded poorly to the one-week treatment with cefoperazone in combination with metronidazole. He had no other notable medical history. He reported a trip to Hainan Province in 2005 but no trip to Africa or Southeast Asia. He denied having undergone blood transfusions. Since the onset of the illness, he had a normal spirit and regular excretory habits but a compromised appetite and sleep. He had lost about 5 kg in the past 9 months.

2.8.1 Physical Examination

On admission, he was febrile (temperature, 38.5 °C). He appeared ill but conscious. There was no remarkable finding on physical examination with the exception of pallor and splenomegaly (palpable at about 1cm below the left costal margin, with tender texture, rough edge, and no pain on palpation).

2.8.2 Diagnosis and Treatment

Initial laboratory tests revealed the following: white blood cell count: 6.61×10^9/L, of which 82% were lymphocytes; hemoglobin: 92 g/L; platelet count: 51×10^9/L; and reticulocyte percentage: 3%. His liver function test results were unremarkable, except for an albumin level of 26 g/L. Findings from feces analysis, fecal occult blood test, urinalysis, renal function tests, and serum tumor markers were unrevealing. ANA and ENA panels, ANCA, CCP antibody, and platelet antibodies were negative. The anti-human globulin tests showed positive anti-IgG but negative anti-IgM and anti-C3. There was nothing remarkable in his peripheral blood immunophenotyping of leukemia, echocardiography, and superficial lymph node ultrasound. Splenomegaly was present on abdominal ultrasonography (diameters: 149 × 55 mm). His peripheral blood smears revealed 8% immature lymphocytes, while the bone marrow aspirate smears showed hyperplasia, along with immuration of granulocytic and megakaryocytic lineages. An increased proportion of lymphocytes, some prolymphocytes, and atypical lymphocytes were present on both peripheral blood and bone marrow aspirate smears, which, associated with flow cytometry immunophenotyping, indicated B-cell lymphoproliferative disorders.

On the third day after admission, the patient had another episode of shaking chills. Immediate investigation of thick and thin blood smears found trophozoites (Fig. 2.7) and schizonts (Fig. 2.8) of *Plasmodium malariae*. The bone marrow aspirate smears also confirmed the presence of *P. malariae*. The patient's regular episodes of intermittent shaking chills, severe fevers, resolution of fever after sweating, and associated symptoms like fatigue once every three days, along with the presence of *P. malariae* on peripheral blood smears detected during the episodes of shaking chills, led to a diagnosis of malaria. Therefore, a total dose of eight dihydroartemisinin + piperaquine tablets (2 tab bid) was prescribed. The patient's

Fig. 2.7 A band-form trophozoite of *P. malariae* without obvious foams in normal-sized RBCs in a blood smear

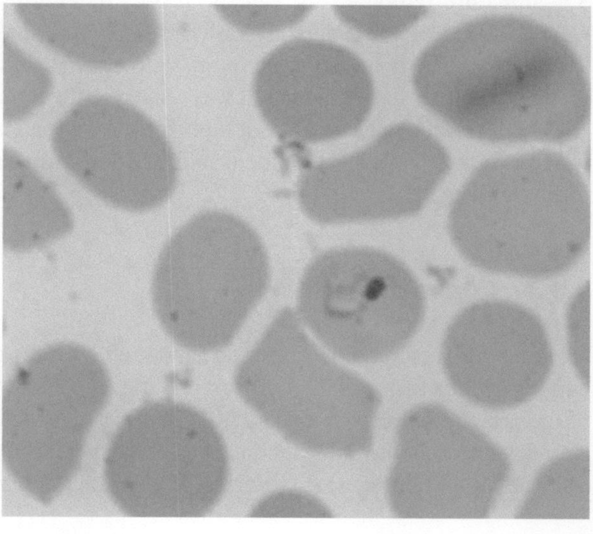

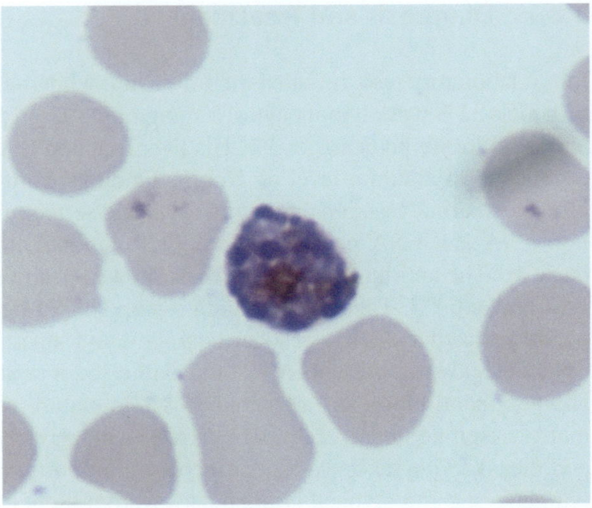

Fig. 2.8 A schizont of *P. malariae* containing about eight merozoites arranged in the periphery of the RBC in a blood smear. Dark brown pigment centered in the RBC

symptoms ceased after completion of the antimalarial treatment. One week after the end of treatment, his laboratory tests revealed the following results: peripheral blood lymphocyte percentage: 63%; hemoglobin: 90 g/L; and recovered levels of platelet, reticulocyte, and albumin. Blood smears yielded negative results. His abdominal ultrasonography revealed significantly alleviated splenomegaly (diameters: 124 × 56 mm). Three months after discharge, the patient recovered well and had no recurrence of the symptoms. Follow-up of his laboratory tests showed 60% of lymphocytes in peripheral blood, a recovered level of hemoglobin, and consistently negative results of blood smears. On follow-up abdominal ultrasonography, the size of his spleen gradually decreased to 112 × 56 mm.

Besides, this patient had developed hyperplasia of peripheral lymphocytes, with 8% immature lymphocytes. But the results of multiple bone marrow evaluations were insufficient for a diagnosis of hematological malignancy. After antimalarial treatment, the body temperature returned to normal, and the lymphocytes decreased gradually, which suggested that it was related to the infection of *P. malariae*, and the lymphocytes could be relatively high in malaria patients. This patient responded well to the antimalarial treatment and had no recrudescence during the 3-month follow-up.

2.8.3 Comments

Malaria is a vector-borne disease transmitted by bites of infected *Anopheles* mosquitoes or transfusion of blood from malaria-infected donors. Major manifestations of malaria are regular onsets of chills, fever, and sweating. Left untreated, patients may develop anemia and splenomegaly. Four species of *Plasmodium* are considered true parasites of humans: *P. malariae*, *P. vivax*, *P. falciparum,* and *P. ovale*. In China,

P. malariae and *P. falciparum* are the predominant species, while the other two species are associated with occasional imported cases.

This case is a local case of *P. malariae* reported in Shanghai, with significant lymphocyte hyperplasia, which resolved quickly after antimalarial treatment. *P. malariae* preferentially invades aged RBC, takes more time for maturation in erythrocytes, and produces fewer schizonts. The density of parasites in the bloodstream is, therefore, quite low. Intracellular parasites are usually present in only 0.01%–1% of a patient's RBC. A low positive rate of blood smear examination thus leads to a higher rate of missed diagnosis. In this case, his thin capillary blood smear was positive for the presence of an intracellular parasite in only 4/1000 of his RBCs. Considering that there have been no local *P. malariae* cases in Shanghai for more than 10 years and the patient has no history of blood transfusion, the source of transmission may have been related to the Hainan travel in 2005 or earlier, but it was not shown due to the persistent low level of infection of *P. malariae*.

References

1. Zhu M, Cai L. Malaria surveillance in Shanghai from 2005 to 2012. Chin J Schistosomiasis Control. 2014 (1):32–7.
2. Jiao Y, Yang G, Xie M, et al. Epidemic characteristics of Malaria in China from 2008 to 2012. Acta Parasitology et Medica Entomologica Sinica. 2013 (2):80–84.

2.9 Immunocompetent *Scedosporium apiospermum* Meningitis

Shao Lingyun, Yu Shenglei, Huang Yuxian and Zhang Wenhong

The 35-year-old patient, male, was a farmer from Kucha County, Xinjiang Province of China. He was admitted to the hospital on August 8, 2014, because of "fever with headache for 3 weeks."

The patient had a fever 3 weeks before admission, the highest temperature being 39.3 °C with chills, and projectile vomiting twice without hematemesis, abdominal pain, diarrhea, rash, blurred vision, etc. He did not go to the doctor in time. On July 19, the patient fell down three times while going to the toilet, and his consciousness was clear without convulsion. Then, he went to the local hospital. No abnormality was found on the CT scan of the head. On July 21, he was transferred to another hospital. Physical examination showed neck rigidity, and the white blood cell (WBC) in cerebrospinal fluids (CSFs) was 1174×10^6/L, protein was 1.46 g/L, glucose was 3.19 mmol/L, and chloride was 114 mmol/L (Table 2.3), and he was considered to have "tuberculous meningitis." On July 22, he was transferred to the Chest Hospital. In the CBC, WBC was 15.07×10^6/L, and N% was 79.6%. Examination of the CSF showed the following: CSF pressure: 180 mmH_2O, WBC: 2805×10^6/L, protein: 1.10 g/L, glucose: 2.67 mmol/L, and chloride: 120 mmol/L (Table 2.3). Pending definitive diagnosis, the initial clinical consideration was

Table 2.3 Summary of patients' cerebrospinal fluid examination and routine blood results

Date	Blood routine		Cerebrospinal fluid								Treatment options	
	WBC (× 10^9/L)	N%	Pressure (mmH^2O)	Number of cells (× 10^6/L)	Apocyte (%)	Monocyte (%)	Sugar (mmol/L)	Synchronized blood glucose (mmol/L)	Chloride (mmol/L)	Protein (mg/L)	Antibacterial drugs	DXM
7.21	–	–	–	1174	–	–	3.19	–	114	1460	Untreated	–
7.22	15.07	80	180	2805	74.9	25.1	2.67	–	120	1100	HRZE+ amikacin Ceftriaxone	–
7.28	–	–	>300	2784	72.7	27.3	2.73	–	120	900		
8.04	–	–	>300	4784	81.3	18.7	1.99	–	123	900	HRZE+ amikacin moxifloxacin + ceftazidime	20 mg/d
8.07	10.24	76	>300	2653	–	–	1.88	–	120	900		
8.11 (after admission to hospital)	9.19	80	>300	1680	68	32	1.9	7.4	119	1080	HRZE+ amikacin Doxycycline	5 mg/d
8.18	8.84	73	200	1420	74	26	1.7	6.0	115	1260	Meropenem + linezolid	7.5-10 mg/d
8.22	–	–	245	1520	62	38	1.7	6.4	111	1510		
9.2	–	–	Unmeasured	1360	23	77	2.6	6.9	116	797	Voriconazole injection	2.5 mg/d
10.14	–	–	Unknown	52	20	80	2.9	–	121	1020	Voriconazole injection	–

Notes: WBC for white blood cells, N for neutrophils, H for isoniazid, R for rifampicin, Z for pyrazinamide, E for ethambutol, and DXM for dexamethasone central nervous system infection, with tuberculous meningitis and pyogenic meningitis identified as the two main differential diagnoses. Accordingly, a combination of antibiotics (isoniazid, rifampicin, amikacin, pyrazinamide, ethambutol, and ceftriaxone) was initiated. The patient's temperature came down to normal on July 27, and the follow-up blood test showed the following: WBC: 9.01 × 10^6/L and N%: 72%. The lumbar puncture on July 28 showed the following: CSF pressure >300 mmH_2O, WBC: 2784 × 10^6/L, protein: 0.9 g/L, glucose: 2.73 mmol/L, chloride: 120 mmol/L (Table 2.3), and no significant improvement. On July 30, he had a fever again and still had the recurrent headache, so ceftriaxone was changed to moxifloxacin combined with ceftazidime on August 1, and the antituberculosis treatment was continued. On August 4, the lumbar puncture showed that the pressure of cerebrospinal fluid was >300 mmH_2O, WBC was 4784 × 10^6/L, protein was 0.9 g/L, glucose was 1.99 mmol/L, and chloride was 123 mmol/L (Table 2.3), and dexamethasone 20 mg qd was added from August 5. The patient had no fever but still had intermittent headache and was admitted to our department for further diagnosis and treatment. Since the onset of the disease, the patient had suffered from fatigue, poor appetite, and sleep and had lost about 10 kg of weight.

2.9.1 Physical Examination

T: 36.8 °C, P: 90 times/min, R: 22 times/min, BP: 100/60 mmHg. Clear mind, normal development, moderate nutrition, answering relevant questions, automatic posture, physical examination cooperation, and he stepped into the ward by himself. Soft neck and no resistance. Heart and lungs (−). The abdomen was soft without rebound tenderness. No edema in both lower extremities. Kernig sign (−), Brudzinski sign (−).

2.9.2 Treatment History

After admission, the relevant tests were completed: blood routine: WBC: 7.95 × 10^9/L, N: 56.6%, L: 33.3%, M: 9.4%, Hb: 138 g/L, PLT: 245 × 10^9/L, ESR: 4 mm/h, CRP: <3.44 mg/L, ferritin: 247 μg/L, and PCT: 0.02 ng/mL. Autoantibodies: negative; tumor markers: CA724: 9.26 U/mL ↑, and the rest were normal; HIV: negative; blood culture: negative; serum cryptococcal latex agglutination test: negative; Brucella antibodies: negative; T-SPOT.TB: positive, antigen A>20 points, antigen B>20 points; EEG: no significant abnormalities; chest CT: left lower lung striae. Cranial MRI enhancement: pia meningeal enhancement, indicating the possibility of infectious diseases (Fig. 2.9).

After admission, the patient continued to receive antituberculosis treatment (isoniazid, rifampicin, pyrazinamide, ethambutol, and amikacin), supplemented by mannitol and dexamethasone for symptomatic treatment. But the patient's headache

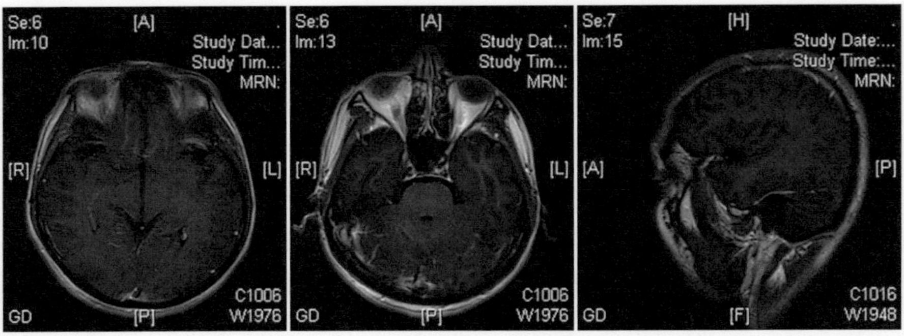

Fig. 2.9 Enhanced MRI image of the patient's head

was not relieved. From August 10, he was given linezolid and moxifloxacin to strengthen the antituberculosis treatment but still had a headache with recurrent fever, with T_{max} 39.5 °C. On August 11, the CSF pressure was >300 mmH_2O, and the WBC count was 1680 × 10^6/L, protein was 1080 mg/L, glucose was 1.9 mmol/L (blood glucose 7.4 mmol/L), and chloride was 119 mmol/L (Table 2.3), with still no significant improvement. The patient was from Xinjiang Province, a high-incidence area of tuberculosis, and T-SPOT.TB was positive, so the suspicion of "tuberculous meningitis" was well-founded. However, after 3 weeks of regular antituberculosis treatment, the symptoms and CSF did not improve significantly. At this time, other possibilities had to be carefully investigated. A careful review of the patient's medical history showed that this was an acute disease, and the blood routine at the beginning of the onset indicated elevated WBC and N%, and the number of WBC in CSF was high, so it was necessary to distinguish the possibility of purulent meningitis. Therefore, we adjusted the antibiotics to linezolid and meropenem on August 12. Ten days later (August 22), the CSF pressure was 245 mmH_2O, WBC was 1520 × 10^6/L, protein was 1510 mg/L, glucose was 1.7 mmol/L (blood glucose: 6.4 mmol/L), and chloride was 111 mmol/L (Table 2.3). The patient tried a variety of treatments, but there was no obvious effect. We felt great pressure. To achieve good results, we had to first identify the pathogen. After admission, the patient received many CSF cultures and other examinations. All were negative. On August 22, we improved the culture method by inoculating CSF into blood culture bottles. Fortunately, on August 27, the bacteriology laboratory told us that the cerebrospinal fluid culture was positive for a filamentous fungus (Fig. 2.10), which was identified as *Scedosporium apiospermum*. Voriconazole 200 mg q12h antifungal treatment was given to the patient immediately, supplemented with 20% mannitol and dexamethasone. The patient's temperature returned to normal the next day, and the headache was significantly relieved. On September 2, the result of CSF was better than before (Table 2.3). The patient was discharged to the local hospital on September 8 and continued treatment with voriconazole, with no fever or headache.

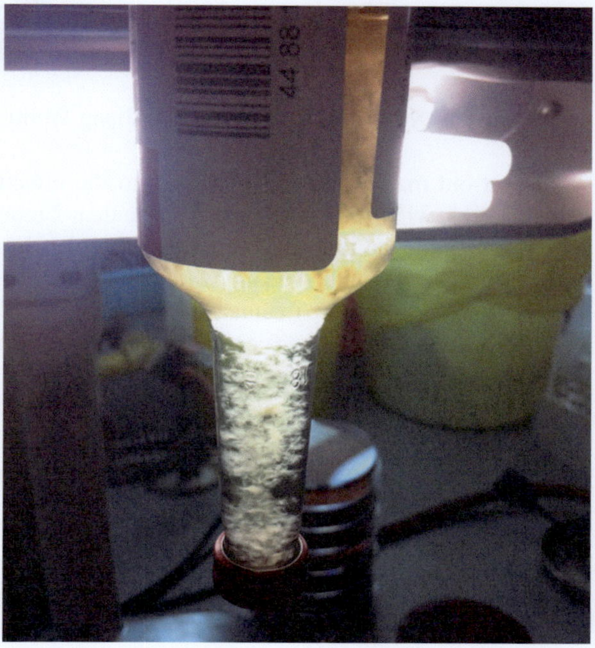

Fig. 2.10 The patient's blood culture bottle of cerebrospinal fluid fungal culture was positive for filamentous fungi

2.9.3 Comments

Cryptococcus is the most common pathogen in the diagnosis of fungal meningitis. *Scedosporium apiospermum* is a relatively rare pathogen with special characteristics in the selection of antifungal therapeutic agents, to which great attention must be paid.

Inoculation of CSF into the blood culture medium can improve the positive rate of pathogen isolation. In this case, the pathogen was identified by morphology as *Scedosporium apiospermum*.

References

1. Weng Xinhua, ed. Selected cases of Incurable fever and clinical cogitation by Weng Xinhua. 2012; Shanghai Science and Technology Press.
2. Zhong YM, Yan Q, Li HL, et al. A case of brain abscess caused by intracranial Scedosporium apiospermum infection and review of the literature. Chin J Lab Med. 2013;36(11):1050–51.

2.10 A Case of Advanced AIDS Confirmed by Nucleic Acid Test After Multiple Negative HIV Antibody Tests

Liu Yuanyuan, Xu Bin, Mao Richeng, and Jiang Weimin

A 22-year-old male freelancer presented to the infectious disease department on July 20, 2015, with recurrent fever for more than 2 months.

The patient began to have fever without any obvious triggers since May 2015, mainly from afternoon to evening, with a body temperature as high as 39.5 °C, and the daily body temperature fluctuates between 38 and 39.5 °C, along with dizziness, fatigue, frequent urination, difficulty urinating, no obvious cough and sputum, chest tightness, shortness of breath, muscle and joint pain. He had no skin rash or conjunctival hyperemia. On July 10, 2015, the local hospital inpatient blood examination routine showed the following: white blood cell: 2.15×10^9/L, neutrophil%: 34.9%, absolute neutrophil count: 0.75×10^9/L, lymphocyte%: 54.4%, hemoglobin: 102 g/L, ESR: 42 mm/h, CRP: 36.9 mg/L, peripheral blood CD3%: 57.8%, CD4%: 25.5%, CD8%: 27.1%, NK%: 13.5%, CD4: absolute count 298/ul, syphilis-specific antibody (+), and HIV antibody (−). B-ultrasound showed mild edema of the ascending colon, ileocecal area, and appendix wall; mesenteric lymph nodes were enlarged; there was a small amount of fluid in the right lower abdomen; and bilateral neck, axillary, and inguinal lymph nodes were enlarged. Gastroscope showed fungal esophagitis and chronic gastritis. Ceftazidime was given for anti-infective treatment of phlegm, liver protection, and defervescence, and recombinant human granulocyte colony-stimulating factor was also given for treatment. Rechecked blood routine showed the following: white blood cells: 7.81×10^9/L, neutrophil%: 75.44%, absolute neutrophil count: 5.89×10^9/L, lymphocyte%: 8.52%, and hemoglobin: 102 g/L. But the patient's symptoms did not improve significantly, and he still had a fever every day. For further diagnosis and treatment, the patient came to our hospital for treatment and was admitted to our department for "fever of unknown origin." He had bronchiectasis previously, which improved after anti-infective treatment in September 2014. He was diagnosed with syphilis in September 2014. His syphilis was determined to be in the active stage and was not given regular treatment. There was no history of trauma, surgery, or blood transfusion; there was a history of allergy to levofloxacin; and the patient denied having bad habits, such as smoking and drinking, or a family history of genetic diseases. He had had five years of homosexual contact.

On examination, the temperature was 37.5 °C, the heart rate was 80 beats per minute, the respiratory rate was 20 breaths per minute, and the blood pressure was 110/80 mmHg. He was somnolent, in good spirits, had normal development and moderate nutrition, and was cooperative with physical examination. The neck was soft, with scattered brown pigmentation on the face, no appearance of anemia, no rash, and no palpable swelling of the superficial lymph nodes. The pharynx was not red, the oral mucosa was seen with thrush, and the tonsils were not enlarged. Breathing sounds of both lungs were clear, with no dry or wet rales; heart rhythm was regular; and no murmurs were heard. The abdomen was soft and slightly distended, and there was no tenderness or rebound pain in the whole abdomen. There was no palpable swelling under the ribs of the liver and the spleen, Murphy's sign was negative, and there was no tenderness at McDonald's point, no tenderness at the ureteral point, no percussion pain in the bilateral kidney region, no bowel sounds, and no swelling of the lower limbs. Physiological reflexes of the nervous system existed, but pathological reflex was not elicited.

2.10.1 Diagnosis and Treatment

The laboratory test results were as follows: blood routine: white blood cell: 1.90×10^9/L, neutrophil%: 78.0%, hemoglobin: 91 g/L, and platelet: 157×10^9/L; CRP: 1.30 mg/L; liver function: ALT 65 U/L, AST 174 U/L, GGT 155 U/L, and others were normal; renal function, electrolytes, myocardial markers, blood lipids, and blood glucose were normal; Hepatitis A virus (HAV) antibody was negative, HBsAg was negative, HBsAb was positive, and Hepatitis C virus (HCV) antibody negative; blood immunoglobulin: total IgE: 6.40 IU/mL, IgG: 10.70 g/L, IgA: 0.24 g/L, IgM: 0.67 g/L; serum complement: C3: 0.76 g/L and C4: 0.26 g/L; autoantibody: ANA: positive and titer: 1: 100; ANCA, dsDNA, ENA, PCNA, PR_3, MPO, and ribosomal P protein were all negative; thyroid function: TSH: 2.38 mIU/L, T4: 108.6 nmol/L, T3: 1.32 nmol/L, FT4: 8.83 pmol/L, and FT3: 3.00 pmol/L; EBV-DNA (whole blood) was negative, and CMV-DNA was positive; Treponema Pallidum Particle Agglutination Assay (TPPA) was positive; HIV antibody was negative; and *Cryptococcus sanguis* latex agglutination test was negative.

Results of computed tomography (CT) of the chest: patches and nodular high-density shadows in the lower lobes of both lungs, probable inflammatory changes, and local dilation of the upper left lobe. Abdominal ultrasound: liver, gallbladder, spleen, pancreas, kidneys, bladder, posterior peritoneum, no obvious abnormalities.

Results of B-ultrasound of the superficial lymph node: The lymph node in the right parotid gland was palpable, and the shape was full. The bilateral submandibular lymph nodes were enlarged, and the reaction might have been proliferative. There were no obvious abnormalities in the bilateral submandibular glands and the left parotid gland. There were no obvious abnormally enlarged lymph nodes in the bilateral neck, bilateral supraclavicular, bilateral axillary, and bilateral groin.

Results of B-ultrasound of the urinary system: There was no dilation of the double ureters and chronic inflammation of the prostate.

Results of the bone marrow smear: The proliferation of bone marrow was mildly active, the granule system had maturation disorder, and some were accompanied by toxic changes. The neutrophil alkaline phosphatase (NAP) integral value had increased. Naive monocytes, lymphoid tissue cells, and hemophagocytic cells could be seen. There were increased macrophages in the hemophagocytic mononuclear tissue.

Results of the bone marrow biopsy: Posterior superior iliac spine biopsy showed more than ten medullary cavities, hematopoietic tissue accounted for about 40%, the ratio of granulocytes to erythrocytes was basically normal, there were six to eight megakaryocytes per HP, plasma cells and mononuclear macrophages proliferated, and the bone marrow regeneration was slightly less effective. Bone marrow flow cytometry: $CD4^+$ T 0.15%; opinion: $CD4^+$ T lymphocytes in the bone marrow were significantly reduced.

Results of the PET-CT: patches in the left lower lung, slightly increased FDG metabolism in bilateral neck, mediastinum, bilateral hilum of lung and bilateral axillary lymph nodes, patches in the right lung, no increase in FDG metabolism was observed, the uneven increase of FDG metabolism in spleen, bone marrow and cerebral cortex was considered to be caused by inflammatory lesions combined with the medical history. Follow-up after treatment was recommended. The rest of the whole-body PET imaging showed no abnormal increase in FDG metabolism. Sinus CT showed bilateral maxillary sinusitis. Gastroscopy showed fungal esophagitis; antral gastritis (hyperemic exudative type, moderate) with bile reflux.

Combined with the oral thrush found in the physical examination after admission, the presence of granulocytosis (leukocyte: 0.57×10^9/L) and the decreased absolute count of CD4 cells as indicated by the blood routine, positive CMV-DNA in blood, bone marrow smear findings (slightly active bone marrow hyperplasia; dysmaturation of granules, some with toxic changes; increased NAP score; infantile monocytes; lymphoid tissue cells and hemophagocytes; and increased macrophages in hemophagocytic monocytes), and the esophageal mucosa *Candida albicans* infection found by gastroscopy, it was considered that the patient had a high possibility of fever caused by secondary opportunistic viral and fungal infections under the state of severe immunodeficiency. However, autoantibodies and PET-CT had no obvious positive results, so autoimmune diseases and tumors were not considered for the time being. Granulocytosis (leukocyte: 0.57×10^9/L) and the reduction in the absolute count of CD4 cells may have been related to a severe viral infection. Therefore, the white blood cells could be raised to normal by subcutaneous injection of recombinant human granulocyte colony-stimulating factor. Cefepime 2.0 q12h intravenous drip was given to prevent infection, and ganciclovir 0.2 bid intravenous drip antiviral therapy was given. Combined with the oral and esophageal mucosal *Candida albicans* infection, the patient was given 200 mg bid oral antifungal therapy with fluconazole. The patient's body temperature came down to normal, and his general condition improved. On August 20, 2015, reexamination of CMV-DNA was negative. After that, the patient still had recurrent low fever, repeated blood routine examination showed significantly lower white blood cells than normal, and physical examination showed multiple leukopleckles in the oral mucosa. Recombinant human granulocyte colony-stimulating factor was given to increase white blood cells; clarithromycin, fluconazole, and compound sulfamethoxazole were given for anti-infective and antifungal treatments; and sputum culture was done. The sputum culture showed *Aspergillus fumigatus* 2+, so fluconazole was stopped, and voriconazole antifungal therapy was given. The patient was discharged from the hospital on September 13, 2015. On September 20, 2015, the patient was admitted to the hospital again with a fever. The blood routine showed that white blood cells were 0.57×10^9/L, and recombinant human granulocyte colony-stimulating factor was given again, and the total number of white blood cells increased to 4.0×10^9/L. Since the patient had a history of homosexual contact for

5 years, the fever was related to opportunistic viral and fungal infections. Although the blood HIV antibody was negative, the possibility of HIV infection was still highly suspected clinically. Was the HIV antibody a true negative or a false negative? Theoretically, the patient had exceeded the window period for HIV antibody testing. If it was not HIV infection, what was the reason for the reduced CD4 cell count in the patient? The patient was diagnosed with HIV infection at the Shanghai Center for Disease Control and Prevention (CDC) on October 14, 2016, with HIV RNA of 10^6 copies/ml and CD4 absolute count of 4/ul, and began highly active antiretroviral therapy (HAART). After treatment, the patient's body temperature came down to normal, the symptoms such as fatigue and discomfort disappeared, and his physical strength recovered. Thrush and other fungal infections disappeared, cough and sputum symptoms disappeared, and the chest CT showed that both pneumonia symptoms had improved significantly.

2.10.2 Comments

HIV belongs to the group of human lentiviruses in the *Lentivirus* genus of the retroviral family. It is a spherical particle with a diameter of about 100 ~120 nm and consists of two parts: the core and the envelope. The core includes two single-stranded RNA strands, core structural proteins, and enzymes necessary for virus replication. Outside the core are viral capsid proteins (P24 and P17). The outermost layer of the virus is the envelope, in which the outer membrane glycoprotein gp120 and transmembrane glycoprotein gp41 are embedded. Laboratory tests for HIV infection mainly include HIV antibodies, HIV nucleic acids, and so on. An HIV 1/2 antibody test is the gold standard for the diagnosis of HIV infection. HIV nucleic acid quantification and $CD4^+$ T lymphocytes are helpful in determining the disease progression, drug selection, efficacy, and prognosis. Among them, HIV RNA testing is helpful in diagnosing HIV infection, but it is expensive in developing countries, so routine testing is not done. For complex and difficult cases (such as those with a history of epidemiology and a significant decrease in CD4 cells), HIV RNA testing is indeed needed to aid diagnosis.

Patients with unexplained fever, a history of male-to-male sex (MSM) epidemics, opportunistic viral infections, and fungal infections should be considered for possible HIV infection. A CD4 cell count test is required for these patients, even if the HIV antibody test is negative. For patients with significantly reduced CD4 cell counts, HIV antibody testing should be repeated. If rapid antibody tests are repeatedly negative, the fourth-generation enzyme immunoassay (EIA) antibody test should be performed (HIV antigen and anti-HIVp24 antibody are simultaneously coated with the carrier to simultaneously detect HIV P24 antigen and HIV antibody in the sample). Theoretically, the window period can be shortened to 4–5 days. If it is still negative, an HIV RNA test should be performed. If the viral load is positive, HAART treatment should be performed.

References

1. Yan Li, Jin-Kou Zhao, Ming Wang, et al. Current antibody-based immunoassay algorithm failed to confirm three late-stage AIDS cases in China: case report. Virol J. 2010;15(7):58.
2. Ortiz de Lejarazu R, Soriano V, Eiros JM, Arias M, Toro C. HIV-1 infection in persistently HIV-1 seronegative individuals: more reasons for HIV RNA screening. Clin Infect Dis. 2008;46:784.
3. Toro C. Absence of HIV-1 antibody response in HIV patients: what is the foe, the virus or the host? AIDS Rev. 2007;9:188.
4. Tang JW, Wong BC, Lam E, Failure to confirm HIV infection in two end-stage HIV/AIDS patients using a popular commercial line immunoassay. J Med Virol. 2008;80(9):1515–22.

2.11 Breast Prosthesis Infection Hidden in the "Coat" of Complicated Urinary Tract Infection

Hu Yuekai and Jiang Weimin

A 55-year-old retired woman was admitted to this hospital because of "repeated fever for more than two months."

The patient had been in her usual state of health until 2 months before this admission, when fevers with temperature as high as 40.0 °C started, along with chills, dizziness, diarrhea, frequent urination, no cough and sputum, no nausea and vomiting, no muscle pain, no joint pain, no rash, etc. The fever subsided after self-moxibustion and diarrhea was relieved, but frequent urination was still an urgency, which was not taken seriously. In the following month, the patient had intermittent fever, with a maximum body temperature of 40.0 °C, accompanied by chills, dizziness, bloating, diarrhea, frequent urination, and urinary urgency. At the beginning of this month, the patient had a fever again, with a body temperature of 39.9 °C, accompanied by chills, nausea, and vomiting. The vomit was mainly stomach contents and no coffee-like liquid, accompanied by diarrhea and back pain, mainly acupuncture-like pain, and the pain continued without relief. The urinary frequency and urgency became worse than before, so she went to the primary hospital to see a doctor. The blood test showed that white blood cells were 15.7×10^9/L and the neutrophil % was 90.2%, and the urinary routine showed occult blood 2+ and white blood cells 2+. The urinary system B-ultrasound showed "right kidney stones, left hydronephrosis and left lower ureteral calculus." After 4 days of emergency infusion (specifically unknown), the diarrhea was relieved, but fever and lower back pain were not relieved. Therefore, she was admitted to the primary hospital for cefodizime 2.0 g qd intravenous infusion. The next night, the patient had a sudden high fever, with a body temperature of 41.0 °C, accompanied by a dry cough and rapid breathing. Considering "sepsis," she was switched to imipenem and cilastatin sodium 0.5 q8h intravenously. After initiating intravenous anti-infective therapy for the patient, he continued to experience fever, recurrent chest tightness, and tachycardia; additionally, his blood pressure showed a downward trend. Further evaluations (including continuous vital sign monitoring, complete blood count, and chest imaging) were conducted to identify the cause of symptom deterioration. Vancomycin 1.0 g q12h was added intravenously. The patient's body temperature did not change significantly, and she was transferred to the ICU on the 4th day after admission. Vancomycin, combined with imipenem and cilastatin sodium, anti-infective treatment was continued, and the body temperature returned to normal the next day, and the stones were discharged by themselves. Two days later, she was transferred to the urology department and continued imipenem and cilastatin sodium anti-infective treatment. The patient's body temperature was normal, frequent urination and urgency were relieved, and dry cough and lower back pain improved. One week after entering the ICU, she changed to cefodizime anti-infective treatment. After that, the patient developed a fever again. With a body temperature of 39.0 °C and skin rash, cefodizime was discontinued, and Tylenol was given 0.5 g q8h intravenously. However, the patient's symptoms did not improve significantly this time, and she still had a fever. The patient was admitted to our hospital for further treatment. Since the illness, she had had poor appetite, good sleep, dry cough, chest tightness, no recent diarrhea, frequent urination, and no significant weight loss. She had undergone right breast fibroma resection more than 20 years ago, and uterine fibroid embolization more than 10 years ago. She had her menarche at the age of 18. Her menstrual cycle was 28 days, with a duration of 5 days per cycle. She had no dysmenorrhea, and her menstruation remained regular thereafter. She denied any history of infectious diseases, smelting tourism, or visiting epidemic areas.

She was somnolent, had normal development and moderate nutrition, was cooperative with physical examination, and had no appearance of anemia, no petechiae, no rash, no palpable swelling of the superficial lymph nodes, no red throat, and no swelling of the tonsils. There was an old surgical scar, about 5cm in length, on the right breast. No discharge was seen. Both breasts were plump, and there was no obvious redness or swelling. Breath sounds in both lungs were coarse, dry and wet rales were not heard, heart rhythm was uniform, grade III/6 systolic murmurs could be heard in the apex area, the abdomen was flat and soft, there was mild tenderness in the right upper middle abdomen, there was no palpable swelling under the liver and spleen ribs, Murphy's signs were negative, McDonald's point had no tenderness, ureteral point had no tenderness, both kidneys had percussive pain, the left side was severe, bowel sounds were not hyperactive, and the lower limbs were not swollen.

The laboratory test results on January 29 showed the following: white blood cells: 5.47×10^9/L, neutrophil%: 68.1%, red blood cells: 2.99×10^{12}/L, hemoglobin: 87 g/L, and ALT: 57 U/L. Urine routine was normal, and stool routine and occult blood were normal. Liver and kidney functions and electrolytes were normal. CRP was 80.50 mg/L, and ESR was 120 mm/h. The electrolyte was normal. Procalcitonin was 0.09 ng/mL. DIC: FDP: 2.4μg/mL, PT: 12.6seconds, APTT: 26.6 s, FIB: 6.41↑g/L, thrombin time: 16.6 s, D-dimer: 0.650, and international standardized ratio: 1.05. Folic acid: 8.70 ng/ml, vitamin B_{12}: 855.00 pg/mL, serum iron:

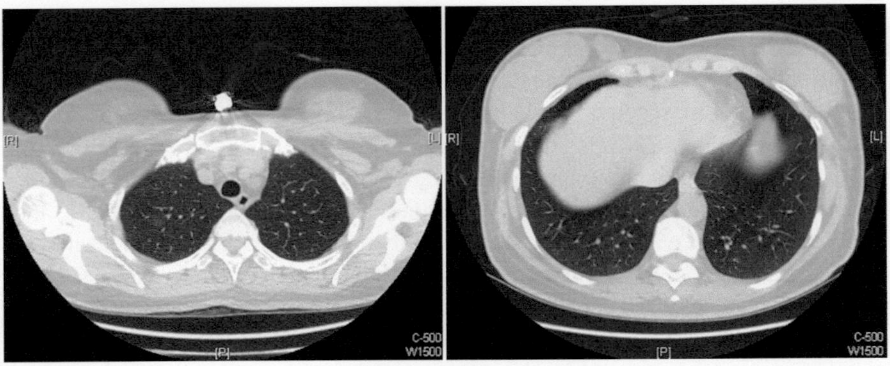

Fig. 2.11 Chest CT scan on January 28, 2016

4.8 μmol/L. SCC: 0.5 ng/mL, AFP: 2.84 g/L, CEA: 3.26, CA125: 25.09 U/ml, CA153: 11.28 U/ml, CY211: 1.57 ng/ml, CA199: 0.65 U/ml, and CA724: 2.10 U/ml. ANA characterization: positive, cytoplasmic granular type: positive (1:100), nucleolar type: positive (1:320), PR3: 3.6 AU/mL, MPO: 1.3 AU/mL, PCNA: negative, ribosomal P protein: negative, anti-ββ body glycoprotein 1 antibody: 5.5 RU/ml, nRNP: negative, SmD1: negative, SS-A/Ro60: negative, SS-A/RO52: negative, PM-Scl: negative, anticentromere B antibody: negative, dsDNA: negative, anti-nucleosome antibody: negative, AMA-M2: negative, dsDNA (qualitative): negative, dsDNA-IgG: <10 IU/ml, anticardiolipin antibody IgG: 2.0 PLIgG-U/ml, anti-histone antibody: negative, Jo-1: negative, Scl-70: negative, SS-B/La: negative, and anti-cardiolipin antibody IgM: <2 PLIgM-U/ml.

Urine culture and blood culture were negative.

On January 28, the results of computed tomography (CT) of the chest showed a ground-glass shadow of the upper lobe of the right lung (Fig. 2.11). It was recommended to review this after treatment.

Results of electrocardiogram: sinus rhythm, electric axis deviation to the right, and clockwise rotation.

Results of cardiac ultrasonography: mild mitral regurgitation and no vegetation.

From the previous clinical manifestations and laboratory examinations, the diagnosis of complex urinary tract infection was established, but the result of poor treatment effect made us consider more situations, such as 1. infection with special pathogens; 2. pathogens entering the blood and bloodstream infections causing infections in other parts (such as heart valves), resulting in insufficient treatment course and repeated illness; 3. urine sensation, combined with other diseases at the same time, i.e., dualism considerations; 4. the cause of complicated urinary sensation being continuous or intermittent, leading to repetition of the feeling of urinating.

Therefore, on the one hand, we actively carried out pathogen culture to search for special infectious agents that may exist, and on the other hand, we did cardiac ultrasound examinations to actively search for possible hidden infections. When I read the chest CT film myself, I found that this menopausal patient had a special chest wall structure, and there seemed to be implants, but the patient had not provided a corresponding medical history. Therefore, we once again consulted the patient about the relevant history and performed a careful physical examination. She informed that breast augmentation was performed at an unknown local clinic 8 or 9 years ago (the material was unknown, and the clinic was closed). She had been suffering from breast swelling and pain in the past two months, and it had become more and more obvious recently, especially one week before admission. She did have tenderness during cardiopulmonary auscultation, but because she paid special attention to privacy protection and other factors, she had not mentioned these problems to the doctor. Further arrangements for breast B-ultrasound and magnetic resonance examinations did not indicate any obvious rupture of the prosthesis. This was different from the clinical judgment. Therefore, we consulted the specialists of the relevant authoritative specialist hospitals. They agreed with our clinical judgment and believed that there was no safe breast augmentation injection currently on the market. Therefore, it was recommended to perform an injection prosthesis removal. She therefore underwent breast augmentation revision surgery at the hospital. During the operation, the original breast augmentation was confirmed to have been performed via injection, and a large amount of yellow pus-bloody gelatinous material was aspirated from the injection cavity. After routine negative pressure drainage, simultaneous culture of the drained fluid was conducted—both cultures were positive, yielding the same bacterium (*Pseudomonas mendocina*). She then continued receiving carbapenem-based anti-infective therapy in the hospital for 2 weeks before being discharged. After being discharged from the hospital, the body temperature did not go up again.

The patient's medical history was not complicated, but she had been in various hospitals for nearly two months. For patients with complex urinary tract infections that have not improved with repeated treatment, on the one hand, it is necessary to obtain the pathogen and drug sensitivity results as much as possible and, as far as possible, find out the susceptibility factors that cause complex urinary tract infections and whether there are anatomical and functional abnormalities. On the other hand, for those who have cleared urine bacteriology after repeated treatments and for whom the susceptibility factors are not complicated, but there is still a high fever, we should consider whether there are other possible causes of fever. Careful medical history inquiry and detailed physical examination are internal medicine's basic skills of diagnosis, which are essential to the diagnosis of fever. In this case, clues were obtained by finding that the chest wall structure was special in the lung CT reading. Obtaining a reliable history of foreign body implantation was the key to diagnosis when tracing the medical history. Although the patient's strict preservation of her privacy prevented the previous doctors from obtaining critical information about the past history, medical history, and physical examination, which caused delays in the diagnosis of her own disease, with our active communication with the patient and repeated medical history inquiry and careful physical examination, it was revealed that there was a possibility of prosthesis rupture infection, and it was this breast prosthesis infection that caused fever for up to 2 months. However, MRI did not indicate a significant rupture of the prosthesis. After communicating with the specialist, it was confirmed that there was an indication of prosthesis removal.

Through the final surgical discovery and pathogenic culture, it was confirmed that the patient had a breast prosthesis infection. This breast implant infection had caused fever for up to 2 months.

References

1. Pu Xingwang, Liu Ning, et al. Clinical diagnosis and treatment standards (Proposed) for complications of polyacrylamide hydrogel (PAHG) injection breast augmentation [J]. Chin J Aesthet Med. 2006;15(10):1153–4.
2. Peng Donghong, Liu Ligang, et al. Clinical manifestations and the impact on imaging diagnosis after polyacrylamide hydrogel injection breast augmentation [J]. Chin J Med Aesthet Cosmetol. 2005;11(3):133–6.
3. Sun Yanhua, Xu Meiquan, et al. Breast lesions after polyacrylamide hydrogel injection breast augmentation [J]. Chin J Tissue Eng Res Clin Rehabil. 2011;15(25):4623–6.
4. Rapsinski GJ, Makadia J, Bhanot N, Min Z. Pseudomonas mendocina native valve infective endocarditis: a case report [J]. J Med Case Rep. 2016;10(1):275–9.

2.12 Acute Rhino-Orbital-Cerebral Mucormycosis

Zhu Haoxiang, Wang Xuan, Lin Jie, and Zhu Liping

The patient, a 28-year-old male, was admitted to the hospital on October 9, 2016, with "left facial numbness with vision loss of the left eye for more than 4 months."

On May 30, 2016, an elevated random blood glucose (16.6 mmol/L) was detected in a local hospital, but the patient did not pay attention to it and gradually developed symptoms such as dry mouth, polydipsia, polyuria, and weight loss, intermittently accompanied by nausea and vomiting, and felt mild left-sided facial pain and numbness, with ptosis of the left eyelid and vision loss of left eye, without chills, fever, or headache. The patient went to the clinic of the local hospital on June 9 because of significantly aggravated numbness and vision loss, accompanied by a small amount of non-purulent nasal discharge. The laboratory tests showed that his blood glucose was 26.8 mmol/L, blood pH was 7.188, urine glucose was 4+, and urine ketone was 4+, and no abnormality was found on the CT scan of the head. Then, he was admitted to the endocrinology department due to "diabetic ketoacidosis." The temperature on admission was 38 °C, and physical examination showed left facial hypoesthesia, and left frontal lines and nasolabial sulcus had become shallow. The upward and outward movements of the left eye were limited, and the left pupillary light reflex was insensitive. Muscle strength and tension of the limbs were normal, and the pathological signs were negative. The patient's condition progressed rapidly after admission, and on June 11, his left eye movement was significantly limited in all directions and worse than before, and the left vision loss was further aggravated. Peripheral blood cell count showed that WBC was 25×10^9/L, N% was 90.6%, and ESR was 84 mm/h. On June 12, his left eye was nearly fixed, and the peak temperature was 38.3 °C. The enhanced MRI of the head showed "cavernous sinus syndrome related to the inflammation of the left maxillary sinus, ethmoid sinus and rhinitis was considered; the left posterior wall of nasopharynx was swollen, and inflammatory edema was considered." Anti-infective agents, including ceftriaxone, levofloxacin, ganciclovir, and meropenem, were given successively, accompanied by insulin to control blood glucose. The ketoacidosis was controlled, and the left eye movement seemed to get better, but the facial numbness did not improve. The cultures of the patient's nasal secretions were positive four times for *Mucor* species, and rhino-sino-orbital invasive fungal disease was diagnosed. Physical examination showed that there was only light perception in the left eye, with left ptosis; the left pupil was 4.5 mm in diameter; and direct and indirect light reflexes and corneal reflexes disappeared. The movement of the left eye was limited in all directions, with no diplopia. The left facial pain and warmth sensation had disappeared, while the sense of touch was normal. Left frontal lines and nasolabial sulcus had become shallow, and the left eye was incompletely closed. Air leaked when he puffed out his cheeks, the corners of his mouth skewed when the teeth were exposed, and the tongue was extended to the left. His hearing, pronunciation, and swallowing were normal, and no abnormality was found on the right side. The pathological signs and meningeal irritation sign were negative. On June 15, a lumbar puncture was performed, and the pressure was 90 mmH_2O, and the cerebrospinal fluid (CSF) test showed that the nucleated cell count was 18 × 10^6/L, glucose was 10.56 mmol/L, and protein was 740 mg/L. CT scan of sinuses showed "inflammation on left maxillary sinus, frontal sinus, bilateral sphenoid sinus and ethmoid sinus." From June 17, he was given liposomal amphotericin B (AmB) (gradually increased from 5 mg qd to 100 mg qd), in combination with dexamethasone 5 mg qd. On June 20, a nasal septoplasty + sinusotomy + bilateral turbinoplasty was performed under general anesthesia, during which a large amount of pus scab-like secretion was seen in the nasal cavity, with a large amount of black mucous membrane in the left nasal cavity, and black middle and inferior turbinates. The pathological nasal and sinus mucosa were removed; the left ethmoid sinus, sphenoid sinus, frontal sinus, and maxillary sinus were opened in turn; and a large amount of pus was seen in the maxillary sinus, which was repeatedly flushed with hydrogen peroxide, saline, and diluted iodophor after removing the diseased tissue from the sinus cavity. On June 27, the lumbar puncture was repeated, and the CSF examination showed a nucleated cell count of 230 × 10^6/L, glucose of 5.98 mmol/L, and protein of 1280 mg/L, with no improvement over the previous one. On July 1, liposomal amphotericin B was increased to 100 mg qd, combined with posaconazole solution 200 mg q6h orally, for antifungal therapy. MRI of the head was repeated on July 6 and showed the following: "Multiple abnormal signals in left frontal lobe, basal ganglia, thalamus, left cerebellar hemisphere and vermis; mucosal thickening of the nasopharynx with postoperative changes in the left sinus; sinusitis of bilateral ethmoid, sphenoid, maxillary sinuses, and left frontal sinus; left mastoiditis was also seen." On July 7, the nasal sinus surgery was performed again, during which the dark brown mucosa of the left middle nasal tract and nasopharynx was seen. The right ethmoid, sphenoid, frontal, and maxillary sinuses were opened sequentially to remove the pathological mucosal tissue. The pathological examination revealed "fungal disease of the sinus mucosa." On September 13 (after 3 months of antifungal treatment), the patient developed renal impairment with the highest increase of blood creatinine to 138 μmol/L. The renal function gradually returned to normal after oral administration of compound α-ketoacid tablets and coated aldehyde oxystarch capsules. During the course of treatment, a lumbar puncture was performed several times, and the CSF was negative for bacteria, fungi, and tuberculosis in smear or culture. And his blood glucose was controlled reasonably. The patient was admitted to our hospital for further diagnosis and treatment because he did not feel any significant relief from the symptoms and had slurred speech, weakness of limbs, and difficulty in walking.

2.12.1 Physical Examination

T: 37.1 °C, P: 84 beats/min, R: 20 breaths/min, BP: 131/84 mmHg, clear consciousness, slurred speech, left ptosis, left frontal lines became shallow, bilateral pupils equal in size and round, no light perception or light reflex in the left pupil, left eye fixed. There was no deformity of the external nose, no pressure pain in the paranasal sinus area on both sides, with the left nasolabial sulcus becoming shallow, and left deviation of the extended tongue. The neck was soft and nonresistant. Breath sounds in both lungs were clear, and no dry or wet rales were heard. The heart rhythm was regular, and no pathological murmur was heard in each valve. The abdomen was flat and soft, there was no tenderness or rebound tenderness in the whole abdomen, the liver and spleen were not touched under the ribs, and there was no percussion pain in the liver and kidney area. There was no edema in either lower limb. The muscle strength and tension of the limbs were normal. The physiological reflexes were normal; the pathological reflexes and the meningeal irritation sign were negative (Fig. 2.12).

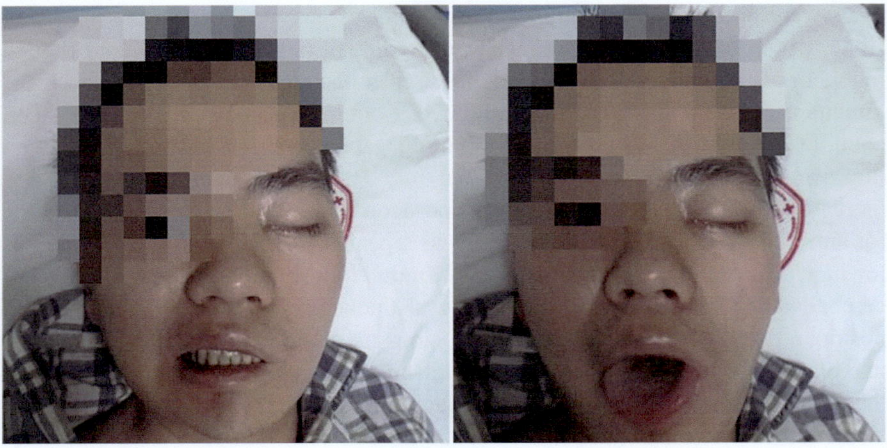

Fig. 2.12 Left ptosis, left frontal lines, and nasolabial sulcus became shallow, with left deviation of the extended tongue

2.12.2 Diagnosis and Treatment After Admission

After admission, the relevant tests were carried out: Lumbar puncture on October 9 showed that the cranial pressure was 150 mmH_2O; CSF test showed that WBC was 50×10^6/L, mononuclear cells were 35/50, glucose 3.6 was mmol/L (synchronous blood glucose was 6.7 mmol/L), chloride was 123 mmol/L, and protein was 1095 mg/L; and CSF was negative for bacteria, fungi, and tuberculosis in smear or culture.

Peripheral blood cell count showed the following: WBC: 5.32×10^9/L, N: 0.77, RBC: 2.7×10^{12}/L, hemoglobin: 79 g/L, platelets: 344×10^9/L, fasting blood glucose: 6.7 mmol/L, and glycosylated hemoglobin: 6.2%. Electrolytes and liver and kidney functions were nearly normal. No significant abnormality was seen in thyroid function and tumor markers. Immunoglobulin examination indicated a mild decrease in IgM and IgG levels. ESR was 44 mm/h, PCT was <0.06 ng/mL, CRP was <3.38 mg/mL., and 1, 3-beta-D-glucan in the plasma was 158.2 pg/mL.

Cranial enhanced MRI on October 11, 2016 showed multiple abnormal signals in the left cerebellar hemisphere, left basal ganglia, left cavernous sinus area, prepontine cistern, and bilateral frontoparietal cortex areas, with local meningeal enhancement, which was considered to be infectious lesions with local abscess and granuloma formation; local loss of bone in the left maxillary sinus wall, for which postoperative changes were considered; and inflammation of the left mastoid, right maxillary, and ethmoid sinuses, and bilateral frontal sinuses. An ophthalmology consultation was requested on October 13, suggesting secondary optic atrophy. The pathological slides from the sinus surgery were examined by our pathology department, which confirmed "acute and chronic inflammation with necrosis, inflammatory cells including lymphocytes, plasma cells, neutrophils and eosinophils. Irregular, hyaline and partially right-angle branched hyphae without separation could be seen disorderly arranged in the tissue. Some areas showed coagulative necrosis, and fungal invasion of blood vessels could be seen around the necrosis (Fig. 2.13)."

Based on the clinical features and histopathological findings, the patient was diagnosed with acute rhino-orbital-cerebral mucormycosis. It took about two weeks from the onset of symptoms to diagnosis. After admission, the patient was given amphotericin B (gradually increased from 5 mg qd to 30 mg qd, and the patient's weight was 60 kg) intravenously, combined with posaconazole solution 400 mg bid orally, for antifungal therapy, and aggressive glycemic control and symptomatic support therapy were also given. The patient's condition gradually improved. His speech was clearer than before, with mental improvement. He could walk independently, and his body temperature dropped to normal. There were no adverse effects, such as nausea or vomiting. Lumbar puncture was repeated on December 8, 2016,

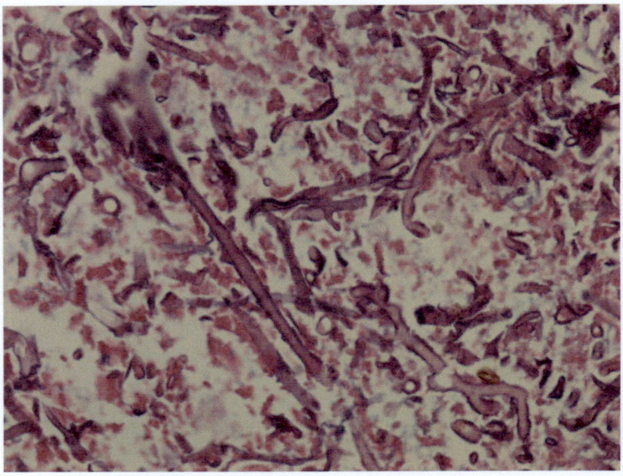

Fig. 2.13 Histopathology of pathological sinuses

with a cranial pressure of 160 cmH_2O, and the CSF test was apparently improved. The WBC count was 9×10^6/L, glucose was 3.6 mmol/L (synchronous glucose 5.8 mmol/L), chloride was 123 mmol/L, and protein was 720 mg/L. On December 9, 1, 3-beta-D-glucan in the plasma decreased to 84.48 pg/ml. The ophthalmology consultation suggested optic atrophy of the left eye, and an electrical auscultation was performed in an otolaryngology consultation, which showed total deafness of the left ear. A repeat cranial enhanced MRI scan on December 12 suggested multiple abnormal signals in the left cerebellar hemisphere, left basal ganglia, left cavernous sinus area, prepontine cistern, and bilateral frontoparietal cortex areas, with local meningeal enhancement, which suggested infectious lesions with local abscess and granuloma formation, with slightly smaller lesions than before (October 11, 2016). Later, the dosage of amphotericin B was reduced to 25 mg qd on January 29, 2017, due to the development of renal impairment, and it was discontinued on February 5, with a cumulative dosage of 3510 mg of amphotericin B (without liposome). Thereafter, oral posaconazole 400 mg bid was continued and was not yet discontinued, with a follow-up in May 2017. Lumbar puncture was repeated on May 5, 2017, with a cranial pressure of 165 mmH_2O. The CSF was colorless and clear, WBC was 2×10^6/L, glucose was 4.2 mmol/L (synchronous glucose was 10.7 mmol/L), chloride was 124 mmol/L, and protein was 735 mg/L. The 1, 3-beta-D-glucan in the plasma was 11.65 pg/mL. The lesion on cranial MRI was significantly improved on May 4, 2017. The patient is still blind in the left eye and has left-sided facial paralysis (Fig. 2.14).

2.12.3 Comments

Mucorales rank third among the common pathogens of invasive fungal infections. The incidence of invasive mucormycosis is increasing, especially in immunocompromised populations, and the mortality is extremely high. The most common site

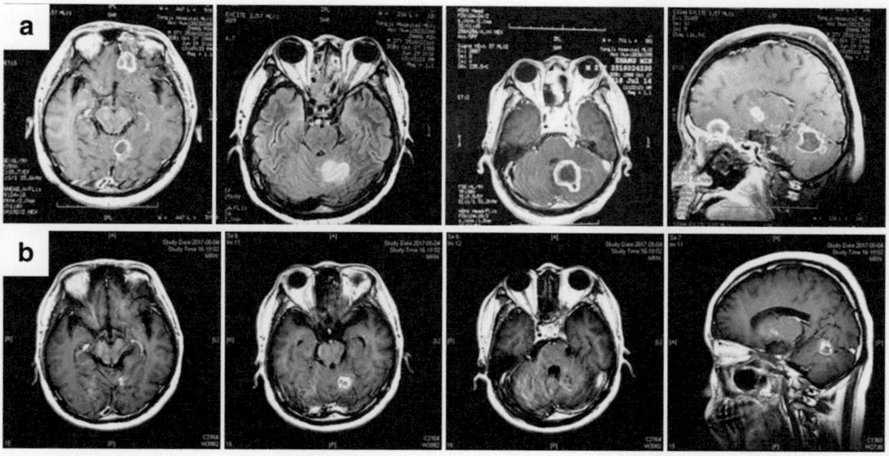

Fig. 2.14 Enhanced MRI of the head before and after treatment. (**a**) Images taken in June 2016 and (**b**) images taken in May 2017

of involvement in patients with diabetes and poor glycemic control is the sinus, and further invasion of adjacent tissues by the infection can lead to rhino-orbital-cerebral mucormycosis. In this case, the patient had a diabetic base, with poor glycemic control, complicated by ketoacidosis, from which acute rhino-orbital-cerebral mucormycosis developed. The diagnosis of this disease depends on the histopathological examination of the lesion or direct microscopic examination of sterile samples, and early diagnosis and reasonable antifungal treatment are crucial for the prognosis.

Mucormycosis of the central nervous system is uncommon clinically. In this case, the patient developed an acutely progressive rhino-orbital-cerebral infection after diabetic ketoacidosis, which was pathologically confirmed as *Mucor* infection. His condition improved after adequate surgical debridement and timely antifungal treatment using amphotericin B, combined with posaconazole. But amphotericin-related renal adverse effects were observed, so posaconazole monotherapy was continued. There is no uniform standard for the antifungal duration of central nervous system mucormycosis, and individualized treatment is needed. In general, therapy should continue until there is clinical resolution of the signs and symptoms of infection, as well as resolution of radiographic signs of active disease; therapy should also continue until the reversal of underlying immunosuppression.

References

1. Chakrabarti A, Das A, Mandal J, et al. The rising trend of invasive zygomycosis in patients with uncontrolled diabetes mellitus [J]. Med Mycol. 2006;44(4):335–42.
2. Roden MM, Zaoutis TE, Buchanan WL, et al. Epidemiology and outcome of zygomycosis: a review of 929 reported cases [J]. Clin Infect Dis. 2005;41(5):634–53.

3. Pagano L, Ricci P, Tonso A, et al. Mucormycosis in patients with haematological malignancies: a retrospective clinical study of 37 cases [J]. GIMEMA Infection Program (Gruppo Italiano Malattie Ematologiche Maligne dell'Adulto). Br J Haematol. 1997;99(2):331–6.
4. Ribes JA, Vanover-Sams CL, Baker DJ. Zygomycetes in human disease [J]. Clin Microbiol Rev. 2000;13(2):236–301.
5. Lanternier F, Sun HY, Ribaud P, et al. Mucormycosis in organ and stem cell transplant recipients [J]. Clin Infect Dis. 2012;54(11):1629–36.
6. Spellberg B, Walsh TJ, Kontoyiannis DP, et al. Recent advances in the management of mucormycosis: from bench to bedside [J]. Clin Infect Dis. 2009;48(12):1743–51.
7. Chakrabarti A, Denning DW, Ferguson BJ, et al. Fungal rhinosinusitis: a categorization and definitional schema addressing current controversies [J]. Laryngoscope. 2009;119(9):1809–18.

2.13 Multiple Liver Infections with Intermittent Fever for 15 Years in Immunosuppressed Patients After Kidney Transplantation

Dong Minhui, Zhu Beidi, Yang Feifie, Wang Xinyu, Li Qian, and Zhang Jiming

A 43-year-old male patient was admitted to our hospital on September 1, 2017. His chief complaint was recurrent fever of 2 months' duration, with a past medical history of renal transplantation performed 15 years earlier. The patient underwent "right kidney transplantation" because of "chronic kidney disease and bilateral renal atrophy" in 2003 and was treated with antirejection drugs for a long time after the operation. The patient developed fever after overwork in July 2017 and had a fever every night. His highest body temperature reached 39 °C at night, and his body temperature would return to normal in the early morning of the second day, with chills and no abdominal pain, diarrhea, cough, expectoration, headache, or other discomfort.

He was admitted to the local hospital on July 10, 2017. The local abdominal ultrasound examination on July 15 showed that there was an irregular mixed-echo mass in the anterior lobe of the right liver with a size of about 27 × 24 × 31 mm. A small liquid dark area could be seen inside, and the echo of blood flow could be detected, and an abscess was possible. Piperacillin/tazobactam, metronidazole, biapenem, and teicoplanin were given successively for anti-infective treatment, but the body temperature did not decrease after the reduction of immunosuppressants. On July 25, 2017, imipenem/cilastatin sodium, combined with linezolid, was used for empirical anti-infective therapy, and the body temperature returned to normal. Three weeks later, abdominal B-ultrasound showed "changes after treatment of right liver abscess." Linezolid was discontinued on August 14, 2017, and imipenem/cilastatin sodium was given to fight infection. About 10 days later, the fever occurred again. The body temperature fluctuated between 38 and 39 °C, the highest temperature

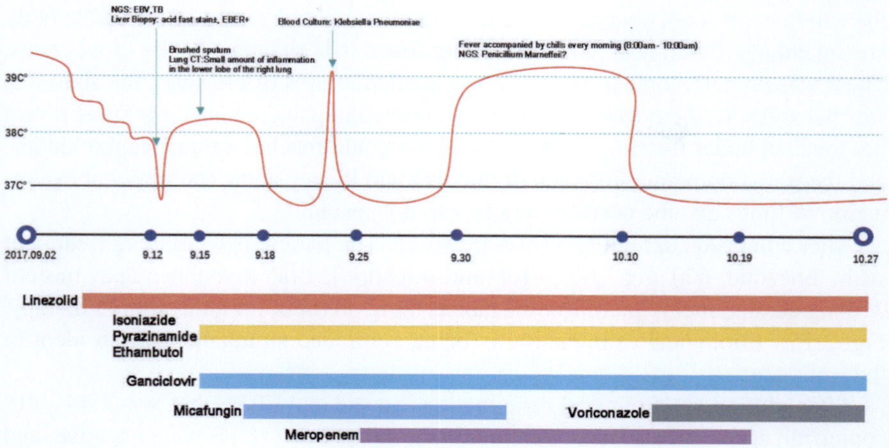

Fig. 2.15 The course of admission, diagnosis, treatment, and the change of body temperature

was 39.6 °C, and the fever type was basically the same as before (Fig. 2.15). Cefoperazone sodium/sulbactam sodium, combined with linezolid, was used to fight infection, and there was still a high fever and chills.

On August 27, 2017, he visited a hospital in Shanghai and was given imipenem/cilastatin sodium to fight infection. The patient still had a high fever and chills. On August 29, 2017, ultrasound-guided percutaneous liver puncture showed no purulent fluid, other abnormal fluid collections, or space-occupying lesions. A liver biopsy was performed, which showed patchy degenerative and necrotic tissue, a small amount of inflammatory fibrous connective tissue around, and no obvious atypia of hepatocytes.

2.13.1 Past History

The patient used to have diabetes and hypertension. At present, the patient is taking oral medications: gliquidone and acarbose for blood glucose control, and valsartan for blood pressure control. In 2003, right kidney transplantation was performed because of "bilateral renal atrophy." After the operation, mycophenolate mofetil and methylprednisolone tablets were used for antirejection therapy. Total thyroidectomy plus bilateral six-zone lymph node dissection was performed for thyroid cancer in 2012, and he had been taking the remaining thyroid sodium tablets after the operation until the time of consultation.

2.13.2 Admission for Physical Examination

T: 36.8 °C, heart rate: 111 per minute, respiration rate: 18 per minute, and BP 132/79 mmHg. Clear mind, withered spirit, underweight, the skin and mucosa of the whole body is not abnormal, and the superficial lymph nodes of the whole body are not enlarged. Soft neck, thick breathing sound in both lungs, no dry or wet rales. There was no pathological murmur in each valvular area of the heart, the abdomen was flat and soft, there was no tenderness or rebound pain, the liver and spleen were not touched under the rib, the right iliac fossa could reach the transplanted kidney, and there was no percussion pain in the liver and kidney area. The physical examination of limbs and the nervous system was not special.

After admission, a high fever still persisted. The patient is continuing treatment with: linezolid 600 mg Q12h (for anti-infection), oral mycophenolate mofetil 250 mg qd, and methylprednisolone tablets 6 mg qd (both for antirejection therapy, Fig. 2.15). Etiological examination is being continued simultaneously to identify the pathogen.

After admission, etiological examination showed that EBV-DNA was 1.48×10^4 copies/ml, cryptococcal latex agglutination test and T-SPOT.TB were negative, and there was no obvious abnormality in blood, sputum, cerebrospinal fluid, and bone marrow cultures; liver puncture pathology suggested large areas of coagulative necrosis and chronic inflammatory cell infiltration; in situ hybridization EB Virus-Encoded Small RNAs (EBER) was positive; and liver biopsy tissue second-generation sequencing detected *Mycobacterium tuberculosis*, EBV, *Talaromyces marneffei* sequence. There was a preliminary consideration of liver tuberculosis and EBV infection. On September 12, 2017, the patient was started on antituberculosis treatment with isoniazid, ethambutol, and pyrazinamide. Rifampicin was suspended due to nausea and vomiting after its intravenous infusion. Additionally, ganciclovir was initiated for antiviral therapy, and the dose of linezolid was reduced to 600 mg qd. The body temperature quickly dropped to normal and rose to 38 °C again 1 day later.

At the same time, the patient had increased cough and sputum, the sputum was silk-like, and the chest CT showed a small amount of inflammation in the lower lobe of the right lung, suggesting the possibility of pulmonary fungal infection. Empirical antifungal therapy with micafungin was added on September 15, 2017. The body temperature flattened from September 18, and because of the progressive increase of creatinine to 425 umol/L, the dose of antirejection drugs was increased to mycophenolate mofetil 250 mg bid po and methylprednisolone 20 mg qd intravenous drip.

On September 22, high fever and chills appeared again, suggesting gram-negative bacilli bloodstream infection after enhanced immunosuppression, and *Klebsiella pneumoniae* infection was confirmed by blood culture. After the reduction of mycophenolate mofetil and methylprednisolone, a small dose of 0.5 g q12h of meropenem was given for anti-infective therapy. On September 23, the temperature gradually returned to normal. On September 30, the patient continued treatment with linezolid, plus intravenous isoniazid combined with oral ethambutol and pyrazinamide for anti-TB therapy. In the case of gradual improvement of creatinine and close monitoring of renal function, considering that the bloodstream infection was not completely controlled, meropenem was added to 1 g Q8h after the end of antifungal and antiviral therapy.

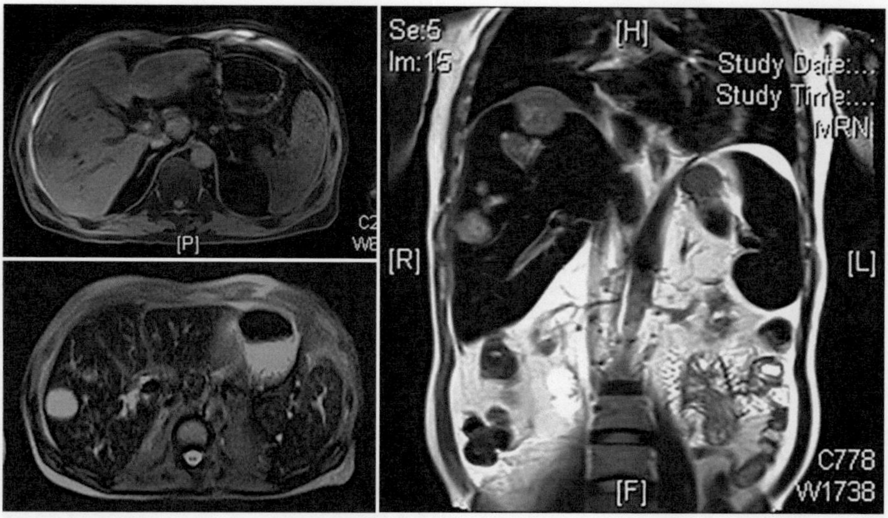

Fig. 2.16 Plain MR scan of abdomen on September 4, 2017

After about a week of stable body temperature, fever and chills appeared at 8–10 a.m. every day after the beginning of October, and the body temperature dropped spontaneously in the afternoon. After adjusting the medication time to eliminate drug fever, *Talaromyces marneffei* was detected, but fungal infection could not be ruled out. Considering the increase in NT-proBNP, itraconazole was not suitable. The body temperature returned to normal by oral administration of voriconazole 200 mg bid on October 13.

Subsequently, linezolid was discontinued in the patient due to limb numbness. Additionally, ethambutol was withdrawn as the patient presented with tarry stools—a clinical manifestation often associated with upper gastrointestinal bleeding. Oral moxifloxacin was then started for antituberculosis therapy. The patient's body temperature was stable, creatinine decreased gradually, and the condition was stable. The patient was discharged with an oral anti-infective regimen: pyrazinamide 0.75 gqd, isoniazid 0.3 g qd, rifampicin 0.3 g qd, moxifloxacin 0.4 g qd for antituberculosis therapy and voriconazole 200 mg bid for antifungal therapy (Fig. 2.16).

The upper left picture shows a T1WI coronal image, and the lower left image shows a T2WI coronal plane. A 35-mm-like round abnormal signal is seen under the capsule of the right lobe of the liver. The boundary is still clear, showing long T1 and long T2 signals, and the rest of the signal is uniform. The image on the right shows a T2WI sagittal position, showing multiple round-like lesions in the liver (Fig. 2.17).

On the left side is the lung window, with thickened texture of both lungs and a small amount of inflammation in the right lower lung; on the right side is the liver plane of the mediastinal window, with multiple low-density foci in the liver, with a maximum diameter of about 4.5 cm (Fig. 2.18).

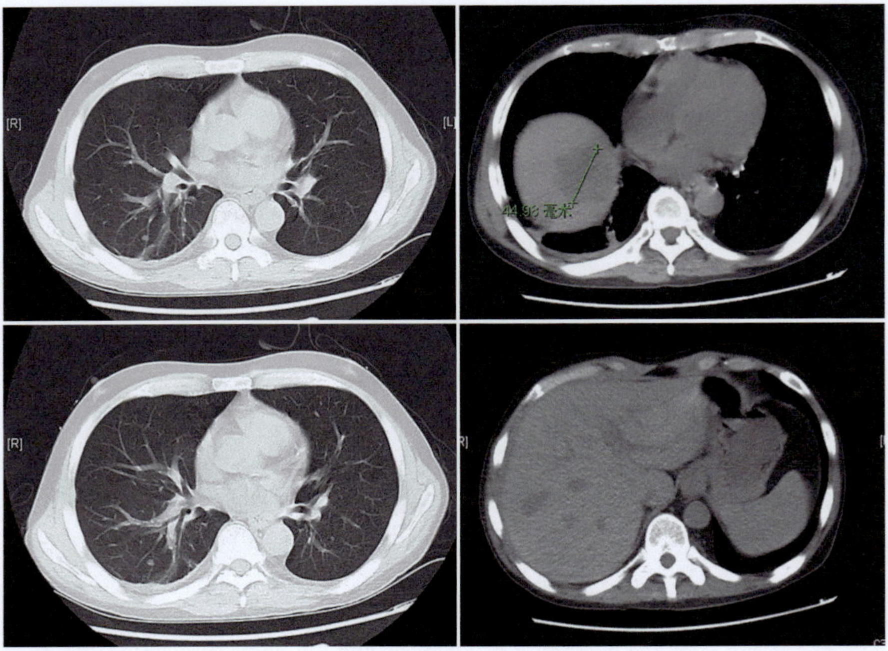

Fig. 2.17 Chest CT on September 11, 2017

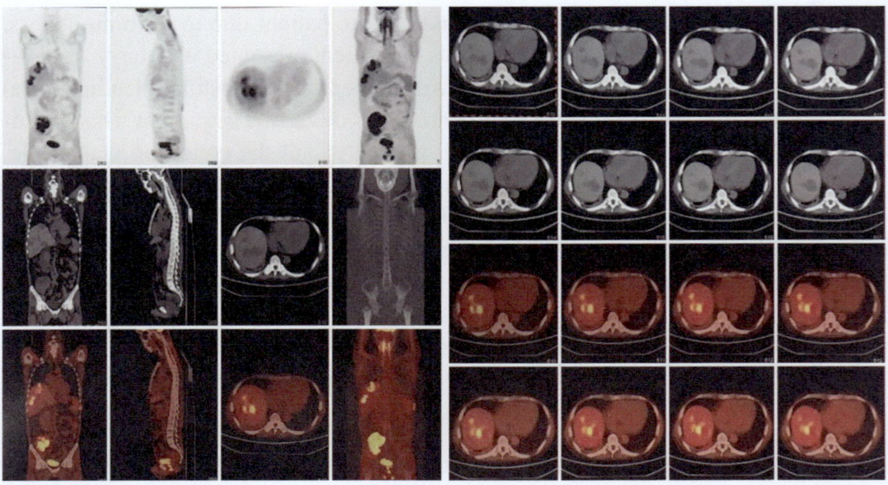

Fig. 2.18 Whole-body PET-CT

There is no evidence of lymphoma for the time being, and multiple metabolic foci of high FDG can be seen in the liver.

On September 8, 2017, second-generation sequencing of the liver tissue detected a list of pathogens (high-throughput gene detection of infected pathogens).

English name	Latin name	The number of sequences detected
Talaromyces marneffei	*Talaromyces marneffei*	5
Human herpesvirus 4 (EBV)	*Human herpesvirus 4*	2868
Mycobacterium tuberculosis complex	*Mycobacterium tuberculosis complex group*	11

Detected sequence number[b]: the number of sequences detected at the genus/species level with strict alignment of the microorganism.

Pathology of liver puncture on September 14, 2017 (Fig. 2.19): A large area of coagulative necrosis was seen in the liver tissue, the portal area of the residual liver tissue was dilated, and a large number of chronic inflammatory cells infiltrated and tended to tuberculosis. Immunohistochemistry: CK7 (small bile duct +), HBsAg (−), HBcAg (−), HCV (−), CD34 (blood vessel +), CK19 (small bile duct +), LCA (+), EBER (+), special staining: MASSON (−), reticular staining (−), special staining Periodic Acid-Schiff Stain (PAS) (−), silver staining (−), and acid resistance (±)

2.13.3 Review

The patient's clinical onset was characterized by acute fever accompanied by a hepatic space-occupying lesion. Additionally, the patient showed poor response to multiple anti-infective treatments administered in other hospitals. Cefoperazone/sulbactam, combined with linezolid, could temporarily abate the fever. Liver puncture suggested inflammatory necrosis changes, so intrahepatic infection lesions had to be considered first, and the possibility of liver abscess was high. At the same time, the patient took antirejection drugs for a long time after kidney transplantation, had a history of diabetes, and was in a state of immunosuppression for a long time. Combined with the positive T-SPOT.TB and effective linezolid treatment in other hospitals, the infection of *Mycobacterium tuberculosis* could not be ruled out, and the infection of other rare pathogens and opportunistic pathogens was also possible.

The types of infections that occur after kidney transplantation and the microbes involved tend to follow a general sequential pattern. Therefore, the differential diagnosis of posttransplant infection based on the time of infection after transplantation is very effective. In the first month after transplantation, infection is most common after general surgery, similar to that in non-immunosuppressed patients who undergo similar surgical procedures. Immunomodulatory viral infections, especially CMV infections, are most important during the 1–6 months after transplantation. In addition to clinical syndromes caused by these viruses, their immunomodulatory properties make the recipient susceptible to opportunistic infections, such as Pneumocystis jirovecii pneumonia, *Listeria monocytogenes*, and *Aspergillus fumigatus*. Other infections that commonly occur during this period include hepatitis,

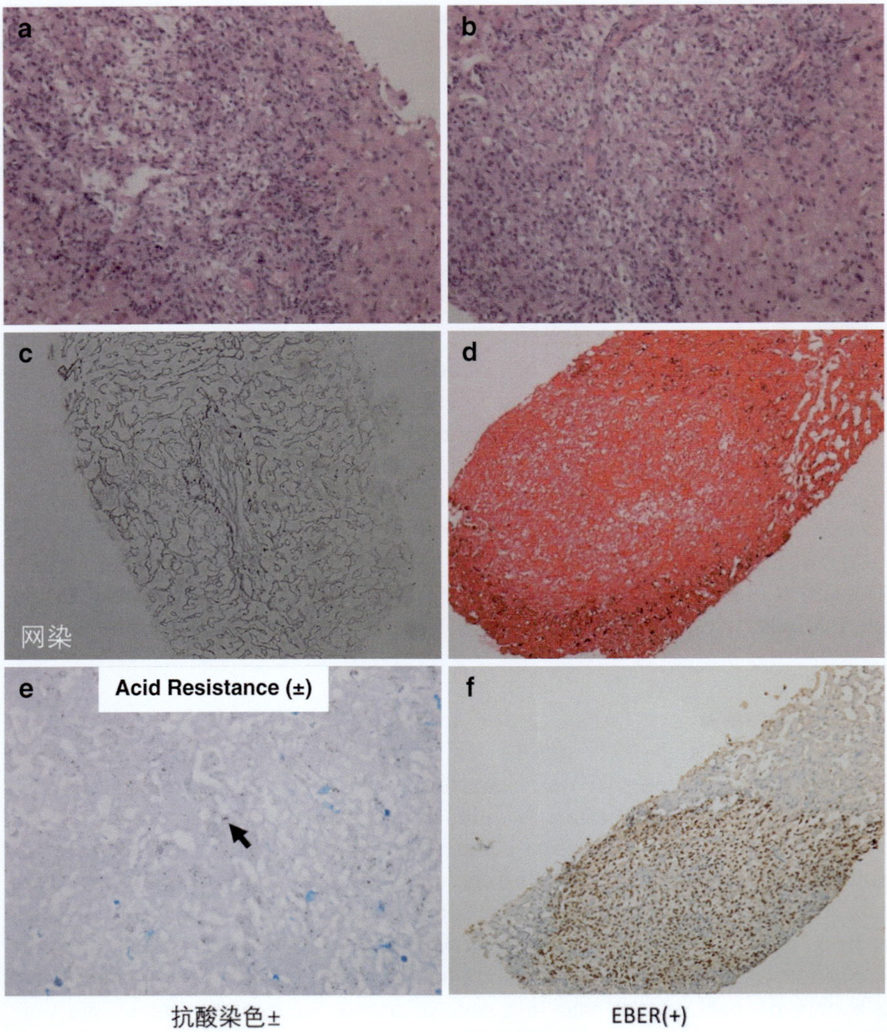

Fig. 2.19 Hepatocentesis pathology. HE staining (**a** and **b**), mesh staining (**c**), silver staining (**d**), acid-fast staining (**e**), and in situ hybridization (EBER +) (**f**). HE staining showed that large areas of coagulation necrosis were observed in the liver tissue and that the portal area of the residual liver tissue was expanded and a large number of chronic inflammatory cells were infiltrated, which were prone to tuberculosis. Reticulate staining (−), silver staining (−), acid-fast staining (±), and in situ hybridization indicated EBER (+)

herpes simplex, herpes zoster, *Mycobacterium tuberculosis*, EBV infection (which can be accompanied by lymphoproliferative disease), and recurrent urinary tract infections. At the later stage of transplantation (more than 6 months after transplantation), most patients have a stable graft function and are treated with minimal immunosuppressive dose maintenance therapy. Most of these patients have infections that are usually similar to those in the general population (influenza, pneumococcal pneumonia, urinary tract infections, etc.). However, about 10–15% of patients have chronic viral infections that are clinically apparent by this time. Examples include CMV infection, choroidal retinitis, lymphoproliferative disease caused by EBV, chronic hepatitis, and clinically acquired immunodeficiency syndrome (AIDS). A small number of patients (5%–15%) have a history of multiple episodes of acute rejection and high levels of immunosuppression. These patients are at risk for serious opportunistic infections that can lead to significant complication rates and mortality, for example, those caused by *Pneumocystis carinii*, *Listeria monocytogenes*, and *Nocardia* asteroides.

The evaluation of diagnostic tests for posttransplant recipient infection generally follows the following principles: (1) The clinical manifestations of host infection may be atypical, or there may be no positive findings on conventional imaging. Because of this, a more sensitive enhanced CT scan or enhanced MRI scan is needed for these patients. (2) The gold standard of microbiological diagnosis includes culture and histology. The detection of proteins, polysaccharide antigens, or nucleic acids is of great value for the diagnosis of transplant patients. (3) Serological tests, which are usually only indicative of past exposure to a pathogen, are valuable for assessing latent infection before transplantation but are not usually used for the diagnosis of acute infection after transplantation. (4) Drug-resistant pathogenic microorganisms are often colonized in transplant recipients, which are often obtained from the hospital environment or anti-infective drug screening.

After kidney transplantation, patients are at risk of acquiring an opportunistic infection with *Mycobacterium tuberculosis*. Due to the hypoxia of the liver tissue, liver tuberculosis is relatively rare in tuberculosis infection, and the prevalence is not higher than 1%. People of all ages are susceptible to it, and it tends to occur mostly in young patients. It is commonly seen in clinically transmitted tuberculosis infection, manifested as diffuse multiple miliary nodules in the liver parenchyma. At present, there is no unified classification standard for hepatic tuberculosis. For the treatment for liver tuberculosis, the WHO tuberculosis treatment plan is also applicable. Currently, there is no unified treatment guideline for this condition, and the recommended treatment course is generally 6 months or longer. For solid organ transplant patients, it is important to note that a TB scheme based on rifampicin may affect the immune inhibitors, as rifampicin can induce cytochrome enzymes P3A4 and reduce the blood concentrations of the immune inhibitors, increasing the risk of rejection. Therefore, the dosage of cyclosporine A, tacrolimus, mortimecofenate, and other drugs should be adjusted appropriately according to the function of the transplanted organ.

The histopathological manifestations of liver EBV infection are varied, with moderate and severe scattered lymphocyte infiltration in the portal area being the most prominent feature. A large number of atypical lymphocytes can be seen, and the diagnosis hints that lymphocytes are arranged in a beadlike manner in hepatic sinusoids. Combined with liver pathology, abnormal liver function, changes in serological antibodies, and EBV-DNA, PCR or in situ hybridization of the liver tissue is of diagnostic value for liver EBV infection, while immunohistochemical staining is not of diagnostic value. Liver EBV infection requires mainly symptomatic support, the benefits of glucocorticoids and acyclovir have not been determined, and the course of disease is usually self-limiting within 2–4 weeks. Ganciclovir can prevent the reactivation of CMV and other Human Herpes Virus (HHV) herpes viruses. For acute EBV-associated liver failure, liver transplantation may be considered. In addition, the immunosuppressant dose should be appropriately reduced at the beginning of treatment for Post - Transplantation Lymphoproliferative Disorders (PTLD), and CD20 mAb or sirolimus-based antirejection therapy should be considered if the response is poor.

References

1. Bosch W, Poowanawittayakom N, Chaikriangkrai K, et al. Tuberculous hepatitis in renal transplant recipients following alemtuzumab induction therapy[J]. Transp Infect Dis. 2013;15(1):E33–9.
2. Le J, Durand C M, Agha I, et al. Epstein-Barr virus and renal transplantation[J]. Transpl Rev. 2017;31(1):55–60.
3. San-Juan R, Manuel O, Hirsch HH, et al. Current preventive strategies and management of Epstein–Barr virus-related post-transplant lymphoproliferative disease in solid organ transplantation in Europe. Results of the ESGICH Questionnaire-based Cross-sectional Survey[J]. Clin Microbiol Infect. 2015;21(6):604.e1–9.
4. Limaiem F, Belkacem O, Bouraoui S. Hepatic tuberculosis[M]. Tuberculosis. 2017.
5. Zakim and Boyers. Hepatology[M]. Liver Disease Associated With Systemic Viral Infection. 2018.

2.14 Dermatomyositis with Scrofula Skin Tuberculosis Infection

Yang Yuling, Yang Feifie, Wang Xinyu, and Zhang Jiming

The patient, a 70-year-old male, was admitted on October 16, 2017, due to erythema on the face and back for more than one year, combined with redness and swelling on the left leg for more than five months.

Since September 2016, the patient had gradually developed red, swollen, and itching rashes on both arms, back, head, and face without any obvious triggers, accompanied by schistose erythema, while no fever and no limb pain were presented. On April 14, 2017, he was treated in the dermatology department of a hospital in Fujian. The antinuclear antibody spectrum was examined as follows: anti-RO-52 antibody (±), anti-JO-1 antibody (±), anti-dsDNA antibody (−), immunoglobulin E: 1610 IU/mL, lactate dehydrogenase (LDH): 268 U/L, and creatine phosphokinase (CPK): 392 U/L. Electromyography showed myogenic damage and partial damage of the right median nerve (could have been carpal tunnel syndrome), which was diagnosed as "dermatomyositis," and the patient was then treated with methylprednisolone. The dosage was as follows: 60 mg/d intravenous for 1 week, then changed to 40 mg/d intravenous plus 12 mg/d orally for 3 days, then changed to 48 mg/d orally for 3 weeks, then changed to 40 mg/d orally for 2 weeks, and then changed to 36 mg/d orally for 2 weeks. The skin lesions improved slightly. On June 25, he developed a fever, accompanied by chills, with the highest body temperature of 39 °C, with mild cough and no sputum, and he had more erythema on the upper limbs and back. Then the patient was admitted to the local hospital and was given higher-dose glucocorticoid (the specific dose is unknown) treatment, and the body temperature came down slightly. Since July 2017, he had presented with left leg and left ankle edema and still had fever (up to 40 °C) with chills, fatigue, headaches, joint pain, and muscle pain. On July 21, PET-CT examination revealed the following: 1. Increased metabolism in multiple muscles, including the right subscapularis, left deltoid, right hemidiaphragm, transverse abdominis, internal oblique, left middle gluteus, gluteus maximus, quadratus femoris, and biceps femoris; 2. Thickening of the right interlobar and costal pleura with increased metabolism; 3. Slightly elevated subcutaneous metabolic activity in the right facial region. Combined with the patient's medical history, dermatomyositis was considered. Lymph nodes with increased metabolism in the right hilum, mediastinum, and right diaphragmatic angle were considered to be possible inflammatory hyperplasia. There was slight inflammation in the middle and lower lobes of the right lung and pleural effusion on the right side. According to the examinations, glucocorticoids and an external cream were prescribed to treat dermatomyositis. However, the left lower limb swelling of the patient gradually aggravated. On August 28, at a hospital in Fujian Province, a blood routine test showed the following: leukocytes: 4.91×10^9/L, neutrophils: 0.952, ESR: 120 mm/h, C-reactive protein: >9 mg/L, and lactic acid dehydrogenase: 353 u/L, and the sputum culture was positive for *Klebsiella pneumoniae* and *Candida albicans*. Cefoperazone/sulbactam, moxifloxacin, linezolid, imipenem/cilastatin, and caspofungin were administered. In addition, the methylprednisolone dosage was adjusted as follows: 80 mg/d for the first week, then reduced to 60 mg/d for the second week, and further adjusted to 40 mg/d for the subsequent treatment course. Ultrasound examination showed a subcutaneous fluid mass of the left lower extremity. On September 8, ultrasound-guided abscess puncture and catheterization were performed, and a thick, yellow liquid could be seen flowing out. The bacterial smear of the pus was of gram-positive bacilli (with phagocytosis), which were branched-shaped. Acid-fast bacilli (+++) were detected by tuberculosis smear, and the diagnosis was "tuberculous abscess (left thigh muscle), dermatomyositis." The patient was treated with isoniazid, rifampicin, pyrazinamide, ethambutol, levofloxacin, amikacin, and clarithromycin for 20 days, and then the rash gradually disappeared, but the left leg was still swollen and painful. The patient was unable to walk and still had intermittent fever with the highest temperature of 40 °C. Therefore, he was transferred to the Department of Infectious Diseases of Huashan Hospital on October 16.

2.14.1 Past History

He was diagnosed with "dermatomyositis" in April 2017 and had been treated with glucocorticoids for more than half a year.

2.14.2 Physical Examinations

Body temperature: 36.5 °C, pulse: 111 beats/min, respiration: 18/min, and blood pressure 120/68 mmHg. He was mentally clear, low-spirited, and skinny. Diffused dark brown pigmentation could be seen on the chest, back, and limbs, and there was no obvious swelling of lymph nodes. Breath sounds in both lungs were clear, dry or wet rales were not heard, heart rhythm was uniform, and no pathological murmurs were heard in each valve. Abdomen was soft, there was no tenderness or rebound pain, the liver and spleen could not be reached, and shifting dullness was negative. The left lower limb was moderately swollen, tender, and restricted in movement. Pathological signs were not elicited.

2.14.3 Case History

When the patient was admitted to our hospital, there was no obvious rash or fever. He had obvious swelling of the right lower limb, with pain, and was unable to walk. Routine blood tests were showed the following: white blood cells: 8.61×10^9/L, neutrophil percentage: 0.812, erythrocyte sedimentation rate: 50 mm/h, creatine phosphokinase: 10 U/L, lactate dehydrogenase: 193 U/L, blood T-SPOT.TB: negative, and antinuclear antibody spectrum: negative. Ultrasound showed multiple small spots in the arteries of both lower extremities, thrombosis in the left calf intermuscular vein, and multiple strips of infection, with a small amount of liquefaction between the muscles of the left thigh; subcutaneous soft tissue infection foci on the right thoracic wall; and no obvious liquefaction. The subcutaneous soft tissue of the right lateral chest wall was infected, and no obvious liquefaction was observed. MR of the thigh showed that the soft tissue infection of the left thigh was likely to form an abscess, an abnormal signal shadow was seen in the lower part of the femur, and femoral osteomyelitis could not be excluded. The right thigh had atrophy; chest CT showed multiple nodules in both lungs, dense shadows in the lower lobes of the lungs, a small amount of pleural effusion on the right, and soft tissue shadows in the right chest wall, indicating the possibility of infectious disease; MRI of the head showed brain changes and brain atrophy, representing elderly brain; and gastroscopy showed gastric antrum and gastric keratitis (uplift and erosion type, moderate) with bile reflux. The patient's left lower extremity thigh was swollen, a subcutaneous bulge was observed in the back of the thigh near the popliteal fossa, and the skin became thin, with pale yellow exudate, and gradually ulcerated. The exudate was collected and stained with acid-fast bacilli (++ + +) (Fig. 2.20). The exudate was

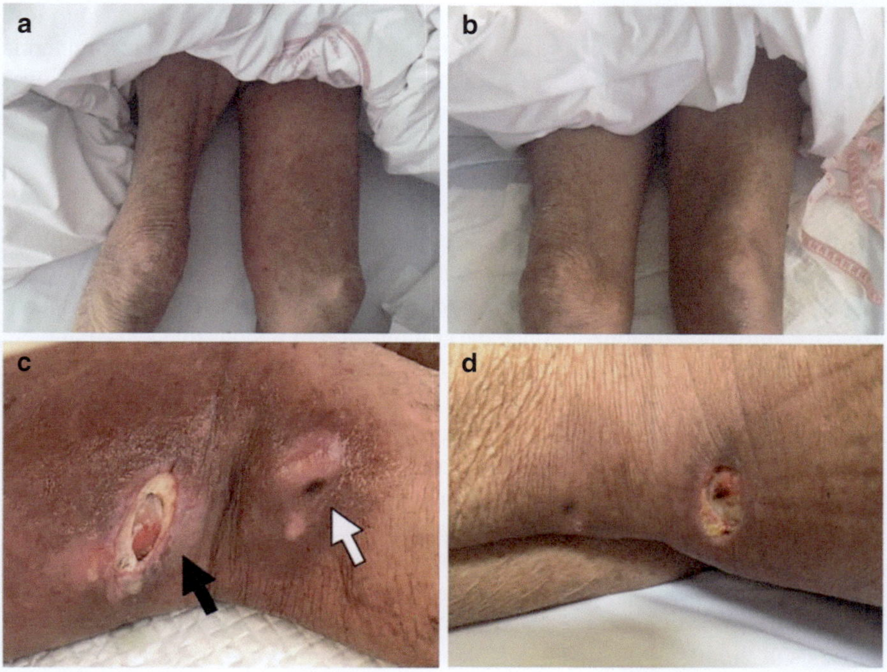

Fig. 2.20 Comparison of the skin appearance of the patient's lower extremities before and after treatment. (**a**) On admission, the patient's left lower limb was significantly swollen, the dorsal thigh skin was flushed, and the right lower limb muscle was atrophied. (**b**) After 40 days of treatment, the swelling of the left lower limb disappeared, and the muscle atrophy of the right lower limb improved. (**c**) Ten days after admission, the skin was swollen and there was local thinning (white arrow), with ulceration and persistent exudation (black arrow). (**d**) After 40 days of treatment, the inflammation of the original ulceration was improved, dry without exudation, and the original thin skin returned to normal

also sent for high-throughput sequencing of infectious pathogens, and the *Mycobacterium tuberculosis* complex was found. The exudate Xpert MTB/RIF assay reported MTB as positive and rifampicin as sensitive, and the exudate was cultured with *Mycobacterium*. Based on the above results, the patient was diagnosed with "tuberculous infection of the soft tissue of the left lower limb."

Then, we administered rifampicin 0.3 g qd, isoniazid 0.3 g qd, pyrazine amide 0.5 g tid, ethambutol 0.75 g qd, and amikacin 0.6 g qd for antituberculosis therapy. As the wound of the patient was open, glucocorticoid therapy was still applied, and since secondary gram-positive bacterial infection had to be prevented, linezolid 0.6 g q12h was added for both antibacterial and antituberculosis treatments. The patient had no fever, but the left lower extremity puncture site continued exudation, and the patient still had severe edema in the left lower extremity and difficulty in movement, and he gradually developed nausea and vomiting, poor food intake, poor mental state, and albumin as low as 25 g/L. Considering how tuberculosis infection is a state of high consumption, the exudation at the puncture site continued to lose protein, poor eating led to insufficient nutritional intake, and hypoalbuminemia could also aggravate edema and exudate, active albumin supplementation was given. When the patient's albumin increased to more than 32 g/L, the edema of the left lower limb was significantly reduced, and the exudation became less.

Fever occurred again 3 weeks after the antituberculosis treatment, the blood culture was negative, and the percentage of white blood cells and neutrophils was slightly increased. Sputum smear reported a yeast-like bacterium, and the culture was positive for *Candida albicans* several times. Other fungal infections could not be excluded due to the immunosuppressed state of this patient, so we added fluconazole for antifungal treatment. Since the combination of fluconazole and rifampicin could lead to an area-under-the-curve (AUC) decrease by 25% and a half-life-period decrease by 20% and since rifampicin might easily cause drug fever, we discontinued rifampicin. Antibiotic therapies were adjusted to "isoniazid, pyrazine amide, ethambutol, amikacin, linezolid oxazole amine, fluconazole azole," and the patient then had no fever. After rifampicin withdrawal, the patient's gastrointestinal symptoms were significantly reduced, and his appetite improved.

After discontinuing the infusion of albumin, the patient's left lower limb edema and increased exudation reappeared. The maximum leg circumference of 15 cm above the left lower limb patella was 48.5 cm, and the albumin was as low as 28 g/L. On the basis of actively supplementing albumin and improving colloidal penetration, we treated the patient with hydrogen peroxide debridement of ulcerations once a day. After significant improvement in lower limb edema and exudation, the leg circumference decreased to 38 cm (Fig. 2.21). The general condition of the patient improved, and he could walk with help. Upon discharge from the hospital, the lower limb MRI (Fig. 2.22) and chest CT (Fig. 2.23) were reexamined, and the infection was obviously controlled.

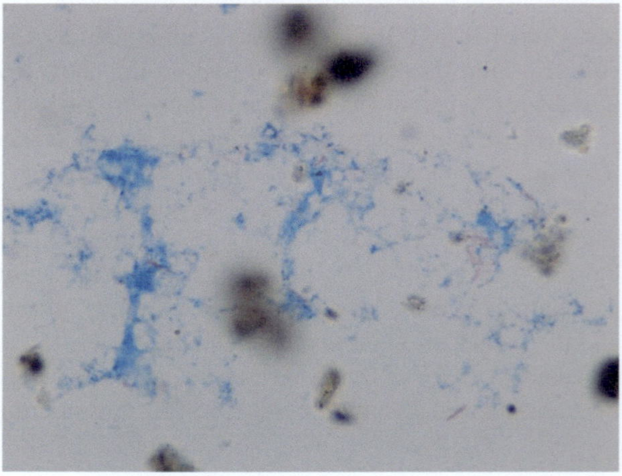

Fig. 2.21 Acid-fast staining of the patient's wound surface exudation. Acid-fast staining (++++) on admission

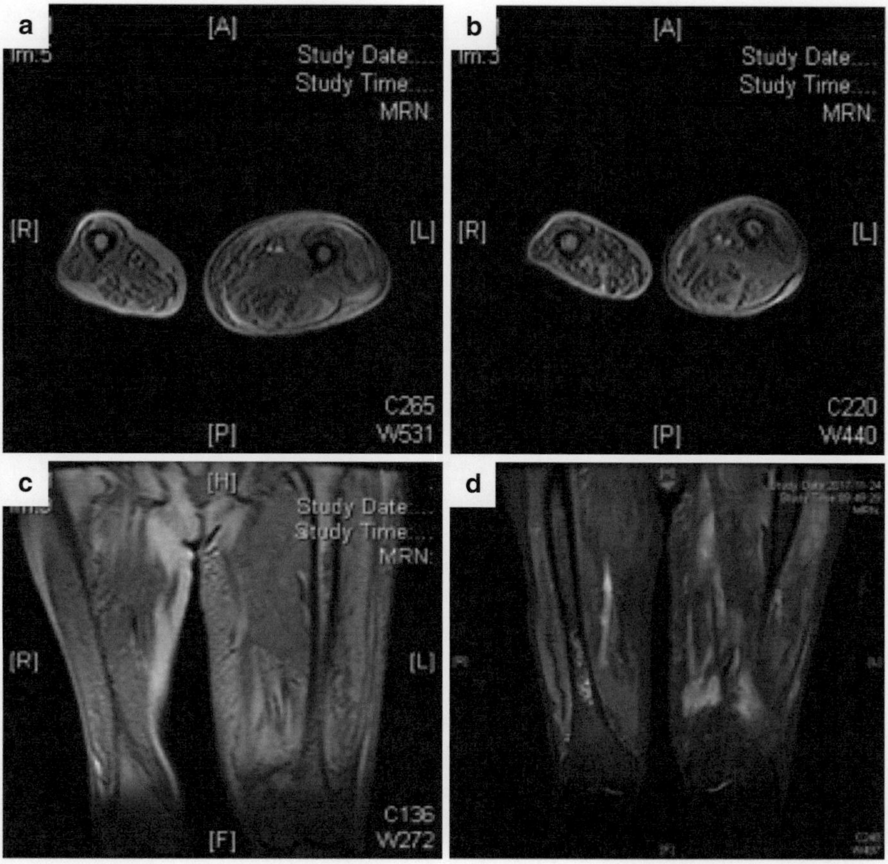

Fig. 2.22 Comparison of thigh MRI before and after treatment. (**a** and **c**) lower limb MRI on admission. (**b** and **d**) lower limb MRI after 40 days of treatment

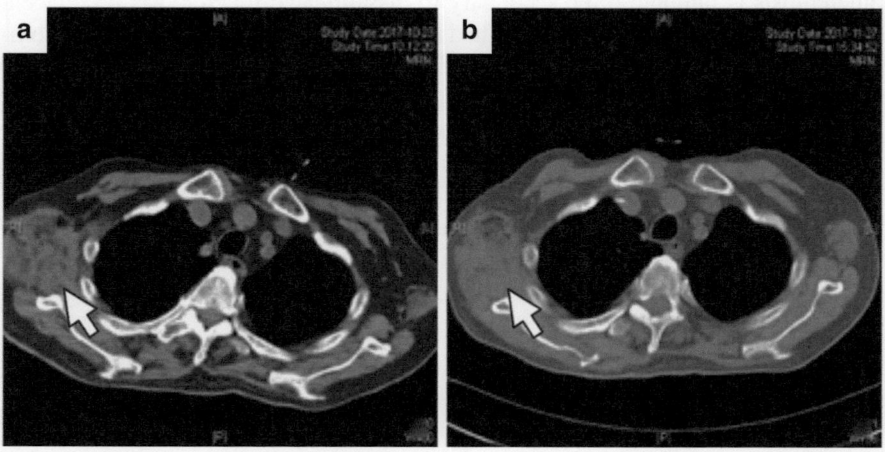

Fig. 2.23 Comparison of chest CT before and after antituberculosis treatment. (**a**) Chest CT on admission showed a soft tissue shadow on the right chest wall. (**b**) The soft tissue shadow was significantly reduced after 40 days of treatment

2.14.4 Discussion

Scrofulous skin tuberculosis (also called liquefied skin tuberculosis) is a type of skin tuberculosis that used to occur much more frequently before effective antituberculosis treatments were developed. The disease is caused by an infection of deep constitutions (e.g., lymph nodes, bones, joints, or epididymis), extending directly to the overlying skin. Scrofulous skin tuberculosis can occur at any age, but it occurs most frequently in children, adolescents, and elderly individuals. Clinically suspected scrofulous skin tuberculosis should be differentiated from purulent nodules of other causes, including atypical mycobacteria, sporotrichosis, actinomycosis, coccidioidomycosis, venereal lymphogranuloma, syphilis, severe acne conglobata, and hidradenitis suppurativa.

This patient was an elderly male with a history of dermatomyositis and long-term use of glucocorticoids. Methylprednisolone was used for more than 1 month at a dose of 40–60 mg; thus, this was a high-risk factor for tuberculosis infection. The patient had no history of tuberculosis, and T-SPOT after glucocorticoids could have had false negatives, so the fever in the early stage with swelling of the right lower limb had not been diagnosed in time, resulting in a prolonged and worsened condition. After admission to Huashan Hospital, although T-SPOT.TB was still negative after reexamination, the exudate was strongly positive for acid-fast staining. The Xpert MTB/RIF assay had a positive result, so the diagnosis of right lower limb soft tissue tuberculosis infection was clear. Although the body temperature was stable in the early stages of treatment, the effect of local soft tissue infection and exudation of the right leg had not decreased. Considering the patient's poor nutritional status and insufficient local tissue antituberculosis drug concentration, we administered nutritional support and strengthened local debridement and dressing care. In addition, the use of glucocorticoids had to be minimized under the premise of controlling dermatomyositis in a stable condition. Scrofulous skin tuberculosis is rare and often secondary to disseminated tuberculosis or adjacent deep-organ tuberculosis. The patient had no history of tuberculosis, and after completing imaging examinations of the brain, chest, abdomen, etc., no tuberculosis infection lesions were found, so we considered simple scrofula skin tuberculosis. Therefore, the long-term use of glucocorticoid therapy for rheumatic diseases affecting the skin should be routinely screened for tuberculosis infection. If local skin and soft tissues are red and swollen and if the efficacy of common antibiotics is not effective, we should be alert to the possibility of tuberculosis infection. At this time, the dosage of glucocorticoids should not be increased. In addition, a combination of multiple detection methods should be used to improve the sensitivity of tuberculosis diagnosis.

References

1. Lindi VZ, Jeanetta DP, Joe V. Cutaneous tuberculosis overview and current treatment regimens [J]. Tuberculosis. 2015;95:629–38.
2. Santos JB, Figueiredo AR, Ferraz CE, et al. Cutaneous tuberculosis: epidemiologic, etiopathogenic and clinical aspects-part I [J]. An Bras Dermatol. 2014;89(2):219–28.
3. Amir KR, Luis GC, Laurence EB, et al. Chest wall soft tissue tuberculosis: a protracted course over a 10-year period [J]. Scand J Infect Dis. 2006;38(2):129–30.
4. Puttick MP, Stein HB, Chan RM, Elwood RK, How AR, Reid GD. Soft tissue tuberculosis: a series of 11 cases. J Rheumatol. 1995;22:1321–5.
5. Wang Yanping, Zuo Xiaoxia, Luo Hui, et al. Clinical analysis and literature review of 6 cases of diffuse connective tissue disease with skin and soft tissue tuberculosis [J]. Chin J Rheumatol. 2009;13(10):701–4.
6. Airio A, Kauppi M, Kautiatinen H, et al. High association of mycobacterial infections with polymyositis in a non-endemic country for tuberculosis. Ann Rheum Dis. 2007;66:1404–5.
7. Nicholas TV, Julie S, Jane B. Prevalence, screening and treatment of latent tuberculosis among oral corticosteroid recipients [J]. Eur Respir J. 2014;44:1373–5.
8. Erika B, Synne S, Morten R, et al. Prednisolone treatment affects the performance of the QuantiFERON gold in-tube test and the tuberculin skin test in patients with autoimmune disorders screened for latent tuberculosis infection [J]. Inflamm Bowel Dis. 2011;17(11):2340–9.
9. Jia Chi Yu. Tuberculous wound – a neglected and noteworthy clinical problem [J]. Chin J Injury Repair. 2014;9(4):9–11.

2.15 Fever with Bilateral Adrenal and Multiple Intracranial Masses: Lymphoma or Tuberculosis Infection

Zhang Shu, Li Tao, Zhu Zuiyun, and Li Ning

A 33-year-old female patient was admitted to the hospital on August 16, 2017, due to “fever for more than 4 months.”

After a cesarean section on April 6, 2017, the patient began to experience fever, T_{max} 39 °C, and the body temperature would only return to normal after taking ibuprofen, but the body temperature would rise 1 or 2 days later, accompanied by chills, cough, and no sputum or other special discomfort. She was hospitalized in a local hospital in Enshi, Hubei Province. Her T-SPOT.TB test was positive (antigen A hole: 80 points; antigen B hole: 21 points). A contrast-enhanced CT of her pelvic cavity and adrenal gland showed double adrenal mass lesions, which could not be excluded as metastatic tumor; retroperitoneal lymph node enlargement; and a space-occupying lesion in the right lobe of the liver, possibly a hemangioma. With anti-infective treatment with cefoxitin, ornidazole, and meropenem, the patient’s fever was not relieved, with T_{max}: 38.5 °C mainly in the afternoon, without night sweats or fatigue.

On May 16, the patient was transferred to a tertiary hospital in Hunan Province. Head MRI enhancement showed multiple enhanced nodules in the brain parenchyma, indicating a high possibility of metastasis. There was no obvious abnormality in the cerebrospinal fluid biochemical and routine results of lumbar puncture. PET-CT examination showed increased FDG uptake in the following lesions: 1. Bilateral adrenal glands; 2. Multiple enlarged lymph nodes in the retroperitoneal para-aortic region; 3. Multiple cerebral nodules with peripheral edema. All of these findings were highly suggestive of lymphoma.

The patient then underwent adrenal mass puncture and bone marrow biopsy. Pathological results of adrenal puncture showed epithelioid cell nodules and multinucleated giant cells, a small amount of caseous necrosis, and negative acid-fast staining, indicating a high possibility of tuberculosis. Bone marrow biopsy indicated that bone marrow hyperplasia was active, and no other obvious abnormal pathological cells were observed. On June 8, she was transferred to a designated pulmonary tuberculosis hospital in Changsha, where she began to receive isoniazid, rifampicin, ethambutol, and pyrazinamide (HREZ) diagnostic antituberculosis treatment, and at the same time, she was given supportive treatment. However, the patient requested to be discharged because she still had a low-grade fever. The treatment was changed to the HREZLFx (levofloxacin) quintuplet regimen when she was discharged, and the antituberculosis treatment was continued without interruption. Since the illness, the patient had been in good spirits, with normal appetite and sleep, normal urine and feces, and no significant weight loss.

2.15.1 Past History and Personal History

The patient was in good health, there was nothing special in any of the systematic reviews, and she denied any history of hypertension, diabetes, heart disease, or other chronic basic diseases. The patient was a medical worker who had been exposed to tuberculosis patients for a long time.

2.15.2 Physical Examination on Admission

T 37.0 °C and HR 80 bpm. Mind was clear, there was no anemic appearance, no rash or mucosa was observed in the skin of the whole body, and no swelling was observed in the superficial lymph nodes. The neck was soft without resistance, and the double lung breathing sound was clear. The abdomen was flat and soft, and there was a 10-cm surgical scar in the middle of the lower abdomen, which had healed well. There was no tenderness or rebounding pain in the whole abdomen, no swelling under the liver, spleen, or costal area, and no tapping pain in the liver and kidney area.

2.15.3 Workup After Admission

Her blood T-SPOT.TB test was strongly positive after admission (antigen A hole: >60 points; antigen B hole: >20 points), and a reexamination of head MR enhancement showed "scattered spotty enhancement foci in brain parenchyma, considering the clinical conditions, it was likely to be the lymphoma infiltration" (Fig. 2.24). A reexamination of the adrenal CT showed "bilateral adrenal mass (left lesion, $d \approx 6.4$ cm; right lesion, $d \approx 3.32$ cm), possibly the neoplastic lesions" (Fig. 2.25).

However, a reexamination of the lumbar puncture showed normal CSF pressure and no obvious abnormality in CSF routine and biochemical tests. CSF cytological examination and pathological biopsy of the adrenal mass puncture of the patient in another hospital showed no tumor in consultation with the Department of Pathology, Fudan University, Shanghai Cancer Center. To eliminate drug fever caused by rifampicin, we changed the antituberculosis regimen to isoniazid, ethambutol, pyrazinamide, and levofloxacin (HEZLfx). The temperature had dropped briefly but soon returned to low-grade fever of around 37.5 °C–38 °C, which did not improve by adding amikacin 600000 U qd IVGTT or linezolid 600 mg q12h. On August 31, the patient began to experience persistent dull pain in the left renal region, which could be elicited by percussion of the area of the back overlying the left kidney. A reexamination of the adrenal gland by B-ultrasound on September 4 showed that "parenchymal space occupied in bilateral adrenal areas (the right adrenal area was 66 × 39mm clear low-echo area, irregular shape; in the left adrenal gland, there was a clear low-echo area of 95 × 43 mm with full shape)," both of which were significantly larger than before (Fig. 2.26).

Since early June 2017, the patient has received standard antituberculosis treatment. However, the patient still had intermittent low-grade fever, worsening dull pain in the left renal region, and enlarged bilateral adrenal lesions. This indicated a poor response to antituberculosis therapy, and the possibility that the adrenal space-occupying lesions were extranodal lymphoma could not be ruled out. On September 12, another biopsy was performed on the left adrenal gland, and the pathological diagnosis showed "(puncture biopsy of the left adrenal mass) adrenal granulomatous inflammation with coagulative necrosis." Therefore, the possibility of lymphoma was excluded, and HEZLFx quadruplet antituberculosis therapy was continued. The patient's condition improved, and she was discharged on September 13.

After being discharged, the patient developed a fever of 39 °C again due to a cold, accompanied by coughing and coughing up yellow-green sputum, and felt that the left lower back pain was aggravated. After 5 days of oral administration of azithromycin, the patient's body temperature dropped to 37.5 °C, and the left lower back pain was relieved, so she stopped azithromycin voluntarily and changed to oral roxithromycin treatment until September 26. During this period, the patient still had a low-grade fever (below 38 °C), with no chills, night sweats, weight loss, or other symptoms. Additionally, the patient had a mild cough without sputum and no obvious left lower back pain. The patient returned to our department for hospitalization again on September 27, 2017.

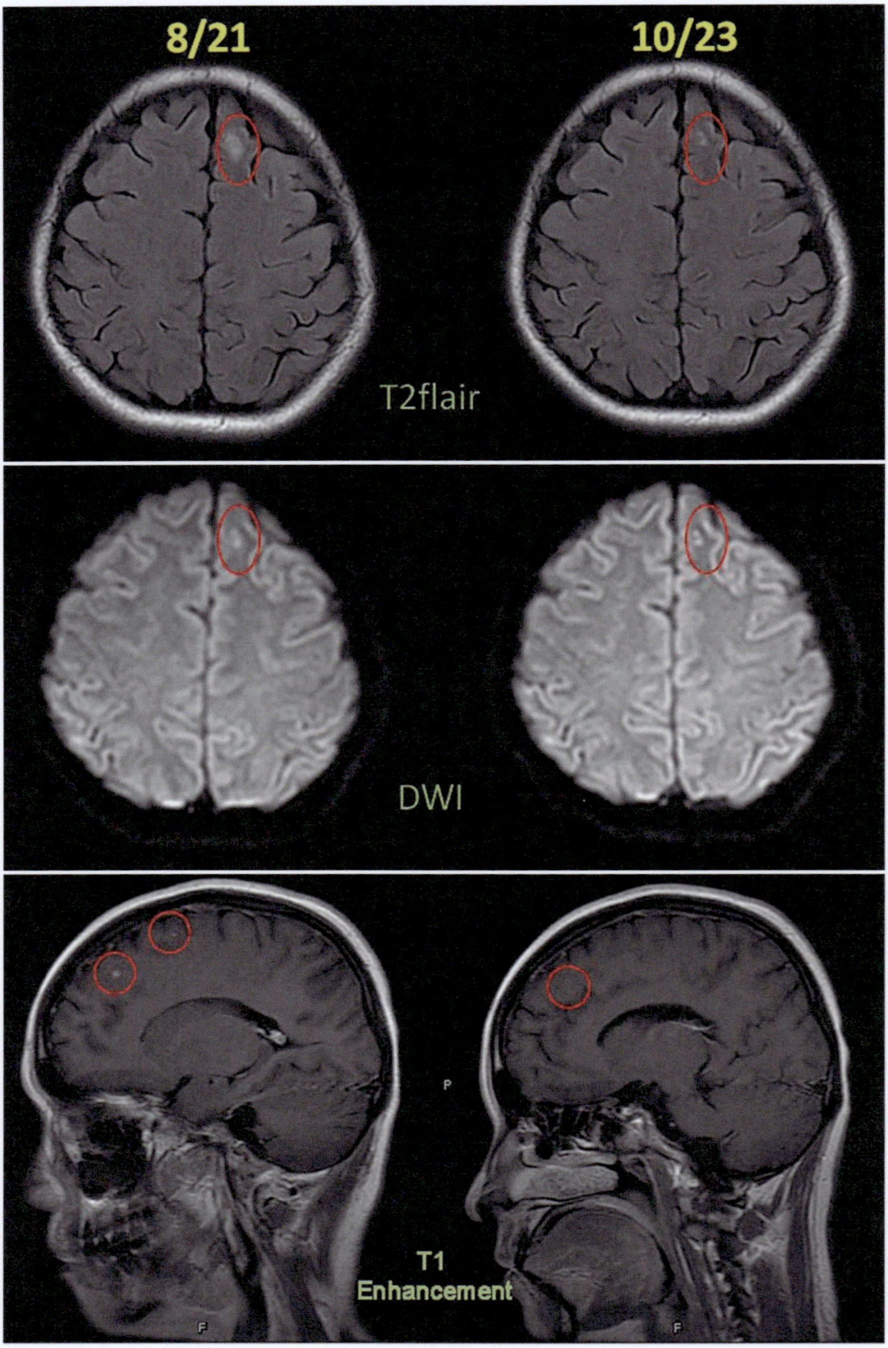

Fig. 2.24 Brain MRI enhancement before and after comparison. August 21: Scattered dotted abnormal signals in the brain parenchyma, T2 flair showed peripheral edema, and DWI showed a hypersignal, which was significantly enhanced after enhancement. October 23: Spotted T2 Fluid Attenuated Inversion Recovery (FLAIR) hyperintensity shadow in the left frontal lobe, hyperintensity in the DWI lesion, and suspicious ring enhancement in the lesion after enhancement

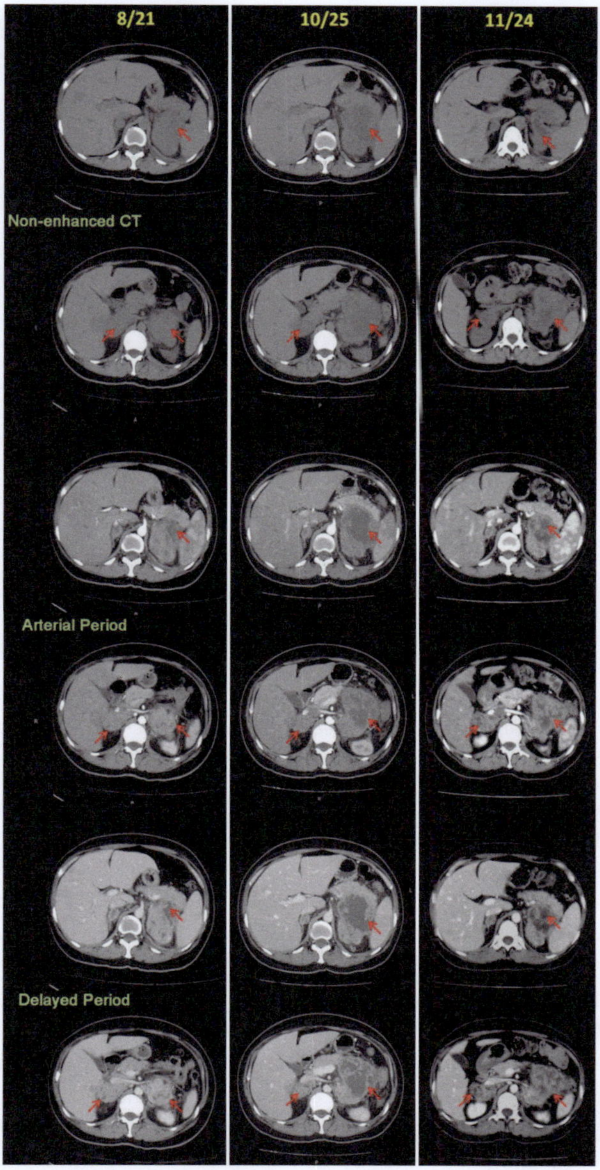

Fig. 2.25 Adrenal gland CT enhancement before and after comparison. As shown on August 21, a soft tissue mass shadow was observed in both adrenal areas. The diameter of the lesion on the left was about 6.4cm, and the diameter of the lesion on the right was about 3.32 cm. The density of the lesions was uneven, and both lesions showed moderate enhancement on contrast-enhanced scan. As shown on October 25, irregular masses were seen anterior to bilateral adrenal glands, about 6.4 × 9.5 cm (left) and 3.3 × 4.2 cm in size (right). Segmentation and cystic density were seen inside. The lesion showed internal septations and cystic density. The bilateral adrenal glands exhibited compressive changes, and the masses showed significant inhomogeneous enhancement on contrast-enhanced scan. After the puncture and abscess extraction on November 24, the results showed that multiple nodules were fused in the adrenal areas on both sides. The maximum range on the left side was about 6.2 cm, with uneven internal density and multiple low-density shadows. After enhancement, multiple annular enhancement areas and multiple liquefaction necrosis areas were observed

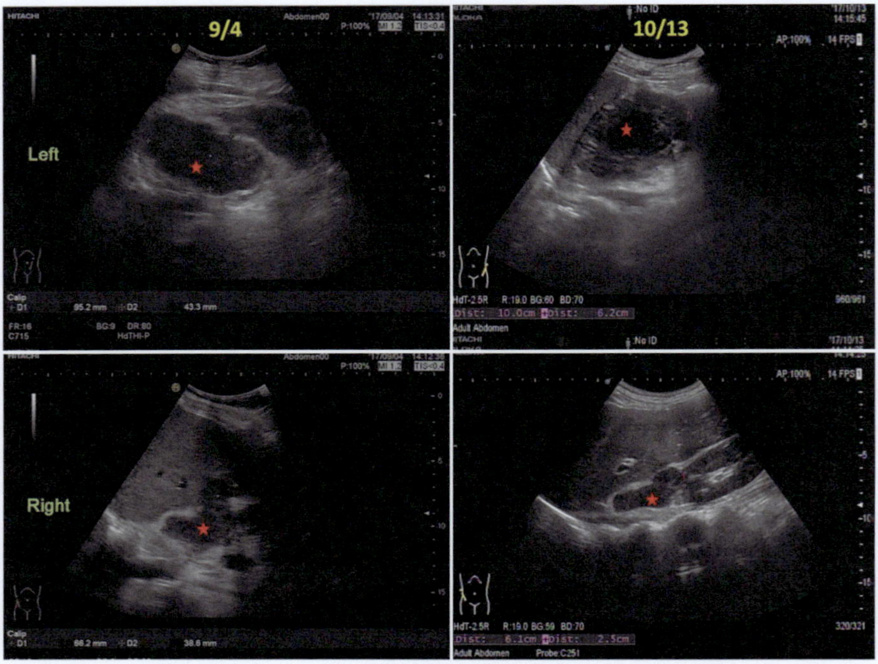

Fig. 2.26 Comparison of adrenal B-ultrasound. On September 4, the left adrenal gland showed a 95 × 43-mm low-echo zone with a clear boundary and full shape. In the right adrenal gland, a 66 × 39 mm demarcated hypoechoic area is seen, which is irregular in shape and closely related to the liver. On October 13, it was shown that the left adrenal gland was a mixed-echo area with a size of about 100 × 62 mm and mainly low-echo, with a clear boundary and irregular shape. A 61 × 25-mm hypoechoic area was seen in the right adrenal gland

After the second admission, considering the effectiveness of oral azithromycin, we considered the possibility of drug-resistant TB or non-*Mycobacterium tuberculosis* infection, therefore adjusting the regimen to rifampicin 0.6 g qd po + ethambutol 0.75 g qd po + pyrazinamide 0.5 g tid po + clarithromycin 0.5 g bid po + levofloxacin 0.5 g qd IVGTT + amikacin 600000 U qd IVGTT + linezolid 0.6 g q12h IVGTT. After 2 weeks of treatment, the patient's body temperature decreased gradually from 38.4 °C to normal, and there was still a mild percussion pain in the left kidney region.

However, ultrasonography showed no substantial reduction in the adrenal mass (on September 29, the right adrenal mass was 59 × 27 mm, and the left adrenal mass was 98 × 61 mm with mixed mass; On October 13, imaging showed a solid hypoechoic space-occupying lesion in the right adrenal gland, measuring 61 × 25 mm, and a mixed-density space-occupying lesion in the left adrenal gland, measuring 100 × 62 mm). Therefore, we sent two adrenal puncture pathological slides again to the Department of Pathology, Public Health Clinical Center, Fudan University, to read the film to find acid-fast bacilli. Pathologic consultation returned the following observation: [the left adrenal gland puncture 1, before the chemotherapy treatment] Inflammatory cell infiltration, fibrous tissue hyperplasia, epithelioid granuloma formation, complete coagulative necrosis 1–2 positive bacteria were found in acid-fast staining, PAS (−), indicating tuberculosis. [the left adrenal puncture 2, 3 months after antituberculosis treatment] inflammatory cell infiltration, fibrous tissue hyperplasia, epithelioid granuloma formation, complete coagulative necrosis, acid-fast staining + (a few L-type bacteria), indicating tuberculosis (Figs. 2.27 and 2.28, provided by Feng Yanling, director of the Department of Pathology, Shanghai Public Health Clinical Center). At this point, the diagnosis of adrenal *Mycobacterium* infection was established, so we continued to give the patient the original seven regimens of antituberculosis treatment.

After 1 month of treatment (October 23), the patient's enhanced head MR reexamination showed "lesion in the left frontal lobe (punctate T2-FLAIR hyperintensity shadow in the left frontal lobe, hyperintensity in the diffusion weighted imaging (DWI) lesion, suspicious ring enhancement in the lesion after enhancement), and infectious lesion was possible." Compared with the intracranial lesion on August 21, there were fewer lesions (Fig. 2.24). It seemed to suggest that the anti-infective treatment was effective.

Compared with the previous images, the adrenal abscess lesion of the patient in adrenal CT enhancement on October 25 was considered to have obvious liquefaction necrosis (Fig. 2.25), so the left adrenal abscess was punctured twice under the guidance of ultrasound on November 9 and November 16, and 50 ml and 46 ml, respectively, of yellow-white bloody pus were extracted (Fig. 2.29).

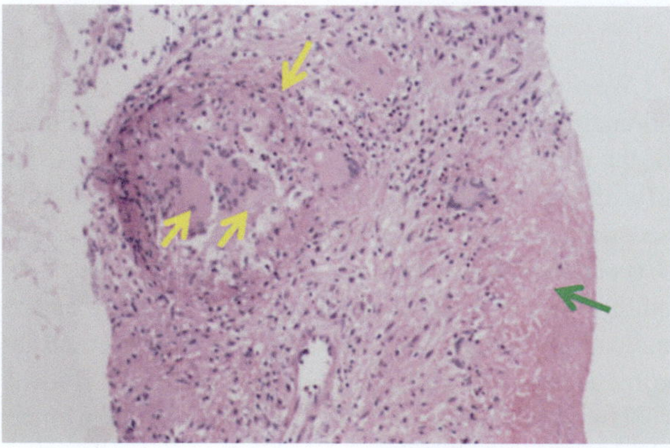

Fig. 2.27 Inflammatory cell infiltration, epithelioid granuloma, and multinucleated giant cell formation (yellow arrow) and complete coagulation necrosis (green arrow) in the adrenal gland tissue

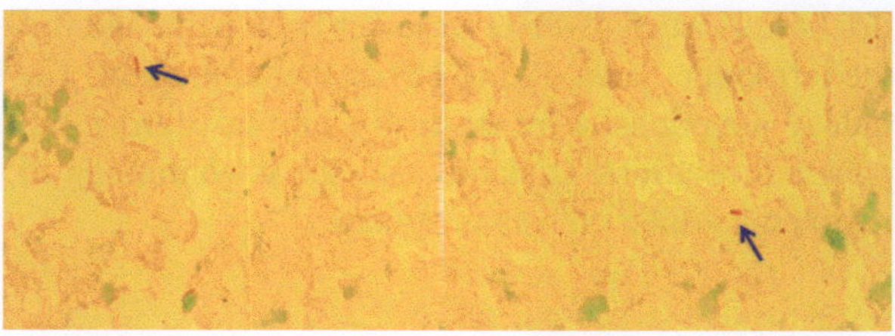

Fig. 2.28 Two strains of *Mycobacterium tuberculosis* were found under the microscope (shown by blue arrow); acid-fast staining × 1000

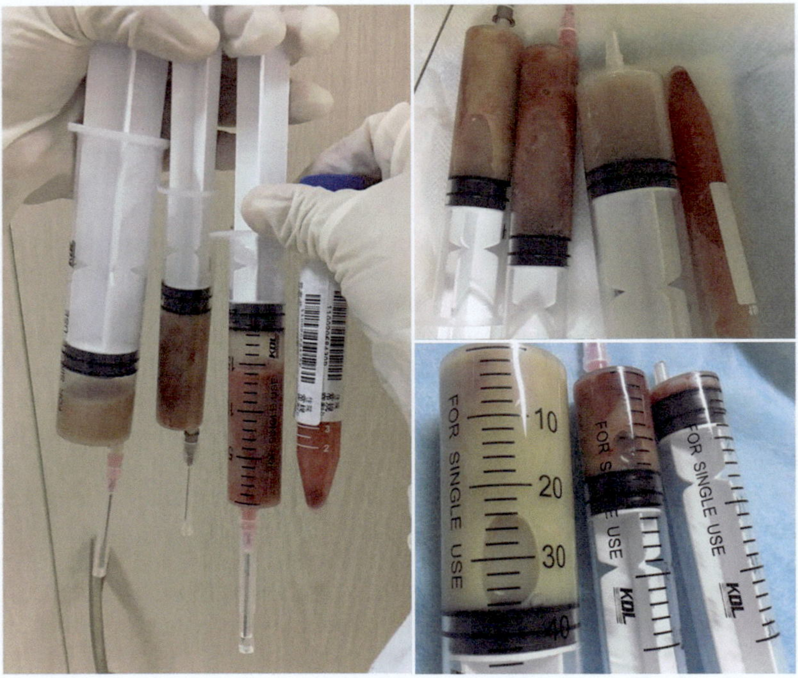

Fig. 2.29 Under the guidance of B-ultrasound, 50 ml and 46 ml of yellow-white bloody pus were extracted from the left adrenal abscess twice by puncture

We did not perform aspiration on the right side as the liquefied area of the right adrenal abscess was not obvious. Xpert MTB/RIF and Xpert MTB/RIF Ultra tests of the pus samples on the next day were the first to report positive nucleic acid of *Mycobacterium tuberculosis* and sensitivity to rifampicin. At the same time, the second-generation sequencing technology reported that six sequences of the *Mycobacterium tuberculosis* complex group were detected in the pus, and the pus culture results a few weeks later were also *Mycobacterium tuberculosis*–positive, indicating that they were sensitive to first-line antituberculosis drugs, which was consistent with the nucleic acid test results and clinical diagnosis.

The patient's adrenal CT enhancement on November 24 showed that the adrenal abscess was smaller than one month ago (see Fig. 2.25), indicating that the treatment was effective. By the time of discharge on November 28, the patient had no discomfort, such as fever or lower back pain, and there was no percussion pain in the left kidney area during physical examination. The blood routine and liver and kidney functions were basically normal during the follow-up. At present, the patient's condition is stable, and she is continuing the HREZ standard quadruple regimen antituberculosis treatment.

2.15.4 Comments

Adrenal tuberculosis is rarely seen clinically, and most patients may first seek treatment in the urology department due to the discovery of an adrenal mass. In case reports, the onset of the disease is insidious, and there are usually no clinical symptoms in the early stage. For some patients, this is accompanied by fever, fatigue, night sweats, cough, and other systemic symptoms of tuberculosis, while some patients may not have fever. Chest imaging may not show old or active pulmonary tuberculosis, there may be no pulmonary nodules, and sputum culture and other tests are mostly negative. CT scans of the adrenal glands typically show bilateral adrenal enlargement with peripheral ring enhancement and central necrosis, with or without calcification. MRI images show hypointensity or isointensity at T1 and hyperintensity at T2. Ultrasound examination may indicate mixed echogenicity or hypoechogenicity in lesions. PET-CT examination can detect an abnormal increase in glucose metabolism in the adrenal mass, which can be misdiagnosed as a metastatic tumor. Other nonspecific indicators include increased erythrocyte sedimentation rate, C-reactive protein, and specific positive T-SPOT.TB test. In the end, the definite diagnosis is made by pathological and etiological detection after mass puncture or resection.

The patient was a young woman of childbearing age with a chronic course of disease. The main clinical features of the patient were two: first was the long-term, recurrent afternoon low-grade fever, for which ordinary anti-infective treatment was ineffective; second was the presence of multiple mass lesions in multiple locations, mainly involving bilateral adrenal glands and intracranial lesions. The auxiliary examination showed that the index of inflammation was increased, and there was mild anemia. On imaging, in addition to multiple space-occupying lesions, there was also retroperitoneal lymph node swelling, not excluding the possibility of metastatic tumors.

If monism is used to explain the etiology of fever with occupying space, we first consider two directions: tumor invasion or low-virulence pathogen infection. Therefore, while we began to refind the patients' previous adrenal puncture pathological films to send to the relevant authorities for reading consultation, we mobilized the patient to find experienced experts for adrenal focus puncture biopsy again and finally obtained the pathological and etiological basis of tuberculosis. In the case that the diagnosis is correct, but the targeted treatment is ineffective, the clinician should not only keep calm and "let the bullet fly a little longer" but also make full use of professional advantages to do enough work on the treatment details, such as adjusting the anti-infective treatment plan based on the evidence and timely and actively puncture and drainage for abscess lesions. The key to the diagnosis of this case was the overall view of the infectious diseases specialist in the diagnosis and analysis and the unremitting pursuit of the etiological results.

References

1. Chinese Antituberculosis Association. Guidelines for the chemotherapy of drug-resistant tuberculosis. Chin J Antituberculosis. 2015;37(5):421–69.
2. Tuberculosis Branch of the Chinese Medical Association. 2012 Expert consensus on the diagnosis and treatment of nontuberculous mycobacteria disease. Chin J Tuberc Respir Dis. 2012;35(8):572–80.
3. Zhang Daoxin, Wang Wenying, Zhang Lujia, et al. Diagnosis and treatment of adrenal tuberculosis. Int J Surg. 2016;43(6):405–7.
4. Upadhyay J, Sudhindra P, Abraham G, et al. Tuberculosis of the adrenal gland: a case report and review of the literature of infections of theadrenal gland. Int J Endocrinol. 2014,2014:876037.
5. Denny N, Raghunath S, Bhatia P, et al. Rifampicin-induced adrenal crisis in a patient with tuberculosis: a therapeutic challenge. BMJ Case Rep. 2016,2016. pii: bcr2016216302.
6. Kumar R, Dey P. Fine-needle aspiration cytology of non-neoplastic adrenal pathology. Diagn Cytopathol. 2016,44(6):472–6.

2.16 Disseminated *Nocardia* Infection Following Treatment for Membranous Nephropathy

Wang Xuan, Wang Xinyu, and Jiang Weimin

A 57-year-old man was admitted to our hospital due to "membranous nephropathy for 11 months, fever accompanied by headache for more than 2 months" on April 1, 2017.

In May 2016, the patient underwent examinations, which showed the following results: 24-hour urinary protein: 5.09 g; serum albumin: 23 g/L; serum cholesterol: 7.87 mmol/L in Huashan Hospital due to edema of lower limbs and eyelid for half a year. On May 10, a kidney puncture biopsy was performed, and the pathology showed membranous nephropathy. Lipid-lowering, hypotensive, and diuretic treatments were given. Due to no significant remission of the disease, Cyclophosphamide (CTX) 0.8 g pulse therapy was given from December 6, together with oral prednisone 60 mg qd. After that, the patient received CTX 0.8 g pulse therapy again on January 7 and February 7, 2017, respectively, with a cumulative dose of 2.4 g CTX.

On the second day after the third CTX pulse treatment (February 8, 2017), the patient developed fever, chills, headache, and poor appetite. Antimicrobial agents, including piperacillin, ceftazidime, azithromycin, and ampicillin, were given successively in another hospital, but the symptoms had no obvious improvement two weeks later. Therefore, the patient was admitted to the Department of Nephrology of our hospital again on February 22. Laboratory examinations showed that blood WBC was 13.62×10^9/L, N% was 90.9%, CRP was 75.6 mg/L, PCT was 0.39 ng/mL, serum creatinine was 131umol/L, and albumin was 24.5 g/L; urinalysis showed 3+ protein, and chest CT suggested (February 22) "increased bilateral lung markings, multiple nodules, mild mediastinal lymphatic enlargement with calcification and thickening of the pericardium" (Fig. 2.30). Meropenem, moxifloxacin, ganciclovir, caspofungin, and compound sulfamethoxazole were given, and methylprednisolone 20 mg q12h IVGTT was also administered.

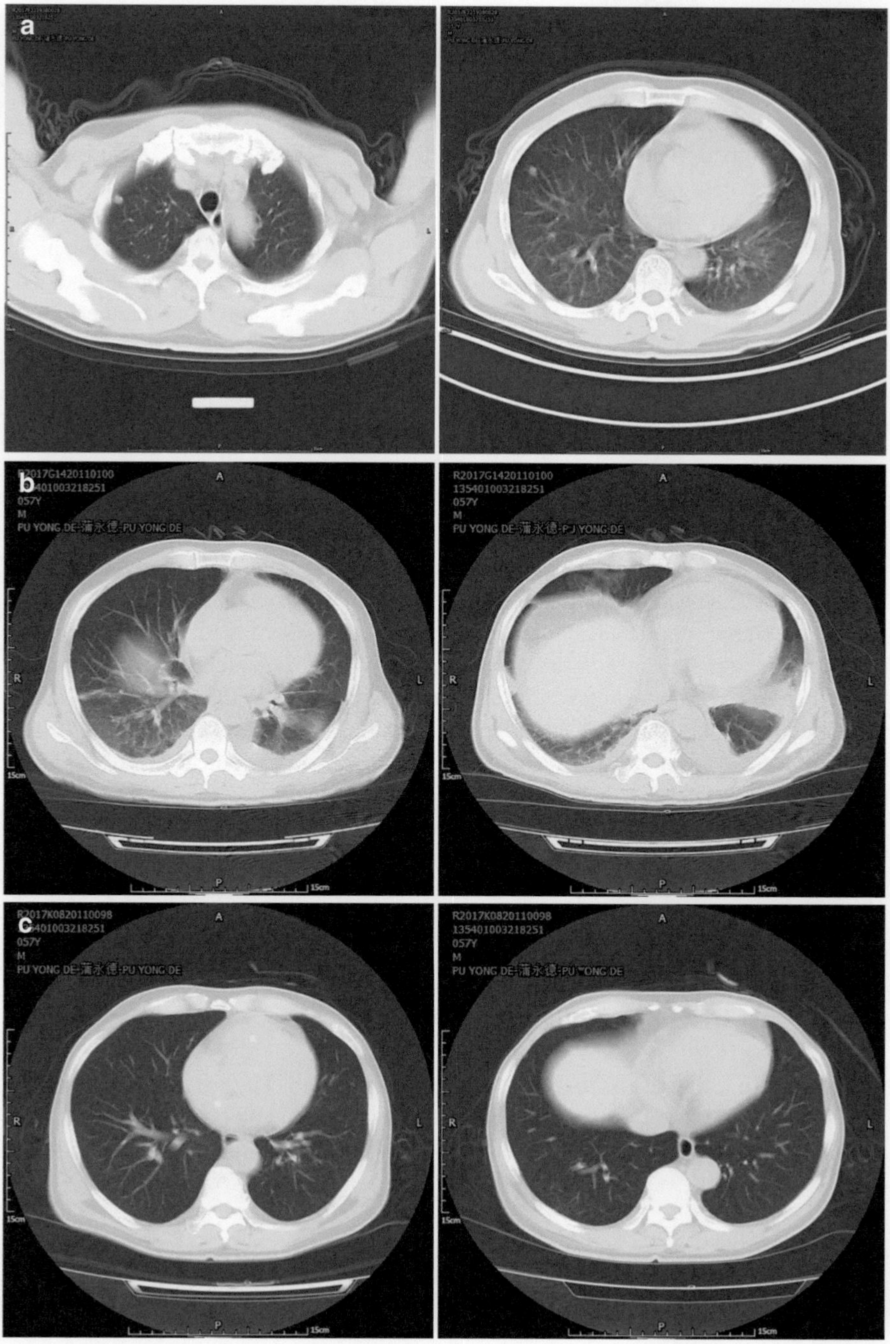

Fig. 2.30 Lung CT follow-up: (**a**) February 22, (**b**) March 14, and (**c**) May 8

On February 28, bronchoalveolar lavage was performed, and fungal spores and gram-positive cocci were identified in his lavage fluid. Compound sulfamethoxazole and caspofungin were discontinued, linezolid 600 mg q12h IVGTT as well as voriconazole 200 mg q12h IVGTT were added, meropenem was added to 1.0 q12h IVGTT, and the glucocorticoid was reduced to prednisone 15 mg qd po on March 1. The peak body temperature dropped and returned to normal on March 3. Thereafter, the dose of prednisone was gradually reduced, and the use of ganciclovir, meropenem, linezolid (due to the presence of pancytopenia), and moxifloxacin was gradually discontinued. The reexamination of the lung CT on March 14 showed no significant change compared with before (Fig. 2.30). The recheck results of CRP and PCT were not elevated. Monotherapy with voriconazole was used from March 17. However, after that, the peak body temperature increased slightly, with the highest axillary temperature of 37.2 °C, and no obvious discomfort was presented. The CRP and PCT were monitored and did not increase significantly, and the peripheral blood cell count gradually increased.

On March 20, the patient developed fever and headache again after taking a bath. Peripheral blood cell count showed that WBC was 3.9×10^9/L and N% was 57.4%. The peak body temperature gradually increased to 39.2 °C, accompanied by severe headache, while the meningeal irritation sign was negative. A reexamination of the chest CT showed obvious absorption of the lesion compared with before. Voriconazole was discontinued due to elevated aminotransferase, and hepatoprotective therapy was given. The patient's liver function gradually improved, but the fever and headache remained unchanged. On March 30, the head MRI plain scan showed "punctate abnormal signals in bilateral frontal lobes, with high DWI signal, not excluding the new infarction." On March 31, a lumbar puncture was performed, and the pressure was normal; the CSF test showed that WBC was 490×10^6/L, mononuclear cells were 70%, glucose was 3.15 mmol/L, protein was 0.44 g/L, and chloride was 116 mmol/L. Bacteria, fungi, and tuberculosis smears were negative. On the morning of April 1, the patient's temperature was 38 °C, and he still had a severe headache. He was admitted to our department for further diagnosis and treatment. Since the disease started, the patient had been in poor spirits and had a poor appetite, unremarkable sleep, less urine volume, foam urine, and dry stool than before. No significant weight loss was reported.

2.16.1 Past History and Personal History

The history of tuberculosis and close contact was denied. The patient had hypertension for more than one year. At the time of admission, his blood pressure was controlled by oral administration of valsartan, furosemide, and spironolactone, and the blood pressure was 95/62 mmHg on admission. He denied having any heart or respiratory problems or diabetes.

2.16.2 Physical Examination

The patient was clear of mind, had medium nutrition, was cooperative with physical examination, had scattered brown pigmentation on the face, and no rash was seen. The superficial lymph nodes were not palpable for swelling. The neck was soft and without resistance. The breathing sound of both lungs was clear, no rales were heard, the heart rate was regular, and no murmur was found. The abdomen was soft. There was no tenderness or rebound pain in the whole abdomen. There was no swelling of the liver and spleen under the ribs, no percussion pain in the bilateral kidney area, and no edema in both lower extremities. The neuropathological signs were negative.

2.16.3 Diagnosis and Treatment After Admission

The patient had obvious symptoms of headache and fever after admission on April 1, 2017. Meropenem 2.0 q8h IVGTT for antimicrobial treatment and 20% mannitol 250ml q8h IVGTT to reduce the intracranial pressure were administered, and prednisone 10 mg tid po was continued. At the same time, we actively carried out relevant examinations. The patient's blood T-SPOT.TB test returned positive results (well A >20; well B >20). Considering that the diagnosis of tuberculous meningitis could not be excluded, meropenem was discontinued, and five diagnostic antituberculosis therapies were initiated on April 7: isoniazid 0.6 qd IVGTT, rifampicin 0.45 qd IVGTT, pyrazinamide 0.5 tid po, ethambutol 0.75 qd po, and levofloxacin 0.5 qd IVGTT. At the same time, the glucocorticoid was gradually reduced to prednisone 10 mg qd po. During the treatment, the patient's temperature was still fluctuating. On April 14, prednisone was added to 10 mg bid po, and then his headache and fever were significantly improved.

Lumbar puncture was performed again on April 19, and the intracranial pressure was 260 mmH2O; the CSF test showed that WBC was 360 × 10^6/L, mononuclear cells were 100%, protein was 0.51 g/L, glucose was 2.53 mmol/L (synchronous blood glucose was 6.86 mmol/L), and chloride was 121 mmol/L; and no obvious abnormality was found in the etiological examination. Prednisone was reduced to 5 mg bid po on April 24. On May 4, the CSF test of lumbar puncture was further improved, WBC decreased to 50 × 10^6/L, protein decreased to 0.27 g/L, glucose decreased to 2.19 mmol/L (synchronous blood glucose was 7.84 mmol/L), and chloride decreased to 118 mmol/L. Routine urine examination during this period indicated the presence of urinary tract infection, and a clean middle urine culture indicated the *Nocardia* genus, which was further identified by molecular

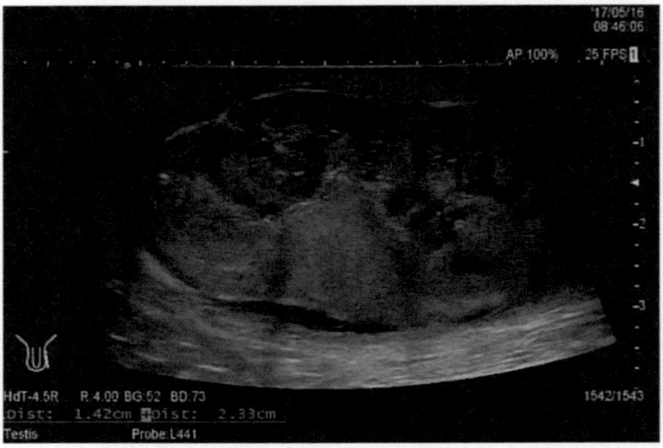

Fig. 2.31 Ultrasonography of the epididymis

identification as *Nocardia terpenica* species. The patient complained of swelling and pain in the testis, and fever occurred again, with body temperature fluctuating between 37.5 and 38.4 °C. An ultrasound of the reproductive system performed on May 2 suggested left epididymitis (Fig. 2.31). On May 11, a clean middle urine culture still indicated the *Nocardia* genus.

On May 11, 2017, rifampicin, isoniazid, pyrazinamide, and ethambutol were discontinued, and compound sulfamethoxazole 2# tid po, ceftriaxone 2.0 q12h IVGTT, and levofloxacin 0.5qd IVGTT were administered. The patient's body temperature gradually dropped to normal, swelling and pain in the testis improved, and no other new symptoms appeared. The reexamination of lumbar puncture on May 18 showed that the intracranial pressure had decreased to 70 mmH2O, WBC of CSF was reduced to 27×10^6/L, protein was 0.25 g/L, glucose was 2.66 mmol/L (synchronous blood glucose was 5.98 mmol/L), chloride was 120 mmol/L, and cerebrospinal fluid etiology was negative. On May 18 and later, the clean middle urine culture remained negative.

We further conducted a drug sensitivity test on the cultured Nocardia species. According to the drug sensitivity results (Fig. 2.32) (susceptible to amikacin, gentamicin, and linezolid; intermediate to ceftriaxone, ciprofloxacin, and sulfamethoxazole; and resistant to ampicillin and ampicillin sulbactam), the anti-infective agents were changed to ceftriaxone 2.0 q12h IVGTT, levofloxacin 0.5 qd IVGTT, and amikacin 400,000 U qd IVGTT on May 24. The patient had a normal temperature and was discharged to the local hospital to continue the anti-infective regimen. Later, the patient's testis gradually enlarged, accompanied by pain and fluctuating feeling. He received a puncture and drainage in another hospital on June 9 and returned to our hospital for reexamination on July 14 and October 16, respectively. No obvious abnormality was found in either lumbar puncture. The pain and swelling in the testis subsided 1 month after puncture and drainage, and the ulcer healed. After discharge on October 20, the anti-infective regimen was changed to levofloxacin 0.5 qd po, compound sulfamethoxazole 2 # bid po, and cefixime 100 mg bid po.

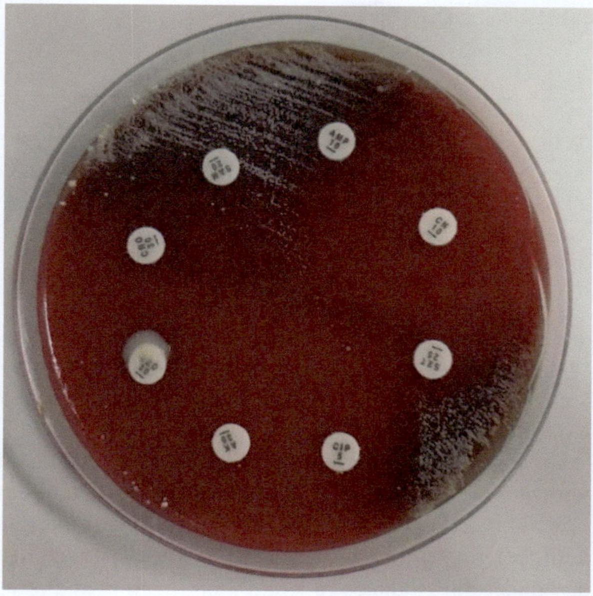

Fig. 2.32 Drug sensitivity test (disc diffusion method). (Note: In clockwise direction, abbreviations stand for the following: *AMP* ampicillin, *CN* gentamicin, *SXT* compound sulfamethoxazole, *CIP* ciprofloxacin, *AK* amikacin, *LZD* linezolid, *CRO* ceftriaxone, *SAM* ampicillin sulbactam)

2.16.4 Comments

Nocardiosis is an uncommon gram-positive bacterial infection caused by aerobic actinomycetes of the genus *Nocardia*. Some species of the genus *Nocardia* could cause local or systemic suppurative diseases in humans and animals. Nocardiosis is often treated as an opportunistic infection, but about one-third of those infected are immunocompetent. Nocardiosis is characterized by its ability to disseminate to almost any organ (especially the central nervous system) and by its tendency to relapse or progress despite appropriate treatment. It should be noted that *Nocardia* is a large genus of aerobic actinomycetes, and there is significant heterogeneity among different species in this genus. Different patterns of antimicrobial susceptibility can be found among these species. For instance, diverse characteristics can be seen among *Nocardia brasiliensis*, *Nocardia otitidiscaviarum*, and *Nocardia transvalensis*, which were once thought to be very homogeneous species. Because of these, sulfonamide should not always be the first choice of treatment for nocardiosis caused by any species. Second, because of the variable antimicrobial susceptibility patterns, identification of species level and drug sensitivity test should be applied to all the isolated strains, which is of great significance for efficacy.

This patient had a membranous nephropathy case with pulmonary, central nervous system, and genitourinary system infections after high-dose glucocorticoid and CTX pulse therapy. Considering the positive results of T-SPOT.TB and the control of the disease by antituberculosis treatment, it was easy for clinicians to make the diagnosis of pulmonary tuberculosis concurrent with tuberculous meningitis. However, the evidence for the diagnosis of tuberculosis infection was not sufficient

Table 2.4 Lumbar puncture follow-up

Date	March 31, 2017	April 19, 2017	May 4, 2017	May 18, 2017	July 14, 2017	October 16, 2017
Pressure	/	260	/	70	120	135
WBC	490	360	50	27	8	5
Mononuclear cells	70%	100%	98%	100%		
Glucose	3.15	2.53	2.19	2.66	2.5	3.1
Synchronous blood glucose	/	6.86	7.84	5.98	5.5	5.2
Protein	0.44	0.51	0.27	0.25	0.51	0.38
Chloride	116	121	118	120	121	123

since T-SPOT.TB positivity can indicate prior or latent infection but cannot be used to confirm current infection.

In consideration of repeated positive clean middle urine culture twice, together with symptoms and signs of genitourinary system infection, disseminated *Nocardia* infection can, in the monistic view, explain all these presentations. Therefore, the antituberculosis therapy was discontinued. The application of anti-*Nocardia* therapy under the guidance of strain identification and drug sensitivity test was the key to the cure of this case. Finally, it should be emphasized again that in the case of disseminated nocardiosis, especially with central nervous system involvement, a combination therapy and intravenous administration is required, and the course of treatment should be individualized based on the patient's immune status (Table 2.4).

Acknowledgments
We thank Dr. Yu Xu from the Clinical Laboratory of Huashan Hospital North and Dr. Yaojie Shen from the Department of Infectious Diseases for their hard work in the isolation and identification of strains and in vitro drug sensitivity test.

References

1. Brown-Elliott BA, Brown JM, Conville PS, et al. Clinical and laboratory features of the Nocardia spp. based on current molecular taxonomy. Clin Microbiol Rev. 2006;19(2):259–82.
2. Peleg AY, Husain S, Qureshi ZA, et al. Risk factors, clinical characteristics, and outcome of Nocardia infection in organ transplant recipients: a matched case-control study. Clin Infect Dis. 2007;44(10):1307–14.
3. Pintado V, Gómez-Mampaso E, Cobo J, et al. Nocardial infection in patients infected with the human immunodeficiency virus. Clin Microbiol Infect. 2003;9(7):716–20.
4. Lederman ER, Crum NF. A case series and focused review of nocardiosis: clinical and microbiologic aspects. Medicine (Baltimore). 2004;83(5):300–13.
5. Uhde KB, Pathak S, McCullum I Jr, et al. Antimicrobial-resistant nocardia isolates, United States, 1995–2004. Clin Infect Dis. 2010;51(12):1445–8.

2.17 A Case of Coccidioidomycosis Easily Misdiagnosed as Miliary Tuberculosis

Hu Yuekai, Li Yuxin, Wang Chao, and Chen Mingquan

A previously healthy 28-year-old male seafarer presented to our hospital with a two-month history of rash and cough and one month of fever.

The patient's manifestation began with systemic erythema multiforme (Fig. 2.33) during navigation on October 23, 2017. The erythema was not pruritic; triamcinolone acetonide ointment and antihistamine could relieve it. Ten days later, he developed a paroxysmal cough with a small amount of white sputum. In the middle of November, he developed a fever of 39 °C. The blood routine showed the following: WBC: 18.6×10^9/L and N% 78.9%. The patient received anti-allergic drugs and cephalosporin for presumed urticaria. A few days later, the rash substantially resolved, with some pigmentation left. However, the respiratory symptoms remained, accompanied by fatigue and night sweats. The chest CT on November 30 exhibited bilateral miliary nodules, consolidations in the right lower lobe, and

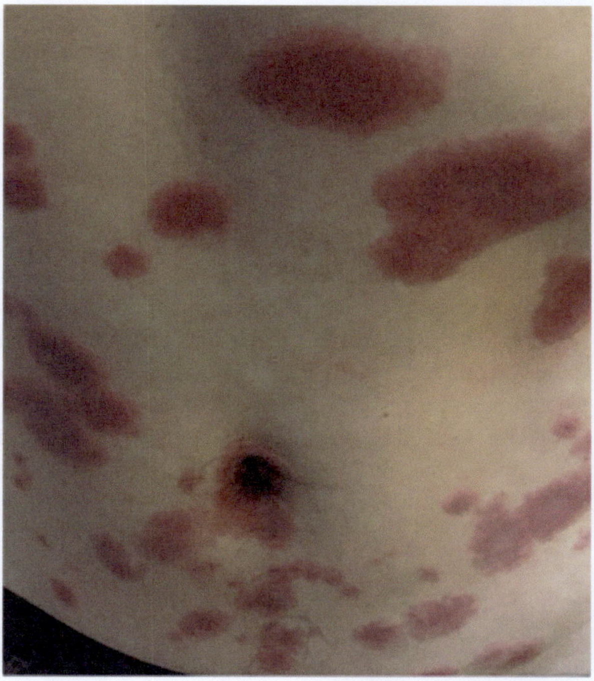

Fig. 2.33 Systemic erythema multiforme on October 23, 2017

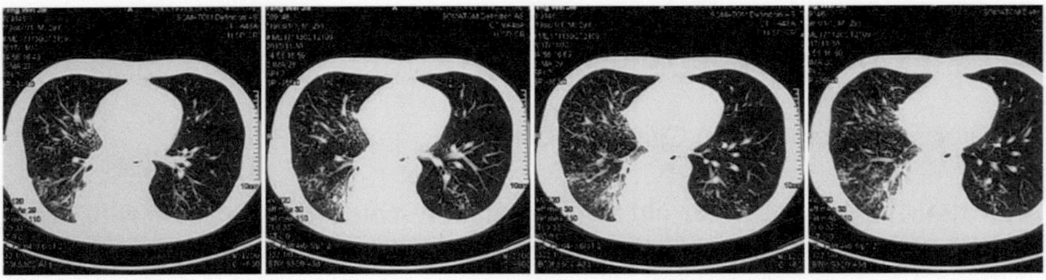

Fig. 2.34 Chest CT on November 30

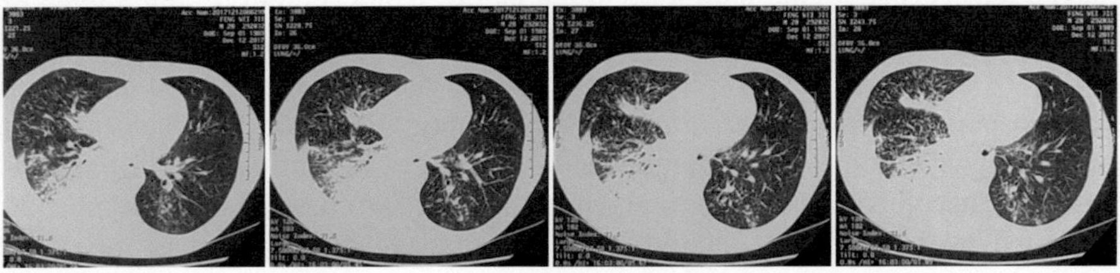

Fig. 2.35 Chest CT on December 12

multiple lymphadenectasis around the right hilum, mediastinum, right supraclavicular fossa, and right diaphragmatic crus, along with right pleural effusion (Fig. 2.34). Ultrasound imaging also showed pleural effusion and multiple lymphadenectases. Another blood routine showed elevated levels of WBC and neutrophils. The patient underwent antibiotic therapy of moxifloxacin and meropenem. G test was 551.8 pg/ml. GM test and ANA were negative. T-SOPT.TB was positive.

On December 8, the right clavicular lymph node biopsy revealed granulomatous inflammation and necrosis. SMZco and voriconazole were added to treat potential fungal infection. However, the bronchoalveolar lavage fluid (BALF) did not exhibit acid-fast bacilli under the microscope. Parasitic infection was also suspected, but the specific antibody could not be confirmed. The culture of bacteria and fungi also yielded negative results. Both the GM test and the anti-fast bacilli nucleic acid test for BALF were negative. Chest CT reexamination on December 12 demonstrated atelectasis in the right lower lobe, multiple lymphadenectasis in the mediastinum, and a small amount of pericardial effusion (Fig. 2.35). The consolidation in the right lower lobe was considered an infectious change and the bilateral miliary nodules an outcome of tuberculosis.

On December 14, the patient was transferred to the tuberculosis specialty. The diagnostic antituberculosis therapy consisted of isoniazid, rifampicin, ethambutol, and pyrazinamide. Piperacillin and tazobactam were also initiated for presumed bacterial infection. Without apparent improvement, the patient was transferred to another hospital. The laboratory analysis showed that WBC was 16.78×10^9/L, N% was 73.8%, ESR was 68 mm/h, and G test was 53.4 pg/mL. Antituberculosis antibody was negative. Blood and sputum cultures were negative. Thoracentesis and drainage tube placement were performed. Pleural biochemical analysis showed the following: chlorine: 102.9 mmol/L, glucose: 5.88 mmol/L, and total protein:

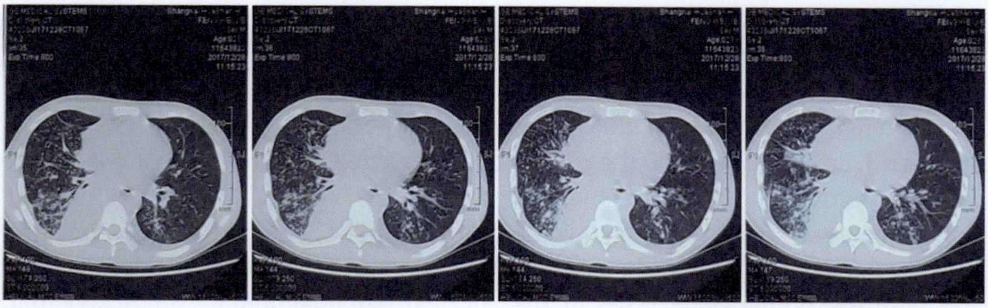

Fig. 2.36 Chest CT scan on December 28, 2017

40 g/L. The pleural histopathology did not report malignant cells. The blood T cell immune response to *M. tuberculosis* was negative, interferon-γ release assay was 0, lymphocyte culture + interferon (baseline N) was 0.08, lymphocyte culture + interferon (stimulating level T) was 0.079, and blood sample smear for tuberculosis was also negative.

The chest CT on December 28 demonstrated consolidation and atelectasis in the right lower lobe, bilateral miliary nodules, multiple lymphadenectasis and fusions in the neck and mediastinum, partial constriction of the superior vena cava, and right pleural effusion, which compressed the left lobe (Fig. 2.36). The patient's body temperature still fluctuated between 38 °C and 39 °C. He was then admitted to our hospital.

The patient was listless and anorexic. Since the onset of symptoms, he had lost about 5 kilograms.

2.17.1 Physical Examination

T 37.6 °C, P 100 bpm, R 20/min, BP 107/73 mmHg, height 170 cm, and weight 50 kg. A chest tube was placed in the right thorax. Multiple hard, swollen lymph nodes with fusions and poor mobility were palpable in the left supraclavicular fossa and right cervix. The lymph nodes had formed adhesions to the surrounding tissues. A decreased breath sound in the right lower lobe was found on auscultation. No significant dry or moist rales were auscultated in either lung.

2.17.2 Diagnosis and Treatment After Admission

On admission, the blood routine revealed the following: WBC: 20.52 × 10^9/L, N%: 84.4%, L%: 8.7%, eosinophils: 1.7%, subtypes of lymphocytes: 5.51% (total), CD3+: 72%, CD4+: 26.33%, CD8+: 36.33%, NK+: 20.44%, CD19+: 5.89%, and CD4/CD8: 0.72. T-SPOT.TB test was negative. G test showed 166.8 pg/ml. The biochemical analysis of hydrothorax showed pale yellow and blurred pleural fluid, RBC was 610 × 10^6/L, karyocytes were 1600 × 10^6/L, N% was 25%, L was 70%, mesothelial cells were 5%, and protein was 34 g/L. The hydrothorax smear and culture were both negative. The repeated Xpert MTB/RIF Ultra tests reported

TRACE. The ultrasound imaging revealed several swollen lymph nodes, partially fused in the cervix and supraclavicular fossa, where the largest was 32 mm in diameter. The antituberculosis therapy continued, and rifampicin was substituted to avoid drug fever (isoniazid 0.3 qd, ethambutol 0.75 qd, pyrazinamide 1.5 qd, moxifloxacin 0.4 qd, and linezolid 600 mg q12h). However, the cough and body temperature did not improve.

On January 6, 2018, the patient went through a PET-CT (Fig. 2.37). The imaging indicated consolidations in the right lower lobe, bilateral miliary patchy nodules, and multiple lymphadenectases in the cervical, submandibular, supraclavicular, axillary, mediastinal, hilar, and inguinal areas, with increased FDG uptake. Taking the medical history into consideration, it suggested malignancy, which required pathological confirmation.

From the clinical perspective, lymphoma seemed reasonable for the extensively swollen lymph nodes and nodules in the lungs. Just when it seemed that only lymphoma was a suitable diagnosis, the patient told us the specific sailing route of his cargo ship: It broke down in Los Angeles on September 30, arrived in Los Angeles on October 6 to unload, left on October 13, docked in Stockton on October 15, departed for Vancouver on October 20, broke down in Vancouver on October 24,

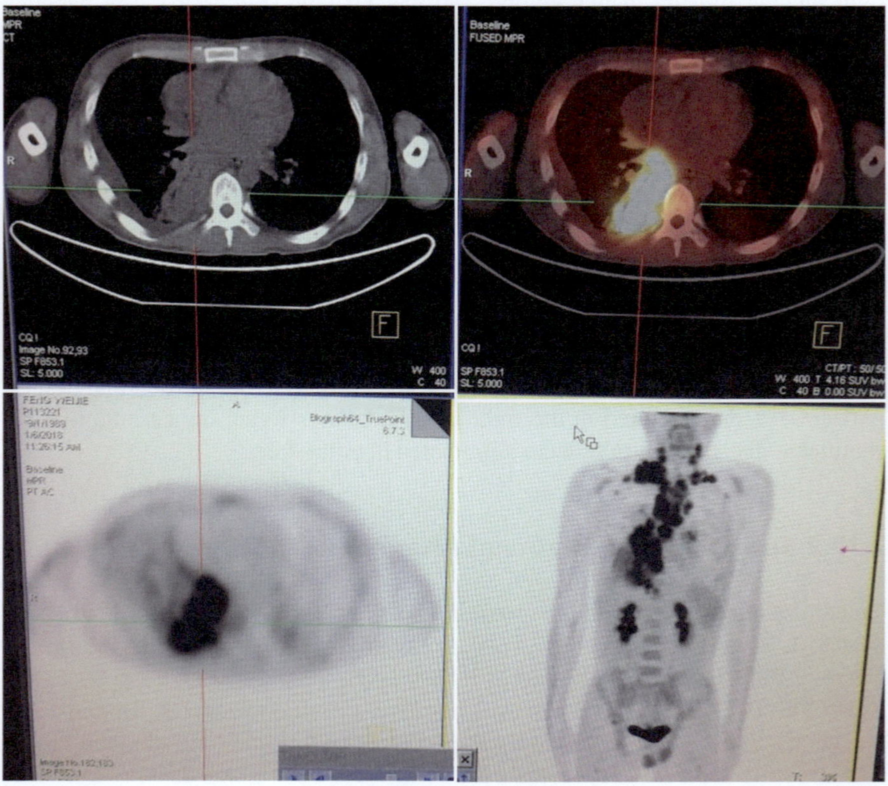

Fig. 2.37 PET-CT showed consolidation of the lower right lung and abnormal imaging of systemic lymph nodes

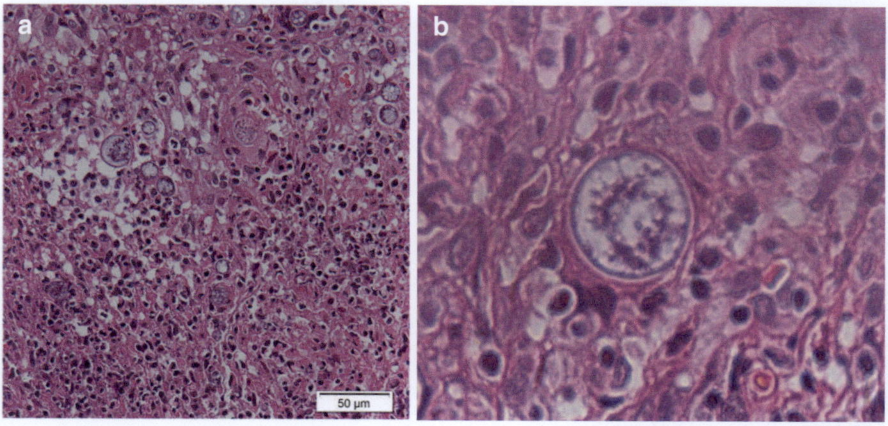

Fig. 2.38 Lymph node biopsy found *Coccidioides immitis* spores with thickened walls. (**a**) Low-power field. (**b**) Spore in the high-power field

docked on October 26, departed Vancouver on October 29, arrived in Japan on November 16, and reached Tokyo Bay on November 19. We identified an important clue: 1–2 weeks prior to the rash onset, the patient had traveled through an area potentially linked to the rash's etiology—specifically California, located on the west coast of the United States.

The possibility of coccidioidomycosis was then considered, considering his travel history and the features of chest CT. One week of intravenous itraconazole treatment successfully controlled the body temperature and respiratory symptoms. Further investigation of the lymph node biopsy found spores with thickened walls (Fig. 2.38). The culture and identification of *Coccidioides immitis* required a BSL-3 laboratory facility, which was not available in our institute. We thus collected specimens from peripheral blood, hydrothorax, lymph nodes, and the fluid in the skin blisters for next-generation sequencing. Finally, sequences compatible with *Coccidioides immitis* were obtained from the newly occurred blister in the chest.

The diagnosis of disseminated coccidioidomycosis was established with the skin, lymph nodes, and pulmonary involvement. Considering guidelines and personal economic factors, the antifungal therapy was adjusted to fluconazole 400 mg q12h iv. But the patient's body temperature rose again, and the cough became intense on the second day of adjustment, so itraconazole was administered. With the alternative administration of itraconazole oral solutions and injections, the body temperature dropped, and the respiratory symptoms were apparently relieved (Fig. 2.39, and Table 2.5).

After treatment, we checked the T cell subtype and immunoglobulin level: TBNK: CD3+: 86%, CD4+: 41%, CD8+: 39%, CD19+: 5%, NK: 9%, IgG: 20.7 g/L, IgA: 2.5 g/L, and IgM: 0.49 g/L. The normal CD4+ T cell count after treatment suggested that the immunocompromised status on admission was related to *Coccidioides immitis* infection.

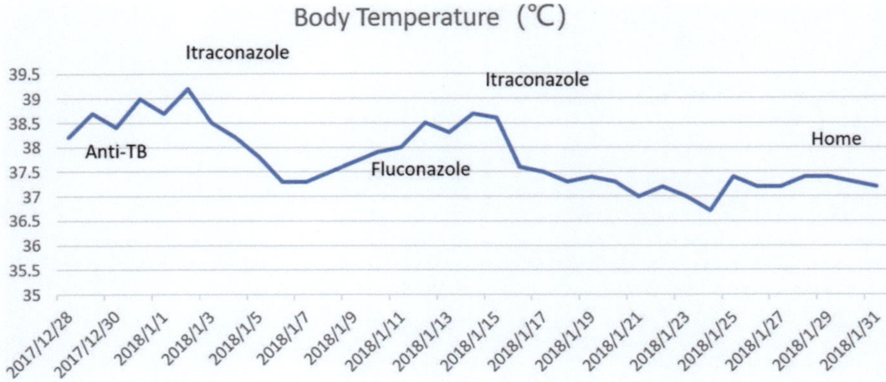

Fig. 2.39 Figure of body temperature

Table 2.5 Erythrocyte sedimentation rate (ESR) and C-reactive protein gradually returned to normal levels

	December 29, 2017	February 9, 2018	February 19, 2018	March 6, 2018
ESR (mm/h)	62	36	25	15
CRP (mg/L)	127	33.9	15	7.9

2.17.3 Comments

Disseminated disease is the worst form of coccidioidomycosis that occurs in less than 1% of cases (the rate can reach up to 11% in hospitalized patients). The classic pulmonary manifestation includes miliary nodules caused by hematogenous dissemination. The primary consolidation occurs occasionally, usually along with lymphadenectasis around the hilum and mediastinum. AIDS and immunosuppressed patients are susceptible to acute respiratory distress syndrome (ARDS), which is a rare complication. Although antifungal plus supportive treatment is utilized, the mortality rate remains high, approaching 100% in those patients. Immunocompetent individuals and patients with other comorbidities, including diabetes and renal failure, can also develop ARDS, with a morbidity rate of 40%–60%. The most common sites of extrapulmonary dissemination include the skin, lymph nodes, skeletal system, and central nervous system. Vertebral disease can extend to adjacent soft tissues, leading to paravertebral abscess or lumbar psoas abscess. Despite the correct diagnosis and antibiotic therapy, the mortality rate of homogeneous dissemination is 28%–56%.

The clinical manifestation of disseminated coccidioidomycosis can be confusing. The pulmonary miliary nodules resemble tuberculosis, and the significantly enlarged lymph nodes can lead to the consideration of lymphoma. However, the patient's identity as a seafarer and the navigation route provided the epidemiologic history, which is essential for an experienced mycologist. When the etiological culture was not available due to exposure risks, the molecular diagnostics helped provide solid evidence for a confirmed diagnosis and the following treatment.

References

1. Liang G, Shen Y, Lv G, Zheng H, Mei H, Zheng X, Kong X, Blechert O, Li D, Liu W. Coccidioidomycosis: Imported and possible domestic cases in China: a case report and review, 1958–2017. Mycoses. 2018; 1–8.
2. Jude CM, Nayak NB, Patel MK, Monica Deshmukh, Poonam Batra. Pulmonary Coccidioidomycosis: pictorial review of chest radiographic and CT findings. RadioGraphics. 2014;34:912–25.
3. Wang XL, Wang S, An CL. Mini-review of published reports on Coccidioidomycosis in China. Mycopathologia. 2015;180:299–303.

2.18 Repeated Hyperpyretic Splenomegaly, Bone Marrow Culture of Drug-Resistant *Staphylococcus epidermidis*, and the Final Diagnosis Was Visceral Leishmaniasis

Wang Ting, Jia Wen, Shao Lingyun, and Zhang Wenhong

The patient was a 38-year-old woman, a farmer, admitted to the hospital on April 20, 2017, due to "intermittent fever for more than half a year."

Since September 2016, the patient had developed chills and high fever without any obvious inducement, with a peak value of 41 °C, and the fever continued during the day and night. After taking ibuprofen or other oral antipyretic drugs, the body temperature would briefly drop to normal, accompanied by heavy sweating. But the fever returned a few hours later, and there was no cough, rash, joint pain, or discomfort. The patient visited the local hospital, and blood examination showed a total leukocyte count of 5.49 × 10^9/L, with the proportion of neutrophils being 68.1%, hemoglobin (Hb) being 125 g/L, platelet count (PLT) being 136 × 10^9/L; C-reactive protein being 101 mg/L, erythrocyte sedimentation rate (ESR) being 70 mm/h, procalcitonin (PCT) being 0.54 ng/ml, and abdominal B-ultrasound–indicated splenomegaly (51 × 174 mm). Bone marrow smear showed active granule proliferation. Since two bone marrow cultures suggested that the skin of methicillin-resistant *Staphylococcus* was positive, the local hospital considered the diagnosis of sepsis and gave anti-infective therapy with ceftazidime+tazobactam, vancomycin, meropenem, and datoromycin, successively. But the effect was not good, and the patient still relied on oral antipyretic analgesic agents during the occurrence of red blood cell and white blood cell line decline (leukocytes: 2.67 × 10^9/L, N: 53.2%, Hb: 97 g/L, and PLT: 143 × 10^9/L). After more than 1 month in the hospital, the patient's temperature gradually decreased to normal, and she was discharged. One month after discharge, in December 2016, the patient developed chills and high fever again, and the characteristics, peak value, and subjective feelings of fever were the same as the previous one. The patient was admitted to the local hospital again, and blood routine was rechecked: WBC: 3.11 × 10^9/L, N: 65%, Hb: 96 g/L, PLT: 117 × 10^9/L, ESR: 82 mm/h, and antinuclear antibodies (ANA) was positive (with a titer of 1:320). Reexamination of bone puncture indicated active hyperplasia of granular lines, and bone marrow culture was again positive for methicillin-resistant

Staphylococcus epidermidis. PET-CT examination indicated spleen enlargement, increased glucose metabolism in the whole bone marrow (SUV 3.6), and increased glucose metabolism in the colon and intestinal wall (SUV 5.8). Sepsis was still considered in the local hospital, and the body temperature dropped to normal after anti-infective treatment with linezolid was given. However, one week before admission in the middle of April 2017, the patient developed chills and fever again, with the same nature as the previous ones. In order to seek further diagnosis and treatment, the patient was admitted to our department. The patient had no special history.

2.18.1 Physical Examination at Admission

Vital signs: Temperature (T) 38.7 °C (axillary, default if unstated); General condition: Clear consciousness, flushed cheeks, no specific rash; Respiratory system: Bilateral lung breath sounds clear; Circulatory system: Regular heart rhythm, no pathological murmurs auscultated; Abdomen: Flat and soft, no tenderness or rebound tenderness. Spleen palpable 5 finger-breadths below the left costal margin (≈7–10 cm), firm texture, mild discomfort on palpation. Liver palpable at the costal margin (0 cm below costal margin). No percussion pain over the liver or costal regions; mobile dullness negative; Extremities: No joint swelling, no lower extremity edema.

2.18.2 Laboratory and Auxiliary Examinations

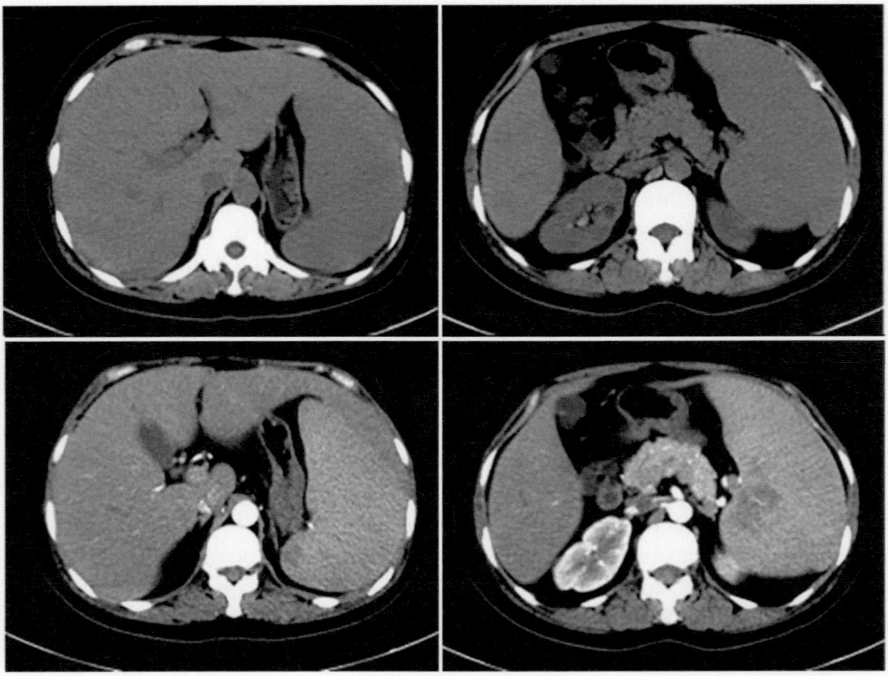

Fig. 2.40 Contrast-enhanced CT images of the patient's upper abdomen. The spleen was visibly enlarged

2.18.3 Diagnosis and Treatment

After admission, blood routine examination was done, which revealed the following: WBC: 2.96 × 10^9/L, NEUT: 67.0%, LYMPH: 28.0%, N: 1.98 × 10^9/L, RBC: 3.67 × 10^{12}/L, HGB: 89 g/L, and PLT: 117 × 10^9/L; CRP: 135 mg/L, ESR: 130 mm/h, SF: 649.2μg/L, and LDH: 491 U/L; hepatorenal function: albumin: 30 g/L, globulin: 62 g/L, and remaining within the normal range; IgG: 46.90 G/L and IgM: 3.44 G/L; and autoantibodies, T-SPOT.TB, *Cryptococcus* sera latex agglutination test, and blood EBV-DNA were negative. Abdominal B-ultrasound showed splenomegaly (209 × 65 mm), and the right kidney calculi, hepatobiliary pancreas, and left kidney were normal. No swelling was observed in the supraclavicular, neck, armpit, submaxilla, groin, and retroperitoneal lymph nodes. Chest CT showed right middle lobe and left lower lung fibrous foci, and CT enhancement of the upper abdomen showed that the spleen was significantly enlarged (Fig. 2.40). Cardiac ultrasound showed mild mitral regurgitation and mild tricuspid regurgitation.

During the patient's body temperature monitoring, a daily high fever of over 39 °C was recorded, with occasional ultra-high fever reaching 40–41 °C. The fever was not self-limiting and required antipyretic analgesics to reduce the temperature. But the body temperature would rise again after 3–6 h of normal temperature; chills were not obvious; often, there was a sudden rise of body temperature (15–30 min up to 40 °C); and there could be two temperature peaks on the same day, as shown in the figure (Fig. 2.41). The fever pattern during this episode matched that of the prior two episodes. After reviewing the fever patterns of all three occurrences, we found

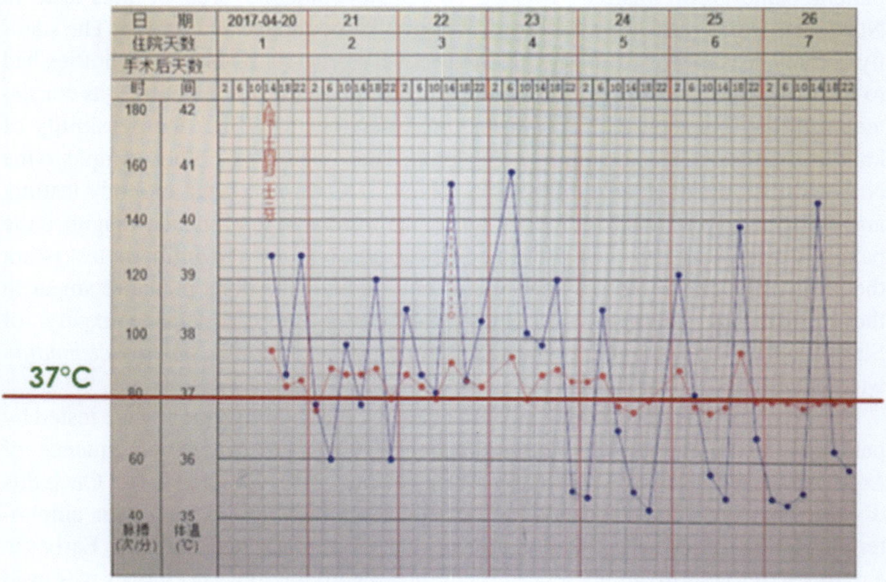

Fig. 2.41 Body temperature of the patient after admission. The patient's peak body temperature reached 40 °C and above, and bimodal fever was observed in some periods

they were largely consistent. This consistency was most likely due to the disease's own inherent features, rather than being a sign of effective anti-infective treatment or a recurrence that developed after stopping the medication. Bone marrow culture results in the local hospital were inconsistent with clinical results, and the possibility of contamination was high. Repeated reexamination of blood culture and bone marrow culture after admission showed no positive results. Therefore, the diagnosis of sepsis could not be considered valid.

In addition to the regularity of fever, another significant clinical feature of the patient was progressive splenomegaly, and the possibility of histoplasmosis and kala-azar had to be taken into account. The results of the bone marrow smear showed that *Histoplasma capsulatum* and *Leishmannia* were not found on the bone marrow smear. A small number of hemophagocytes and atypical lymphocytes were more common, and a small number of juvenile lymphoid cells and their mitotic types were also observed. It was hoped that further clinical examination would eliminate lymphoproliferative diseases. At the same time, there was no abnormality in bone marrow flow, EBV-DNA, or CMV-DNA. All the autoantibodies were negative, and there was no renal involvement, such as proteinuria; no multiserosal effusion; insufficient evidence for connective tissue disease; and no diagnostic evidence for lymphoma or other lymphoproliferative diseases. Based on the clinical features and examination results, we focused on the possibility of infectious diseases. We asked for the history again in detail and got an important clue. One to two months before the onset of the disease (June–July 2016), the patient had engaged in the maintenance of a Chinese prickly ash forest, picking up Chinese prickly ash, living in the mountains for more than a month, where "mosquito" bites were common. The patient came from Shanxi Province (once the epidemic area of kala-azar in Northwest China) and had a history of working in mountains and forests. The sandfly activity season was from May to August every year, so the bites of sandflies had to be considered. In addition, the significantly increased serum globulin was consistent with the characteristics of *Leishmania* infection; therefore, the possibility of kala-azar disease had to be highly considered. Then, we sent the blood sample to the National Institute of Parasitic Diseases, China CDC for kala-azar antibody testing, and the results were positive. At this point, we were able to clinically diagnose the patient's disease as kala-azar. But in epidemic areas, a positive antibody test is not the basis of diagnosis, so we once again sent the patient's bone puncture smear to the Hematology Laboratory of Huashan Hospital and the parasite experts of Shanghai Medical College for repeated consultation and reading, but no *Leishmania* was found.

At the same time, the plasma and bone marrow fluid of the patient were tested by pathogen next generation gene sequencing (NGS), and the gene sequence of *Leishmania* was detected in both of the results (Figs. 2.42, 2.43 and 2.44). Once this disease diagnosis was established for the patient, amphotericin B was given, amphotericin B was administered, and treatment for leishmaniasis was initiated. Early on, a regimen of low-dose amphotericin B combined with low-dose hormones was used to reduce inflammation. One week after treatment initiation, the patient's body temperature gradually returned to normal. Subsequently, the hormone dose was tapered

Type	Name	Coverage	Depth	Unique reads	
				Detection	Relevance
Parasite	*Leishmania infantum*	1.0528	1.78	114	0-2
	Leishmania donovani	0.5532	1.78	18	0-0

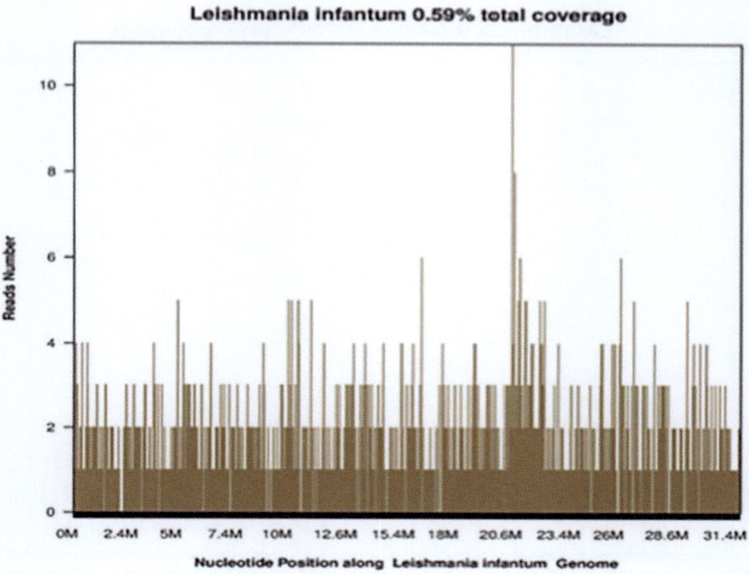

Fig. 2.42 The plasma sequences of *Leishmania infantum* and *Leishmania donovani* were detected by second-generation sequencing technology

step by step, and the patient's temperature remained consistently normal; the spleen also gradually decreased in size (Fig. 2.44 and Tables 2.6 and 2.7). Amphotericin B was discontinued after the total cumulative dose reached 2000 mg, and the symptoms of the patients were not repeated after 3 months of follow-up.

2.18.4 Comments

Kala-azar, or visceral leishmaniasis disease, is a parasitic disease caused by the *Leishmania* spp. The pathogen of visceral leishmaniasis (kala-azar) includes several viscerotropic Leishmania species, mainly Leishmania donovani and *Leishmania* infantum. The protozoa mainly parasitizes the patient's body's macrophages, by the Diptera insects, sandflies, as the vector. The main clinical features are long-term irregular fever, splenomegaly, anemia, emasculation, leucopenia, and an increase in serum globulin. If no appropriate treatment is given, most of the patients will die within 1–2 years after the disease due to complications with other diseases. Remarkably, kala-azar is characterized by a period of normal body temperature, increased appetite, and a slight shrinkage of the enlarged spleen during the course

Type	Name	Coverage	Depth	Unique reads	
				Detection	Reference
Parasite	*Leishmania infantum*	0.0633	1	8	0-35
	Leishmania donovani	0.0282	1	1	0-4

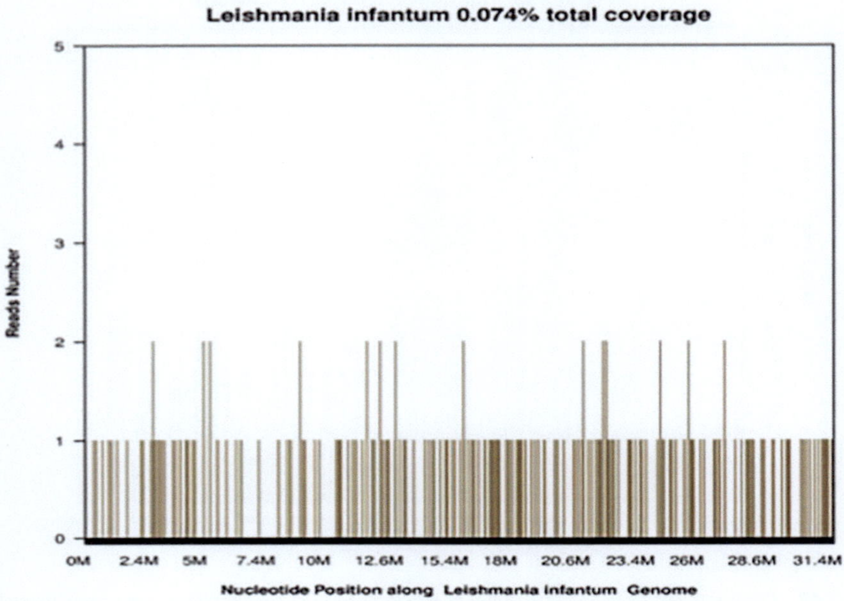

Fig. 2.43 Sequences of *Leishmania infantum* and *Leishmania donovani* were detected by second-generation sequencing technology in the bone marrow fluid of the patient

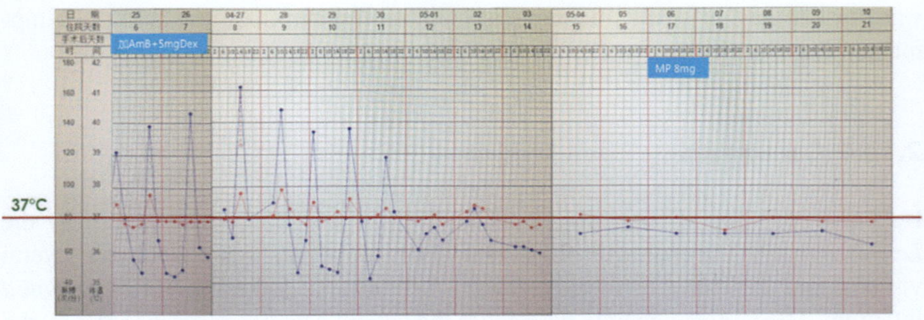

Fig. 2.44 Changes in body temperature after treatment with amphotericin B against *Leishmania*

of the disease. However, after a period of time, the patient developed fever again, and the spleen continued to enlarge. With such repeated episodes of fever and splenomegaly, the patient's condition progressed increasingly, and by the late stage of the disease, the symptoms no longer relieved.

Table 2.6 Changes in spleen size before and after treatment

Date	Long diameter of the spleen (mm)	Transverse diameter of the spleen (mm)	Thickness of the spleen (mm)
4.25	209	71	65
5.12	150	45	50
6.22	139	46	45
7.17	132	38	42

Table 2.7 Changes of hemogram and inflammatory indexes before and after treatment

Date	WBC ($\times 10^9$/L)	HB (g/L)	PLT ($\times 10^9$/L)	CRP (mg/L)	ESR (mm/h)	Globulin (g/L)
4.21	2.96	89	117	130	130	62
4.25	2.51	70	80	89.3	105	55
5.1	2.82	82	80	80	107	53
5.7	3.91	85	118	8.5	67	51
5.17	4.90	102	125	1.9	32	35
5.27	4.83	108	160	1.6	22	30

In this patient, recurrent high fever, accompanied by obvious splenomegaly, was the main manifestation. Laboratory examination showed the decline of two lines of blood cells and a significant increase in polyclonal serum globulin. The possibility of lymphoma and other lymphoproliferative diseases had to be considered after the infection was excluded. Moreover, the patient was a female, with flushed cheeks similar to erythema, repeated course of fever with onset and remission, abnormal blood image, and a polyclonal increase of immunoglobulin, especially with a significant increase in IgG, and her immune system appeared hyperactive, so Systemic Lupus Erythematosus (SLE) and other connective tissue diseases could not be excluded for the time being. The case was diagnosed as "sepsis" for a longer period of time due to multiple positive bone marrow cultures for the same bacteria. However, the poor response to anti-infective treatment and the recurrence of the disease led us to overturn the diagnosis. After a detailed medical history of epidemiology inquiry and summarization of the clinical characteristics, our investigation focused on leishmaniasis. With the help of second-generation sequencing of pathogens, the diagnosis of "kala-azar" was finally confirmed, and the patient was cured after active treatment. The experience gained from this case is that, as a doctor in the Department of Infectious Diseases, we should have the ability to distinguish the false from the true in the diagnostic clues and have a certain understanding of the epidemiological characteristics and unique clinical manifestations of some rare diseases, such as kala-azar and histoplasmosis, so as to identify such suspicious cases in a timely manner.

References

1. National Institute for Parasitic Diseases, Chinese Center for Disease Control and Prevention. www.chinacdc.cn/
2. www.who.int/leishmaniasis/burden/Status_of_endemicity_of_VL_worldwide_2015_with_imported_cases
3. www.who.int/entity/mediacentre/factsheets/fs375/en/

2.19 A Case of Liver Abscess Caused by *Clostridium difficile*

Chen Mingquan

A 68-year-old female was admitted to the hospital on July 16, 2018, 8 months after a simultaneous resection of colon cancer and liver metastasis and after having 7 months of recurrent fever.

In November 2017, the patient's health screening found elevated carbohydrate antigen 199 (CA199) at 218 U/ML and carcinoembryonic antigen (CEA) at 29 ng/ml. Further abdominal CT scan showed an intrahepatic space-occupying lesion, and the possibility of metastatic tumor was considered. Colonoscopy was performed, and an ulcerated space-occupying lesion in the ileocecal area was found. Biopsy pathology revealed adenocarcinoma. PET-CT examination found a 1.1 × 0.8 cm lesion in the ileocecal region and a 1.4 × 2.6 cm bull's-eye lesion in the liver, along with multiple cysts. Therefore, colon cancer with liver metastasis was considered, and the resection of colon cancer and liver metastasis under general anesthesia was performed on December 6, 2017.

Laparoscopic radical resection of the right colon cancer was performed, and intraoperative exploration found a 2 × 1.5-cm mass in the liver segment VIII. Later, specific hepatic segment resection and the incision and drainage of hepatic cysts were performed simultaneously, and liver metastasis of the right colon cancer was diagnosed intraoperatively. On the fifth day after the operation, the patient developed fever with chills and a maximum body temperature of 40 °C. There was a lot of exudation in the surgical incision, and the WBC in the routine blood test increased. Considering incision infection, the incision was opened and sutured, and incision debridement was performed. Meanwhile, ceftriaxone, combined with metronidazole, was given, but the effect was unfavorable. The patient's body temperature dropped slightly but rose again.

No bacterial growth was found in the pathogenic test of the blood and drainage fluid, and vancomycin, combined with meropenem, was administered. Two days later, the patient's body temperature dropped, but she still had low-grade fever, chills, and perspiration. A week later, the antibiotic therapy changed to linezolid, combined with meropenem, and the body temperature dropped to normal, but there was still much exudation from the incision, which could not be sutured. After three weeks of continuous anti-infective treatment, the effusion decreased, and the patient was discharged and continued to have intermittent dressing changes. After discharge, oxaliplatin, combined with Xeloda chemotherapy, was given every 3 weeks. Within 5 months after the operation, the patient occasionally had low-grade fevers, which could be relieved with antipyretic agents. The hemograms were always on the high side, the total number of WBC was between (10–16) × 10^9/L, and the proportion of neutrophils was mostly high.

Six months after the operation, PET-CT found a new lesion (3.7 × 1.1 cm) in the previous intrahepatic operation area, and the SUV value was 13. Further liver MRI examination revealed that the lesion PET-CT indicated was outside the liver capsule and suggested changes in the surgical area. However, based on the abnormal signal area between the right hepatic meridian and the left hepatic vein, combined with the continuously increasing blood tumor indicators, such as CA199 and CEA, over the three months, a new metastatic lesion was suspected. Intrahepatic local radiofrequency ablation was performed. The day after ablation, the patient had a fever again, and the initial temperature was low. Nonspecific inflammatory reaction after radiofrequency ablation was considered, and symptomatic treatment was given. But three days later, the body temperature gradually rose to 40 °C, accompanied by chills, elevated levels of leukocytes (16.3 × 10^9/L), and neutrophils (91%). The liver MRI indicated a liver abscess, so the patient was admitted to our hospital. Since the symptom onset, the patient had been in a status of good spirits, poor appetite, poor sleep at night, occasional diarrhea, and a weight loss of 4kg.

2.19.1 Physical Examination

The body temperature was 40 °C, and the patient was generally fine and had a mildly anemic appearance. No yellow staining in the skin or sclera was observed. No lymphadenectasis was palpable in the superficial lymph nodes all over the body. The heart and lung signs were within normal ranges. The surgical scars could be seen on the abdomen. The abdomen was soft, without tenderness or rebound tenderness. The liver and spleen were not palpable under the costal margins; the hepatic regions were sensitive to percussion. The bowel sounds were normal. No edema in the lower limbs was found.

2.19.2 Diagnosis and Treatment

After admission, liver MR was performed immediately (Figs. 2.45 and 2.49). Liver puncture and drainage were conducted. More than 80 ml of purulent fluid, mixed with blood, was drained (Fig. 2.45), which had no obvious odor. The drainage fluid was sent for bacterial culture and next-generation sequencing. At the same time, levornidazole 0.5 g q12h and imipenem and cilastatin 1.0 q8h were given. After treatment, the patient's body temperature dropped to low-grade, but the hemogram remained high. The BGI test report indicated *Clostridium difficile* (Fig. 2.46), but unfortunately, the bacterial culture was negative.

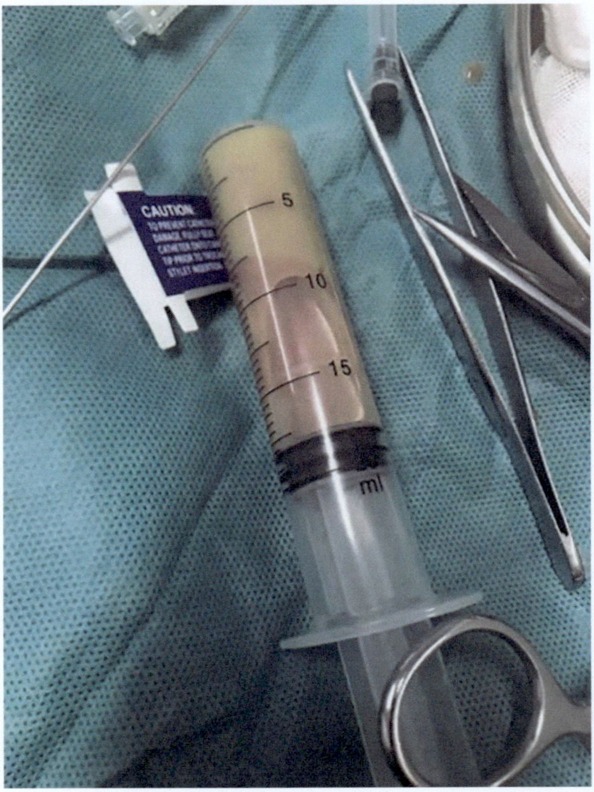

Fig. 2.45 Drained purulent fluid mixed with blood

List of pathogens detected			
Type	Pathogen	Beads	Relative abundance
G+	*Clostridium difficile*	2614	98.94%
List of suspected background microorganisms / contaminated or colonized microorganisms			
Type	Pathogen	Beads	Relative abundance
-	-	-	-

Fig. 2.46 Second-generation sequencing results of the puncture fluid for subphrenic abscess in our hospital on July 22, 2018

The anti-infective regimen was adjusted according to the results. Vancomycin was given at 1.0q12h, and levornidazole 0.5 g q12h was retained. The patient's body temperature returned to normal, and the blood routine showed the following: WBC: 11.15×10^9/L↑, neutrophil %: 77.6%↑, and procalcitonin: 0.07 ng/mL↑. The patient was discharged with medication, taking oral administration of linezolid 0.6 g bid po and metronidazole 0.4 g tid po for anti-infective treatment.

List of pathogens detected				
Type	Pathogen	Beads	Pathogen	Beads
G+	*Clostridioides*	155	*Clostridium difficile*	155

Fig. 2.47 Second-generation sequencing results of the subphrenic abscess puncture fluid in another hospital on September 11, 2018

List of pathogens detected				
Type	Pathogen	Beads	Pathogen	Beads
G+	*Clostridioides*	6	*Clostridium difficile*	6

Fig. 2.48 Second-generation sequencing results of the puncture fluid for subphrenic abscess in another hospital on October 3, 2018

Since discharge, the patient had been suffering from low fever, dull pain and discomfort in the liver area, and repeated fluctuations in body temperature, and the intrahepatic abscess cavity had enlarged again. Therefore, a drainage tube was placed in the cavity of the liver abscess in another hospital for continuous drainage, and normal saline was irrigated. Linezolid, combined with metronidazole, continued to be used, and the drainage fluid was sent to BGI for testing again. The result still showed *Clostridium difficile*. However, the number of gene fragment beads decreased (Figs. 2.47 and 2.48). The culture of drainage fluid showed colony growth, which was suspected to be *Clostridium difficile* based on the odor. Unfortunately, further strain identification and drug sensitivity tests were not done.

After the classic anti–*Clostridium difficile* treatment with vancomycin and metronidazole, the patient still had fever and abscess recurrence, which was considered to be related to host factors, such as postoperative chemotherapy, poor nutritional condition, damaged immune function, and infection associated with bacterial translocation. It may also have been related to the drug resistance of *Clostridium difficile*, but the result of the drug sensitivity test was lacking. Since the patient had been taking vancomycin for a long time, the fever may also have been drug-induced. Subsequently, vancomycin was discontinued and substituted with tigecycline and metronidazole. The next day, the body temperature gradually returned to normal. One week later, antibacterial treatment was stopped, and the drainage tube was removed. The patient was followed up for 7 months, and no disease recurrence was found.

2.19.3 Comments

Clostridium difficile liver abscess is very rare and is usually associated with liver surgery, interventional therapy, and abdominal surgery. Bacterial translocation and colonization set an important basis for infection. Because the clinical manifestations of *Clostridium difficile* liver abscess are difficult to distinguish from ordinary

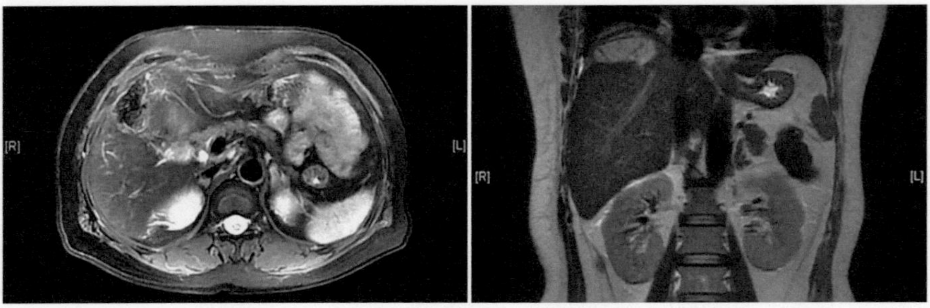

Fig. 2.49 Liver MRI on August 8, 2018

liver abscess, incomplete treatment is likely to lead to recurrence and treatment failure, which should arouse the attention of clinicians.

The possibility of *Clostridium difficile* infection should be considered in all patients with liver abscesses with a history of invasive operation in the liver, bile duct system, or the abdominal cavity. Etiological examination is the key point. The positive rate of *Clostridium difficile* in conventional blood culture is low, but smear and culture of pus or drainage fluid can improve the positive rate. It is particularly important that when considering *Clostridium difficile* infection, adequate communication with the bacterial laboratory is maintained, and specific media are needed to improve the positive rate. At present, the detection of pathogenic genes by second-generation sequencing plays a complementary role to some extent. For example, when there is a clinically suspected infection and the empirical treatment effect is poor, second-generation sequencing can be tried to improve the positive rate of pathogen detection.

The treatment for *Clostridium difficile* liver abscess is similar to the general principle of liver abscess. During the systemic anti-infective treatment, when facing the formation of an abscess cavity, surgery, puncture, and drainage should be performed. For treatment, vancomycin, metronidazole, and other classic antibacterial drugs that are effective against *Clostridium difficile* can be selected. In case of poor efficacy or intolerance in the treatment process, linezolid and tigecycline both have good antibacterial activity against *Clostridium difficile* and can perform as alternative selections. Antibacterial treatment should be individualized, which is related to the degree of damage to the host's basic immune barrier, the degree of necrosis of intrahepatic abscess, and whether puncture and drainage are taken. Generally, 6–8 weeks of antibacterial treatment is recommended, and a short course of treatment is prone to result in recurrence.

References

1. Robach Monique JT, Vernon Jonathan J, Loo Vivian G, et al. Understanding Clostridium difficile colonization [J]. Clin Microbiol Rev. 2018;31(2):e00021–17.
2. McDonald L Clifford,Gerding Dale N, Johnson Stuart, et al. Clinical practice guidelines for clostridium difficile infection in adults and children: 2017 update

by the Infectious Diseases Society of America (IDSA) and Society for Healthcare Epidemiology of America (SHEA) [J]. Clin Infect Dis. 2018;66(7):987–94.
3. Sartelli Massimo, Di Bella Stefano, McFarland Lynne V, et al. 2019 update of the WSES guidelines for management of Clostridioides (Clostridium) infection in surgical patients [J]. World J Emerg Surg. 2019;14:8.
4. Hanson Kimberly E, Couturier Marc Roger, Multiplexed molecular diagnostics for respiratory, gastrointestinal, and central nervous system infections [J]. Clin Infect Dis. 2016;63(10):1361–7.
5. Yimin Zhu, Wenhong Zhang. Application of second generation sequencing in etiological diagnosis of sepsis [J]. J Microbes Infect. 2018; 13(2):97–101.
6. Li JH, Yao RR, Shen HJ, et al. Clostridium perfringens infection after transarterial chemoembolization for large hepatocellular carcinoma. World J Gastroenterol. 2015;21(14):4397–401.
7. Oshima S, Takaishi K, Tani N, et al. Two cases of liver abscess caused by Clostridium perfringens after transcatheter arterial chemoembolization. Cancer Chemother. 2013;40:1795–7.

2.20 A 22-Year-Old Male Patient Was Admitted to Our Department on June 14, 2018, Due to Fever and Lymphadenopathy for 1 Year, with Cough and Sputum for More Than Half a Year

Liu Yuanyuan Liu, Weng Shanshan, Zhu Beidi, Zhu Xiaoxue, Liang Daobin, and Zhu Liping

The patient had bilateral inguinal and cervical lymphadenopathy, successively, in July 2017, and several of them were palpable, with a maximum diameter of 3.5 cm, no pain, no redness, and no swelling. At the same time, he had intermittent fever, with the body temperature fluctuating around 38.5 °C. He went to the local hospital. Blood routine test showed that the white blood cell count was 19.7×10^9/L. No specific treatment was given. In September 2017, the patient reappeared with fever and underwent a biopsy of the right cervical lymph node on October 18, 2017. The pathology showed focal chronic granulomatous inflammation without definite coagulative necrosis. The tissue culture showed the growth of acid-fast bacilli, which was negative in Xpert MTB/RIF. Species identification of the culture was *Mycobacterium* chelonae-abscessus complex. He was diagnosed with *Nontuberculous mycobacteria* (NTM) infection and was given an oral treatment with 0.6 g rifampicin, 0.75 g ethambutol, and 0.5 g azithromycin every day. In December 2017, there was no significant reduction in his lymph nodes during the follow-up visit. In January 2018, the patient developed a fever again, and the anti-NTM therapy was stopped. In February 2018, the patient began to have a cough and yellow sputum. He was examined in a local tertiary hospital on February 19, 2018. The blood test showed that the white blood cell count was 32×10^9/L. The chest CT suggested bilateral inferior pneumonia (Fig. 2.50). Moxifloxacin, meropenem, and

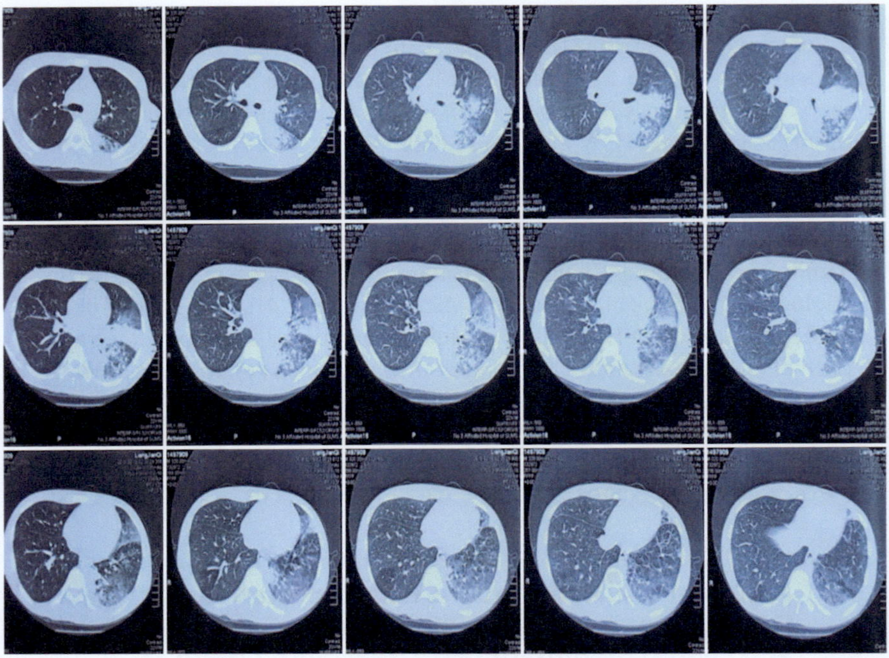

Fig. 2.50 Plain CT scan of the lung (February 19, 2018). Bilateral inferior pneumonia

vancomycin were administered for anti-infective treatment. A reexamination of the chest CT on February 26 showed the following: 1. There were multiple inflammatory lesions in both lungs, especially the posterior segment of the upper lobe and lower lobes of the left lung, and consolidation in some lung tissues, with obvious progress, and nodules in the bronchial wall of the middle segment of the right lung, with little change compared with the former and considered mucus suppository. 2. There was a small amount of effusion in the pericardium and thoracic cavity, showing obvious progress. 3. The bilateral axillary and mediastinal lymph nodes were slightly enlarged than the previous. 4. There were multiple exudations in the subcutaneous fat layer (Fig. 2.51). PET-CT suggested that there were multiple enlarged lymph nodes in the whole body, most of which were slightly active in metabolism. There were multiple metabolically active lesions in the bone throughout the body and in both lungs. The lesions were considered to be inflammatory, but malignant tumors (lymphoma?) could not be excluded. On February 27, bronchoscopy revealed a cauliflower-like mass in the bronchus, which was prone to bleeding on contact. The bone marrow smear showed no abnormality. On March 3, *Talaromyces marneffei* was cultured from the patient's sputum. At the same time, bone marrow biopsy and bronchial neoplasm biopsy suggested a *Talaromyces marneffei* infection. Lymph node biopsy suggested reactive hyperplasia with fibrosis. Then, the anti-infective regimen was adjusted to voriconazole 200 mg twice a day. The patient's body temperature returned to normal, and his cough gradually improved.

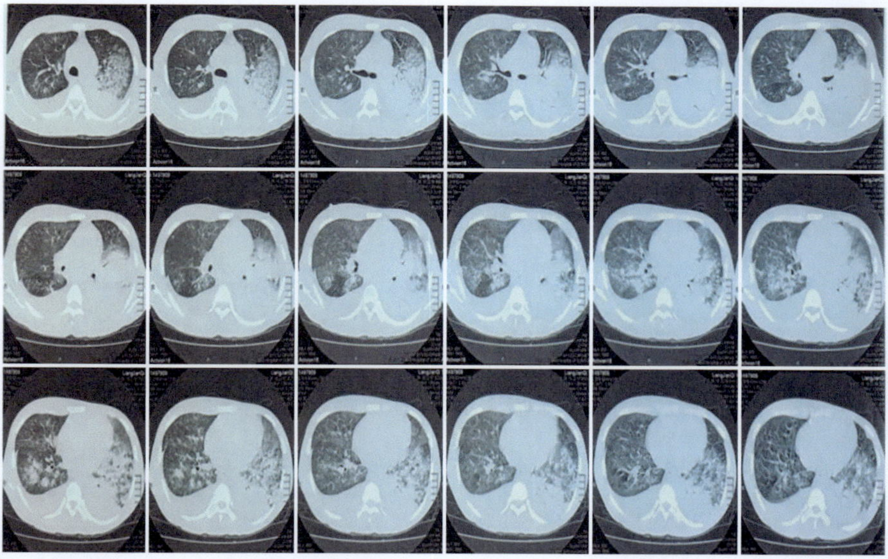

Fig. 2.51 Plain CT scan of the lung (February 26, 2018). Multiple inflammatory lesions in bilateral lungs, mainly in the apical posterior segment of the upper lobe of the left lung and the lower lobe of the left lung, and consolidation in some lung tissues, which were significantly improved

The chest CT results also improved (Figs. 2.52 and 2.53). However, on April 6, the patient reappeared with swollen lymph nodes behind the ears, in the submandibular glands, and in the cervical area, accompanied by obvious tenderness. The ultrasound showed that there were multiple enlarged lymph nodes in the bilateral neck, submandibular glands, and parotid glands, with liquefaction foci observed inside. The blood concentration of voriconazole was monitored to be 0.02 ug/ml. Considering the low blood concentration of voriconazole, the doctors increased the oral dose of voriconazole to 400 mg (8 a.m.) and 200 mg (4 p.m.) to continue with the antifungal therapy. However, on April 20, progressive lymphadenopathy of the left ear, mandible, and neck recurred, accompanied by local tenderness and difficulty in opening the mouth. Considering the poor efficacy of voriconazole, the regimen was changed to amphotericin B on April 21. Treatment with amphotericin B was started with a small dose, and the dose was gradually increased. On April 24, the patient had a fever again, with the maximum temperature reaching 40 °C, accompanied by headache and nausea. Blood culture showed *Salmonella typhimurium*. Then, cefoperazone–sulbactam was added for anti-infective treatment, and methylprednisolone was used for anti-inflammatory treatment. After that, the body temperature gradually returned to normal, accompanied by a significant reduction in the lymph nodes. The dose of methylprednisolone was gradually reduced. On May 15, the patient coughed again, with white foamy sputum, and had a high fever reaching 40 °C. The chest CT showed infections of both lungs, which progressed significantly than before, especially in the left lung. Part of the lung tissue was consolidated. Multiple lymph nodes in the axillary and mediastinum on

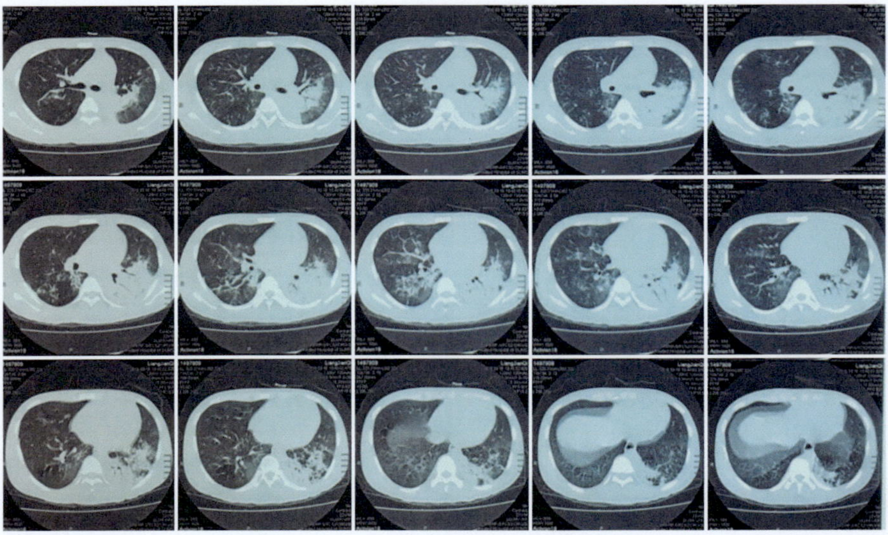

Fig. 2.52 Plain CT scan of the lung (March 9, 2018), better than before

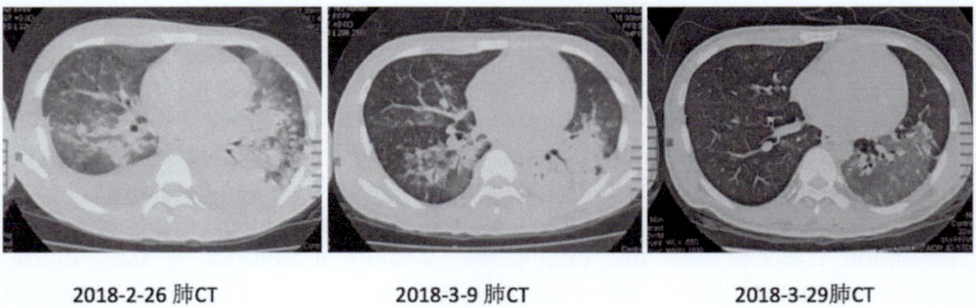

Fig. 2.53 Plain CT scan of the lung (March 29, 2018), better than before

both sides were enlarged, which were significantly larger than before (Fig. 2.54). The symptoms were not improved with amphotericin B liposome, and voriconazole was used for antifungal treatment, cefoperazone–sulbactam for antibacterial treatment, and methylprednisolone 80 mg qd for anti-inflammatory treatment, and immunoglobulin was given. The patient's symptoms improved after 1 week, and the dose of methylprednisolone was decreased. On June 7, the chest CT showed no significant improvement (Fig. 2.54). Voriconazole and methylprednisolone were used up to June 13, by which time the dose of metronidazole had been reduced to 40 mg. For further treatment, the patient was admitted with the diagnosis of disseminated *Talaromyces marneffei* infection. Since the illness, the patient had a clear consciousness, lethargic mentation, normal appetite, poor sleep, normal urine and feces, and no significant weight loss.

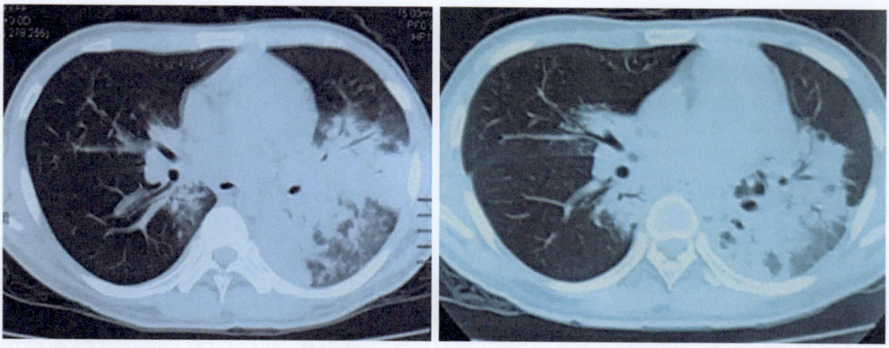

Fig. 2.54 Lung CT plain scan (May 20, 2018). The infection of both lungs was more advanced than before, the left lung was prominent, and some lung tissues were consolidated. The lung CT on June 7, 2018, showed no significant improvement

2.20.1 Past History and Personal History

There was nothing special in the past history and the personal history.

2.20.2 Physical Examination on Admission

The patient had a body temperature of 36.3 °C and a clear mind. A large number of acne-like changes could be seen on the skin all over the body, especially on the face and chest. The left subclavian tissue was slightly swollen, without tenderness. There was no swelling of the superficial lymph nodes throughout the body. Breath sounds in both lungs were coarse, with no dry or wet rales. The abdomen was soft. The liver and spleen were not palpable under the ribs.

2.20.3 The Course of Diagnosis and Treatment

Blood routine examination showed the following: white blood cell count: 31.78×10^9/L↑, neutrophil %: 86%↑, lymphocyte %: 7%↓, hemoglobin: 107 g/L↓, erythrocyte sedimentation rate: 7 mm/h, and C-reactive protein: >200 mg/L↑; HIV: (−) and RPR (−); TBNK: % CD3+ (T cells): 47%↓, % CD3+CD4+ (helper T cells): 12%↓, % CD3+CD8+ (inhibitory T cells): 27%, CD4+/CD8+ ratio: 0.45↓, % CD19+(B cells): 30%↑, % CD16+CD56+ (NK cells): 22%, and % T+B+NK(total lymphocytes): 99%.

B-ultrasonography:The subclavian lymph nodes on the left chest wall were swollen and full; the left axillary and groin lymph nodes were swollen and regular. Combined with the patient's previous sputum culture, bone marrow biopsy and bronchial neopathology suggested the infection of *Talaromyces marneffei*, and the

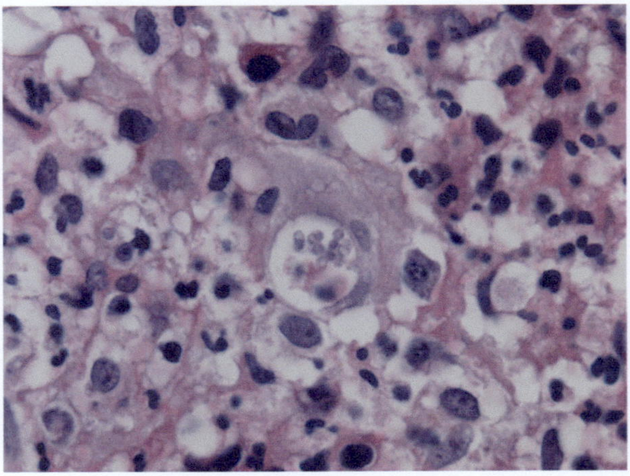

Fig. 2.55 Pathological PAS staining of lung tissue indicates *Talaromyces marneffei* bacteria (in consultation with the Department of Pathology of our hospital)

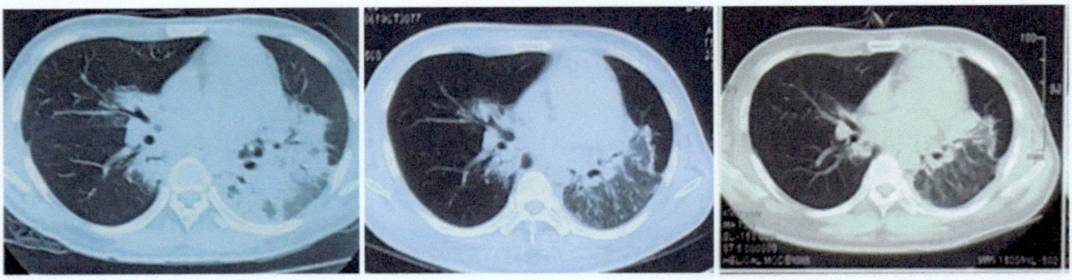

Fig. 2.56 After itraconazole treatment, the absorption of six to 19 lung lesions was better than that of six to seven lesions in other hospitals, and the absorption of six to seven lung lesions was slightly better than that of six to 19 on CT

pathological sections were further sent to our hospital for consultation with the Department of Pathology and a *Talaromyces marneffei* infection was confirmed (Fig. 2.55), so the patient was diagnosed with disseminated *Talaromyces marneffei* infection (lung and bone marrow).

For *Talaromyces marneffei* infections, international guidelines recommend amphotericin B as the first choice. The patient had been treated with amphotericin B, amphotericin B liposome, and voriconazole in another hospital, but the effect was not good.

After admission, a 200 mg q12h load intravenous treatment with itraconazole was given for 2 days, followed by 200 mg qd intravenous treatment of itraconazole. At the same time, the dose of hormones used before admission to the hospital was gradually reduced (methylprednisolone 40 mg qd was reduced to 36 mg qd orally). The patient had no fever, cough, or sputum. The lung CT absorption on June 19 was better than that in the other hospital (June 7) (Fig. 2.56).

On July 4, blood routine examination showed the following: white blood cell count: 23.47×10^9/L↑, hemoglobin: 116 g/L↓, neutrophil%: 89.7%↑, lymphocyte

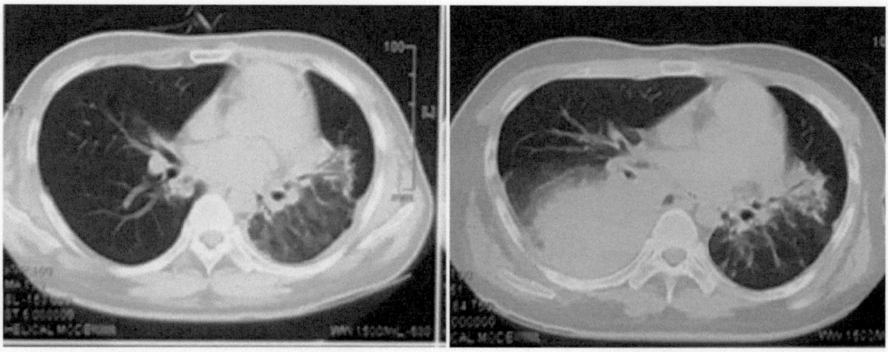

2018-7-6 肺CT 2018-7-23肺CT

Fig. 2.57 Lung CT plain scan (July 23, 2018). Increased lung texture, scattered inflammation in both lungs, and consolidation in the lower lobe of the right lung

%: 3.6%↓; erythrocyte sedimentation rate, C-reactive protein, and procalcitonin were normal; TBNK: % CD3+ (T cell): 47%↓, % CD3+CD4+ (helper T cell): 7%↓, % CD3+CD8+ (suppressor T cell): 29%, CD4+/CD8+ ratio: 0.25↓, % CD19+ (B cells): 28%↑, % CD16+CD56+ (NK cells): 22%, and % T+B+NK (total lymphocytes): 97%. On July 6, the lymph node B-ultrasound and lung CT showed better results than before (June 19) (Fig. 2.56), and he was discharged from the hospital on July 9.

After discharge, the patient regularly took itraconazole oral solution, and the dose of glucocorticoid was gradually reduced. On July 20, 2018, the patient developed chest pain on the right side after fatigue, accompanied by fever (T_{max} 38.5), cough with yellow sputum and sometimes bloody sputum, chest tightness, shortness of breath, and diarrhea with watery stools two or three times a day.

On July 22, he came to the emergency department in our hospital. The blood routine test showed the leukocyte count to be 9.91 × 10^9/L and neutrophil % to be 92.9%. Physical examination findings were as follows: full moon face; superficial lymph nodes could not be touched; rough breath sounds in both lungs, with wet rales in the left lower lung and no breath sounds in the right lower lung; heart rate of 145 beat/min; the liver and spleen could not be touched under the ribs; and no edema in both lower limbs.

On July 23, he was admitted to the hospital again with a body temperature of 39 °C. The chest CT scan showed increased texture in both lungs, scattered inflammation in both lungs, and consolidation in the lower lobe of the right lung (Fig. 2.57). After admission, itraconazole 200 mg qd was given intravenously for antifungal therapy. Imipenem/cilastatin 0.5 g q8h intravenous anti-infective therapy was added because of the return of gram-negative bacteria in the blood culture. The blood culture on July 26 showed the following: *Burkholderia cepacia*. Drug susceptibility results: piperacillin: Susceptible (S); imipenem: S; ceftazidime: S; meropenem: Intermediate (I); ciprofloxacin: Resistant (R); amikacin: R; gentamicin: R. After treatment, the patient's body temperature gradually returned to normal, as did the

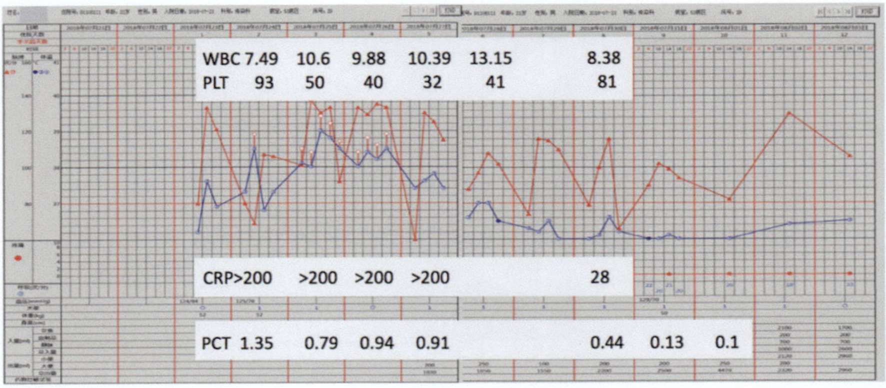

Fig. 2.58 *Burkholderia cepacia* was cultured in the blood, and the body temperature and inflammatory indexes gradually returned to normal after treatment

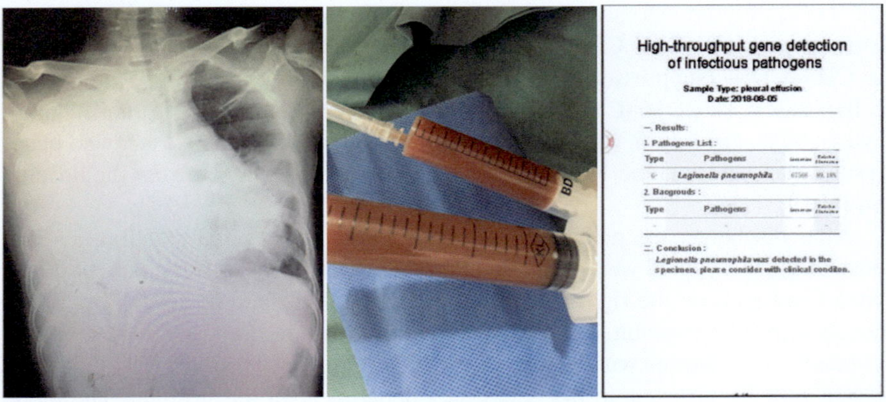

Fig. 2.59 The bedside radiograph showed a large amount of pleural effusion on the right side, and bloody pus was drawn from the pleural cavity. *Legionella pneumophila* was detected by second-generation sequencing of pleural effusion

inflammatory indexes and platelets (Fig. 2.58). In consideration of the patient's multiple infections, methylprednisolone was rapidly reduced.

On July 30, 2018, the patient's temperature was normal, with cough and sputum improved. However, he developed chest tightness and shortness of breath, which were gradually getting worse. He was unable to lie supine and began to have hemoptysis. On August 1, a bedside chest radiograph showed infection of both lungs, with a large amount of fluid in the right pleural cavity. A bedside thoracentesis was conducted, with hemorrhagic pus drained, which was exudate (Fig. 2.59). On August 5, high-throughput sequencing of his pleural fluid reported the following: *Legionella pneumophila* (sequence number 67568; relative abundance 89.18%) (Fig. 2.59). Considering a *Legionella pneumophila* infection, we added doxycycline and levofloxacin for anti-infective treatment. With closed drainage of the right thoracic cavity, the patient's chest tightness and shortness of breath gradually eased. Later, high-throughput sequencing was performed on the sputum of the patient with second-generation sequencing, which showed *Legionella pneumophila* (sequence number 12810; relative abundance 75.45%), and bone marrow sequencing, which showed *Legionella pneumophila* (sequence number 5, relative abundance 0.59%). On August 20, the Shanghai Center for Disease Control and Prevention reported that *Legionella pneumophila* type 1 urine antigen was positive; the sputum culture showed *Legionella pneumophila* type 1. Therefore, the diagnosis of *Legionella* pneumonia was confirmed. The patient had pneumothorax during the course of the disease, but his condition was stable after closed drainage and anti-infective treatment with intravenous itraconazole, imipenem, doxycycline, and ciprofloxacin. Oral methylprednisolone tablets were reduced to 14 mg daily. He was discharged from the hospital on November 2 with stable conditions.

2.20.4 Comments

This patient was a young male. He developed fever with lymphadenopathy, cough, and sputum without any obvious cause. The condition gradually progressed and worsened, and the course of the disease was nearly one year from the onset to the diagnosis. At the early stage of the disease, the anti-NTM regimen in another hospital for 3 months was not effective. Then, the lung lesions appeared, and PET-CT revealed multiple organ involvement throughout the body. The results of sputum culture, bone marrow pathology, and lung tissue pathology confirmed the diagnosis of a *Talaromyces marneffei* infection. Our patient was negative for anti-HIV antibody and HIV RNA. However, the CD4+ T cell count was found to be significantly reduced (Fig. 2.60), which indicated that the patient had idiopathic CD4+ T lymphopenia. During the course of treatment, *Burkholderia* and *Legionella* infections were also found. The patient's condition was fierce and lacked specific clinical manifestations. The culture and identification of pathogenic bacteria were extremely important for the diagnosis of the disease. With the changes in the spectrum of infectious diseases, physicians should be sufficiently cautious and be aware of individuals who are immunocompromised or have immunodeficiency. They should send specimens from infected sites for multiple inspections and use multiple methods to detect pathogens as soon as possible. It is particularly important to choose the treatment regimen based on the results of drug sensitivity.

Fig. 2.60 Peripheral blood CD4+T cell count

DATE	CD4+T Cell Counts（/μL）
2017.09.04	932
2018.05.18	263
2018.06.14	267
2018.07.06	59
2018.08.22	40
2018.09.03	34

References

1. Jin Jialin, Hu Yuekai, Xu Bin, et al. Clinical characteristics analysis of nine cases of Talaromyces marneffei Infection in non-HIV-infected patients and literature review. Microbes Infect. 2017;12(6):333–9.
2. Yi-Min Zhu, Jing-Wen Ai, Bin Xu, et al. Rapid and precise diagnosis of disseminated T.marneffei infection assisted by high-throughput sequencing of multifarious specimens in a HIV-negative patient: a case report [J]. BMC Infect Dis. 2018;18(1):379.
3. Kaplan JE, Benson C, Holmes KK, et al. Guidelines for prevention and treatment of opportunistic infections in HIV-infected adults and adolescents: recommendations from CDC, the National Institutes of Health, and the HIV Medicine Asociation of the Infectious Diseases Society of America [J/OL]. MMWR Recomm Rep. 2009;58(RR-4):1–207. https://www.cdc.gov/mmwr/preview/mmwrhtml/r5804a1.htm.
4. Guidelines for Prevention and Treatment of opportunistic Infections in HIV-Infected Adults and Adolescents [EB/OL]. http://aidsinfo.nih.gov/guidelineson. 5/7/2013.
5. Chun-Hsing Liao, Hou-Tai Chang, Chih-Cheng Lai, et al. Clinical characteristics and outcomes of patients with Burkholderia cepacia bacteremia in an intensive care unit[J]. Diagnos Microbiol Infect Dis. 2011; 70(2):260–6.
6. EI Chakhtoura NG, Saade E, Wilson BM, et al. A 17-Year Nationwide Study of Burkholderia cepacia Complex Bloodstream Infections Among Patients in the United States Veterans Health Administration [J]. Clin Infect Dis. 2017;65(8):1253–9.
7. Lu Feng, Jin Yinlong, et al. Epidemiology of legionellosis. Foreign Med Sci Sect Hyg. 2008;35(2):78–83.
8. Nick Phin, Frances Parry-Ford, Timothy Harrison, et al. Epidemiology and clinical management of Legionnaires' disease [J]. Lancet Infect Dis. 2014;14:1011–21.

2.21 Hemophagocytic Lymphohistiocytosis Induced by Disseminated Histoplasmosis: A Case Report

Yang Feifie, Wang Xinyu, and Zhang Jiming

A 30-year-old man was admitted to the hospital on May 31, 2018, because of "fever with chills and simultaneous peripheral blood cell reduction for a month."

There was no obvious cause of fever since May 1, 2018. Peak temperature reached 40.0 °C, and on May 2, he was treated in the local hospital. Blood routine examination showed that white blood cell count was 2.53×10^9/L, neutrophil ratio was 73.9%, red blood cell count was 3.47×10^{12}/L, hemoglobin was 90 g/L, and platelet count was 83×10^9/L, and blood biochemistry showed that alanine aminotransferase was 4 U/L, glutamic oxaloacetic transaminase was 84. 5 U/L, alkaline phosphatase was 494 U/L, gamma-glutamyl transpeptidase was 101 U/L, albumin was 27.2 g/l, and triglyceride was 1.5 mmol/l. Ferritin was more than 2000 ng/ml. Abdominal color Doppler ultrasound revealed hepatosplenomegaly, a thickened and rough gallbladder wall, and pelvic effusion. Color Doppler ultrasound of other regions showed no abnormalities. Blood culture reported *Staphylococcus hominis* ssp. The patient was considered to have a "bloodstream infection" and given meropenem and levofloxacin for anti-infective treatment, but there was no obvious improvement. The patient presented with high fever and coughed up white sticky phlegm. On May 9, the patient was transferred to the hematology department of another hospital, and his blood culture was negative. Bone marrow smear showed "thrombocytopenia with megakaryocyte maturation disorder; a small number of reticular cells with enhanced phagocytic function." There was no obvious abnormality in the flow cytometry of bone marrow. Testing for 45 leukemia fusion genes and leukemia-related genes in the bone marrow was negative.

Color Doppler ultrasound showed an enlargement of the left cervical lymph nodes. PET-CT showed that "the liver volume increased, and multiple enlarged lymph nodes were found in both submandibular, cervical, hepatic hilar and retroperitoneal regions, all with increased glucose metabolism. Considering the possibility of hematological diseases, neck lymph node biopsy is recommended."

Combined with the patient's history and auxiliary examination, considering "hemophagocytic syndrome," the patient was successively given biapenem, moxifloxacin, vancomycin, and cefoperazone/tazobactam for anti-infective treatment; a glucocorticoid and immunosuppressant for anti-inflammation treatment (May 15 onward methylprednisolone 40 mg q12h, May 19 onward methylprednisolone 40 mg Q8H, May 22 onward dexamethasone 10 mg q12h, and May 25 onward cyclosporine 125 mg bid); and other symptomatic support treatment.

The patient complained that after one week of glucocorticoid use, his body temperature had leveled off for several days, and then he had fever again, with T_{max} 38 °C per day, accompanied by cough and sputum, and the simultaneous peripheral blood cell count was still in progressive decline.

On May 30, he was admitted to the emergency room, and the blood routine test showed the following: white blood cell count: 0.45×10^9/L, platelet count: 15×10^9/L, red blood cell count: 2.64×10^{12}/L, and hemoglobin: 67 g/L. Considering "Fever with Unknown Origin; hemophagocytic syndrome," anti-inflammatory and symptomatic supportive treatment, such as meropenem for anti-infective treatment, caspofungin for antifungal treatment, human immunoglobulin 20 g qd, dexamethasone 15 mg qd, and albumin 10 g qd were given. In order to further clarify the cause of the fever, on May 31, the patient was admitted to our department. The diagnosis and treatment before admission is shown in Fig. 2.61.

Since the onset of the disease, the patient was not in good spirits and was presented as listless, with poor appetite, normal sleep, and normal urine. His weight had decreased significantly by about 10 kg.

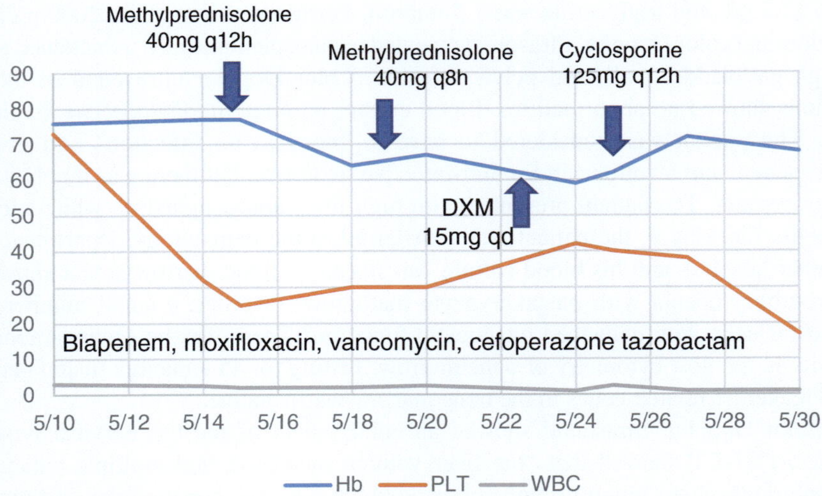

Fig. 2.61 A general picture of the patient's condition before admission

2.21.1 Past Medical History

The patient was healthy in the past. He went to the local hospital in March 2018 for diarrhea. No abnormality was found in the blood routine examination. Gastroscopy showed superficial gastritis, and enteroscopy showed colitis polyps. The symptoms improved after hospitalization.

2.21.2 Physical Examination on Admission

The body temperature was 35.6 °C. The patient was conscious and listless. Swollen lymph nodes could be felt on the bilateral neck, which were about 0.5 cm × 0.5 cm, of medium texture, with no tenderness. There was no subcutaneous bleeding point, and there was an ulcer in the posterior pharyngeal wall. There was no tenderness in the sternum, breath was clear in both lungs, and the abdomen was flat and soft. There was palpable swelling of the liver and spleen, about five fingers below the ribs, of medium texture, with percussion pain. There was mild edema in both lower limbs.

2.21.3 Diagnosis and Treatment Process

On admission examination, blood routine showed the following: white blood cell count: 0.41 × 10^9/L, platelet count: 14 × 10^9/L ↓, and hemoglobin: 66 g/L ↓; liver function showed the following: glutamic pyruvic transaminase: 61 u/L, glutamic oxaloacetic transaminase: 30 U/L, alkaline phosphatase: 229 u/L, gamma-glutamyl

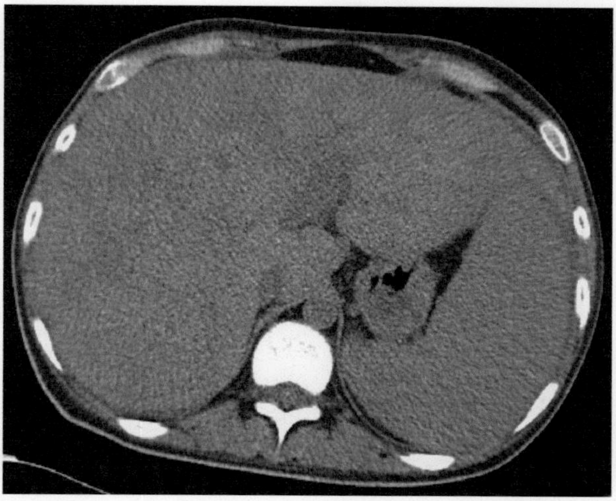

Fig. 2.62 CT of the lung showed obvious hepatosplenomegaly

transpeptidase: 193 u/L, total bilirubin: 23.3 umol/l, lactate dehydrogenase: 554 u/L, albumin: 27 g/L; and DIC showed the following: APPT: 34.6 s, D-dimer: 11.94, fibrinogen degradation products: 32.1 UG/ml, fibrinogen: 2.5 g/L, Pt: 12.2 s, international standardized ratio: 1.07; ferritin: >2000 ng/ml; and lymphocyte subsets: NK + 2.84% ↓.

Lung CT scan showed a little inflammation of both lungs, with bilateral pleural effusion and pericardial effusion; additional findings included hepatosplenomegaly, combined with clinical and other examinations (Fig. 2.62). Ultrasound showed hepatosplenomegaly. There was a small amount of fluid in the pelvic cavity. There were postprandial manifestations of the gallbladder. The pancreas, spleen, kidneys, ureters, bladder, and retroperitoneum were normal. The shape of the lymph nodes in the middle of the left neck was enlarged. No abnormal enlarged lymph nodes were found in the right neck, bilateral supraclavicular, bilateral axillary, and bilateral inguinal areas.

After admission, repeated blood culture examination showed *Escherichia coli* and *Enterococcus faecium*. The next day, a bone biopsy was performed, which indicated "myelodysplasia decreased, especially in megakaryocytic lineage. A large number of pathogens were phagocytized by bone macrophages and neutrophils, especially macrophages." It could be seen that pathogens were phagocytized by neutrophils in the peripheral blood. There was no obvious abnormality in the bone marrow flow cytometry (Fig. 2.63).

Bone marrow biopsy showed that "there were about ten marrow cavities, about 40% of hematopoietic cells, megakaryocytes were easy to see, and there was no obvious abnormality of hematopoietic cells in all lines. Reticular fiber staining shows negative." There was no evidence of lymphoma or other hematological tumors. At the same time, when a smear from a foreign hospital was examined again, a large number of similar pathogens engulfed by macrophages could be observed. Therefore, it was more likely that hemophagocytic syndrome was induced

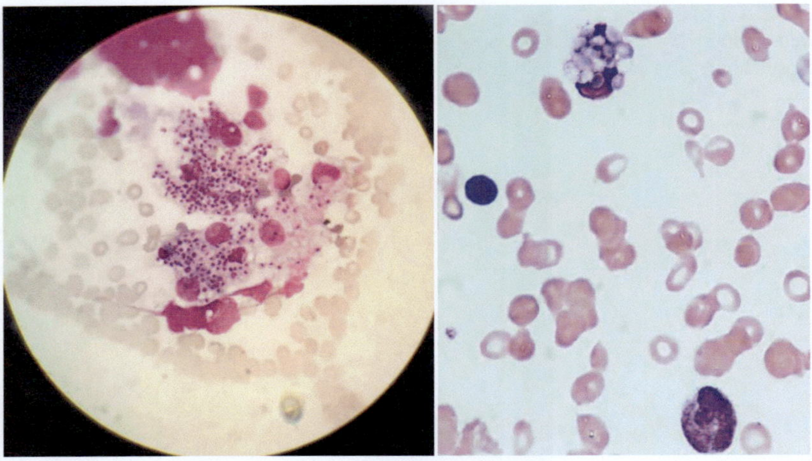

Fig. 2.63 Bone marrow smear and blood smear on admission

genus	sequence number	species	sequence number
Histoplasma	5646	Histoplasma capsulatum	5646
Blastomyces	51	Blastomyces dermatitidis	51
Coccidioides	4	Coccidioides immitis	4

Fig. 2.64 Second-generation sequencing result of bone marrow fluid

by infection. We further tested the antigen of *Plasmodium falciparum* in the peripheral blood and sera of kala-azar and found that they were both negative; we tested the antigen of *Plasmodium falciparum* in the blood and urine, and the results were both positive; second-generation sequencing of bone marrow fluid and plasma (Fig. 2.64) showed that there were 5646 and 190 sequences of *Histoplasma capsulatum*, respectively; the positive results were also reported 3 weeks after the first bone marrow culture (fungal bottle) in our hospital, and under the microscope, it was identified as *Histoplasma* (Fig. 2.65). So far, the diagnosis of the patient was completely clear, and it was considered to be "histoplasmosis; bloodstream infection; hemophagocytic syndrome." After admission, we immediately adjusted the treatment plan: stop cyclosporine, reduce dexamethasone, and adjust the anti-infective plan to "meropenem 1.0 Q8H + vancomycin 1.0 q12h + itraconazole 200 mg QD" intravenously. Even if we made a comprehensive judgment of the patient's condition so quickly and accurately, the follow-up treatment process was still full of twists and turns (see Fig. 2.66).

During the follow-up at about one week, the blood routine of the patient did not improve significantly. While the glucocorticoid continued to be reduced, amphotericin B liposome, combined with antifungal therapy, was added from June 6 (June 6: 10 mg QD, June 7: 20 mg QD, and June 8: 30 mg QD).

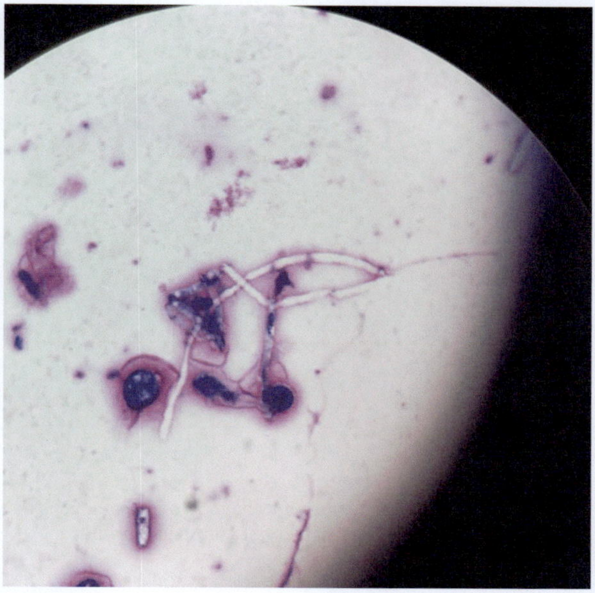

Fig. 2.65 Bone marrow culture showed Histoplasma

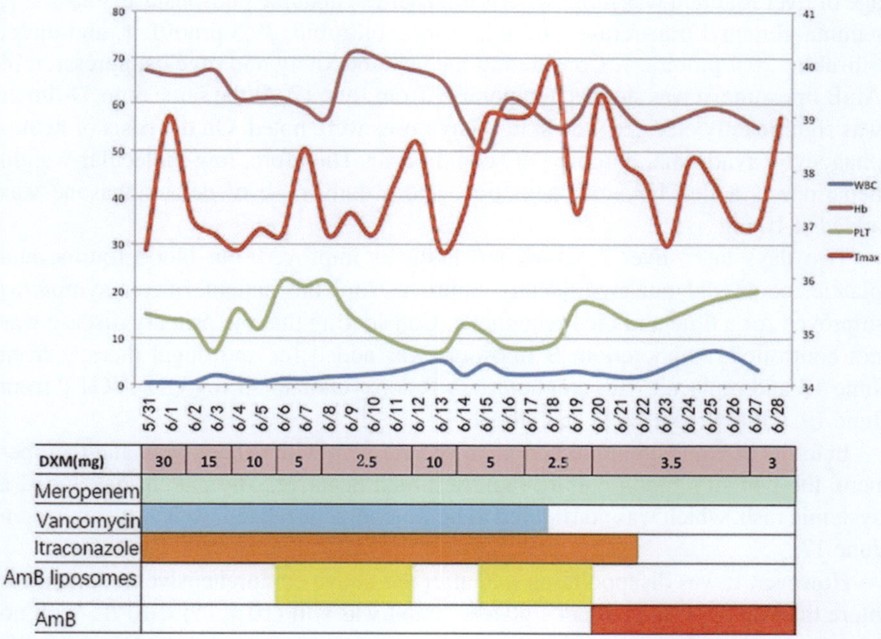

Fig. 2.66 Treatment plan adjustment, hemogram, and body temperature changes of patients in our hospital for 0–4 weeks

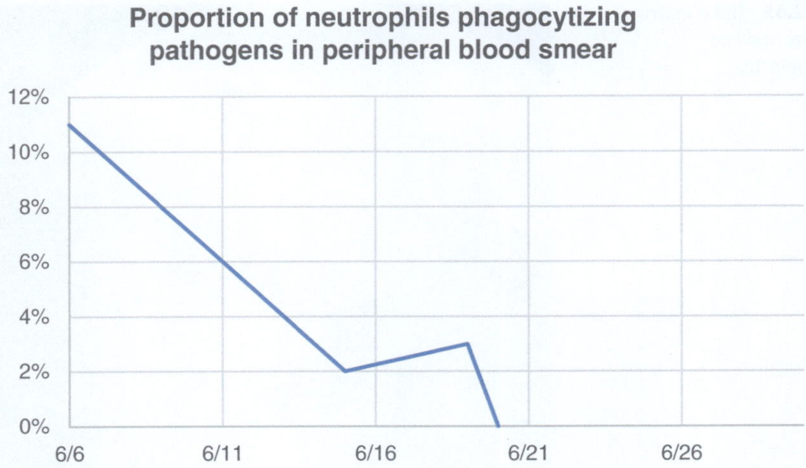

Fig. 2.67 Proportion of neutrophil-phagocytizing pathogens in peripheral blood smear by Mr. Gu Jianfei of the laboratory department of Huashan Hospital

On June 11, the platelet count was still decreasing, only 9×10^9/L, and the damage of liver function was more serious than before: alkaline phosphatase: 428 u/L ↑, gamma-glutamyl transferase: 267 u/L ↑, total bilirubin: 39.5 μmol/L ↑, and direct bilirubin: 20.4 μmol/L ↑. Considering the hepatotoxicity and myelosuppression of AmB liposome, it was stopped temporarily from June 12. At the same time, D-dimer was significantly elevated, and skin ecchymoses were noted. On the basis of hemophagocytic syndrome, chronic DIC could occur. Therefore, low-molecular-weight heparin was added for anticoagulation, and a daily dose of dexamethasone was added at 10 mg.

Two days later, liver function and D-dimer improved, but blood routine and platelet count did not significantly improve. And the patient's fever symptoms improved for a time and then rebounded. Considering that the primary disease was not controlled, amphotericin B liposome was added for antifungal therapy from June 15 and replaced with amphotericin B deoxycholate 25 mg QD IVGTT from June 19, while itraconazole was stopped.

In terms of bloodstream infection, after treatment with vancomycin and meropenem, the patient's blood culture rapidly turned negative. The patient developed a systemic rash, which was considered to be vancomycin-related, so it was stopped on June 17.

However, it was disappointing that after the above comprehensive treatment for more than 20 days, the patient's platelet count was still $(10 \times 15) \times 10^9$/L, with no improvement, and fever symptoms still repeated. When we had doubts about the efficacy of the patient's antifungal therapy and were at a loss for the next treatment, we regained our confidence with a trend chart carefully made by Mr. Gu Jianfei of the laboratory department: The proportion of neutrophils phagocytized by pathogens in the patients' peripheral blood smears decreased significantly (Fig. 2.67). At

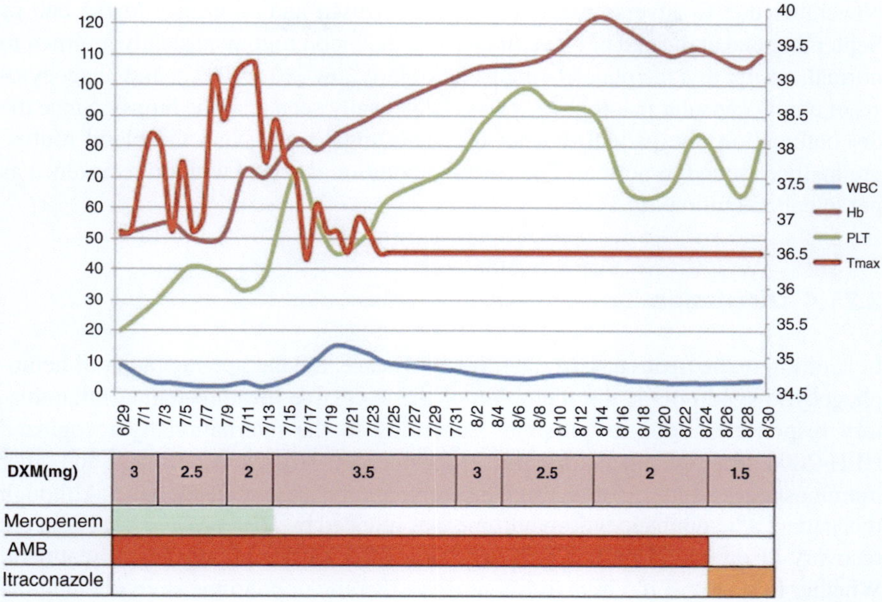

Fig. 2.68 Treatment plan adjustment, blood picture, and body temperature changes of patients in our hospital from 5 to 13 weeks

this time, second-generation sequencing results of the blood also showed that the sequence number of *Histoplasma* was significantly decreased from 190 at the beginning to 8 after 3 weeks of treatment. On June 28, after 4 weeks of antifungal treatment, bone marrow smears showed a significant decrease in the number of phagocytized pathogens, and most of them were empty capsules. Second-generation sequencing showed that the sequence number of bone marrow fluid was reduced to 100. The patient's enlarged liver and spleen retracted significantly from five fingers under the rib to two fingers under the rib. This evidence told us that the antifungal treatment was effective and the overall condition was improving!

Therefore, we continued to give amphotericin B for antifungal treatment and meropenem for anti-infective treatment and gradually reduced the glucocorticoid to 2–4 mg per day. After 7 weeks of treatment, the patient's body temperature was basically controlled, and meropenem was suspended. Second-generation sequencing of bone marrow fluid was negative, and only amphotericin B was given. After 10 weeks of treatment, white blood cells returned to 3×10^9/L to 4×10^9/L, hemoglobin returned to 100–120 g/L, and platelets rose to 80×10^9/L. At the end of August, amphotericin B was stopped, and itraconazole was given intravenously for several days. The patient's condition did not rebound, and he was discharged on August 31 (see Fig. 2.68 for details).

After discharge, the patient was given itraconazole 200 mg QD and methylprednisolone 8 mg QD. Methylprednisolone was gradually reduced by the end of October 2018. Itraconazole was taken orally for 3 months and stopped in late

November due to adverse reactions, such as nausea and vomiting. At the end of September and at the end of November 2018, the blood routine basically returned to normal, except that the platelet count was slightly low (80×10^9/L), and phagocytosis of empty capsular macrophages was occasionally seen on bone biopsy. Since the discontinuation, the patient did not take antifungal drugs, and the blood routine gradually returned to normal. The current condition is stable with no recurrence as per telephone follow-up.

2.21.4 Discussion

In addition to the treatment for the primary disease, the therapeutic target of hemophagocytic syndrome is the inhibition of the excessive life-threatening inflammatory response as soon as possible. According to the internationally recognized HLH-2004 program, glucocorticoids, etoposide (VP-16), cyclosporine A, and other immunosuppressants are often used in combination with gamma globulin. Although this patient's hemophagocytic syndrome was induced by *Histoplasma* infection, the recovery of the blood routine was very slow after sufficient antifungal treatment. Whether to start specific immunosuppressive therapy or continue strengthening the antifungal treatment had become the key to the treatment.

In 2015, Townsend reported 11 cases of hemophagocytic syndrome induced by histoplasmosis in our hospital from 2003 to 2013, of which six cases were of immunocompromised patients (five cases of HIV and one case of renal transplantation). Nine cases were of disseminated infection, and the other two cases were of pulmonary infection. Nine cases received amphotericin B liposome sequential antifungal therapy with itraconazole, one case received antifungal therapy with itraconazole, and another patient's antifungal treatment is unknown. Among the five patients who received the treatment, including gamma globulin and glucocorticoid, four patients died, while among the five patients who did not receive immunosuppressive therapy, only one patient died. At the same time, this article summarizes 27 similar cases reported in the past. Among 14 patients who received antifungal therapy without additional immunosuppressive therapy, 13 patients survived, and one patient died; among six patients who received antifungal therapy and glucocorticoid or gamma globulin therapy, four patients died; among five patients who did not receive antifungal therapy, all died. In addition, two patients' treatment plan and prognosis are unknown. The study suggests that additional immunosuppressive therapy does not seem to benefit patients with such diseases. In April 2019, a new version of the international guidelines on hemophagocytic syndrome was released, which specifically pointed out that hemophagocytic syndrome caused by infection of intracellular bacteria, such as Mycobacterium tuberculosis, *Listeria*, *Rickettsia*, and so on, often does not need strong immunosuppressive therapy but has a good response to specific anti-infective therapy. The successful treatment of this patient in our hospital also confirms this point. For myelosuppression or even hemophagocytosis caused by *Histoplasma* infection, timely and effective antifungal treatment is the top priority.

References

1. La Rosée Paul, Horne AnnaCarin, Hines Melissa, et al. Recommendations for the management of hemophagocytic lymphohistiocytosis in adults. Blood. 2019. https://doi.org/10.1182/blood.2018894618
2. Histoplasmosis. Centers for Disease Control and Prevention. https://www.cdc.gov/fungal/diseases/histoplasmosis/statistics.html
3. Limper Andrew H, Adenis Antoine, Le Thuy, et al. Fungal infections in HIV/AIDS. Lancet Infect Dis. 2017;17:e334–43.
4. Queiroz-Telles Flavio, Fahal Ahmed Hassan, Falci Diego R, et al. Neglected endemic mycoses. Lancet Infect Dis. 2017;17:e367–77.
5. Kauffman Carol A, Histoplasmosis: a clinical and laboratory update. Clin Microbiol Rev. 2007;20:115–32.
6. Joseph Wheat L, Current diagnosis of histoplasmosis. Trends Microbiol. 2003;11:488–94.
7. Zhou Tingyin, Zhang Qiangqiang, et al. Clinical microbiology: diagnosis and illustrations. 4th ed. Shanghai: Shanghai Scientific & Technical Publishers; 2017.

2.22 Gloom of Gallbladder-Preserving Cholelithotomy: A Case of Liver Abscess Mistaken for Simple *Escherichia coli* Infection

Zhou Xian, Hu Yuekai, Chen Shu, and Huang Yuxian

A 42-year-old man was admitted to the hospital on January 15, 2020, because of "dull pain in the right upper abdomen for 5 months, accompanied by recurrent fever for more than 3 months."

On July 15, 2019, the patient developed persistent dull pain in the right upper abdomen with no obvious inducement, accompanied by fever, without chills, nausea, vomiting, or diarrhea. The highest temperature reached 38.5 °C. He was hospitalized in a local hospital, but the fever and abdominal pain did not improve significantly. On July 22, 2019, he underwent an enhanced MRI in the upper abdomen, which showed cholecystolithiasis, cholecystitis, and multiple hepatic cysts. A laparoscopic gallbladder-preserving cholelithotomy was conducted. After the operation, the symptoms of abdominal pain and fever were relieved. At the same time, anti-infective treatment was given, and the patient was discharged one week later. On August 19, 2019, the patient suffered from dull pain in the right upper abdomen again but without fever. He went to an advanced hospital for further examination. An enhanced CT of the upper abdomen showed plaque shadow in the liver area. It was considered a normal reaction in the recovery period after the operation.

On October 15, 2019, he complained that he had dull pain in his right upper abdomen again, which was more severe than before. Seven days later, the patient developed a fever, and the temperature rose to 38.0 °C. He went to the original hospital again for treatment. An MRI of the upper abdomen showed a liver abscess, and the abscess was small. He was ordered to take oral medication, but the patient's symptoms were not significantly relieved. On November 1, 2019, the patient was hospitalized in another hospital and began to receive anti-infective treatment with cefotaxime for 2 weeks. He was discharged after the fever had subsided. After 3 days of discharge, the patient developed fever with right upper abdominal pain again. During readmission on November 20, 2019, the effect of meropenem, cefoperazone–sulbactam, teicoplanin, or imipenem/cilastatin was not good. During repeated examinations of ultrasound (December 3, December 11, and December 16), the right posterior inferior hepatic lesion was getting bigger. On December 14, 2019, a plain MR scan + an enhanced MR + an MRCP of the upper abdomen showed multiple abnormal signals in the liver and abnormal signals in the right abdominal cavity, which were considered inflammatory lesions with local small abscess formation according to the history and were more severe than before. On December 16, the patient underwent liver puncture and abscess extraction, and 1ml of pus was extracted and sent for culture, which reported *Escherichia coli*. Drug sensitivity test showed that it was sensitive to piperacillin–tazobactam, cefoperazone–sulbactam, cefepime, amikacin, imipenem, meropenem, ertapenem, and tigecycline. After treatment with imipenem and amikacin, the patient still had recurrent fever, dull pain in the right upper abdomen, and fatigue. In the past six months, the patient's body weight has dropped by 20 kg.

2.22.1 Past History and Personal History

The patient had a 1-year history of hypertension. The highest blood pressure was 150/100 mmHg. At the time of admission, valsartan was being taken orally qd intermittently, and the blood pressure was controlled stably. There was a history of smoking for 20 years, with an average of 20 cigarettes per day, and he had quit smoking 8 years before. There was a history of drinking for 15 years, averaging 250 g/day, and six months' abstinence.

2.22.2 Physical Examination on Admission

The patient's mind was clear, and there was an appearance of chronic disease, no abnormal skin and mucosa, and no swelling of the superficial lymph nodes. The abdomen was flat and soft. There were three old scars, about 1cm in length, on the upper abdomen. There was no tenderness in the whole abdomen, the Murphy's sign was negative, and there was no percussion pain in the liver and the kidneys.

2.22.3 Diagnosis and Treatment Process

Blood routine examination after admission showed the following: white blood cell count: 6.34×10^9/L, neutrophil%: 77.2%, ESR: 61 mm/h↑, procalcitonin: 0.11 ng/ml, ferritin: 1752.00 ng/ml, and C-reactive protein: 71.80 mg/l↑. On January 16, 2020, liver MR enhancement showed multiple abnormal signals in the liver with irregular enhancement, combined with the history of infection with abscess formation, involving the adjacent peritoneum (Fig. 2.69). On January 17, 2020, the patient underwent a liver biopsy. Second-generation sequencing of liver abscess puncture tissue was negative, and on January 21, 2020, the surgical and pathological examination showed that the liver puncture specimen showed inflammatory fibrous lesions, and neutrophils and new capillaries formed granulation tissue, which was consistent with the purulent membrane structure. The diagnosis was that, combined with clinical examination, it was consistent with liver abscess.

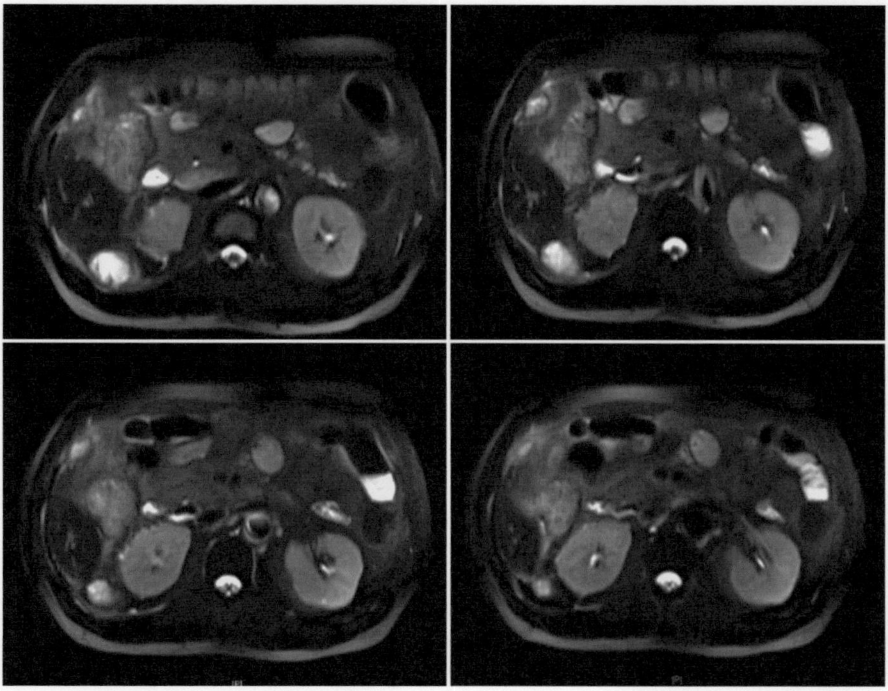

Fig. 2.69 On January 16, 2020, enhanced MR of liver showed round long T1 and long T2 signal shadow, about 12 mm, clear boundary, arterial phase edge enhancement, venous phase, and delayed phase filling enhancement; multiple flaky long T1 and slightly long T2 signal shadow, fuzzy boundary, about 52 × 44 mm, high signal intensity on DWI, irregular enhancement on edge, and honeycomb shape; and abnormal enhancement on peritoneum after enhancement

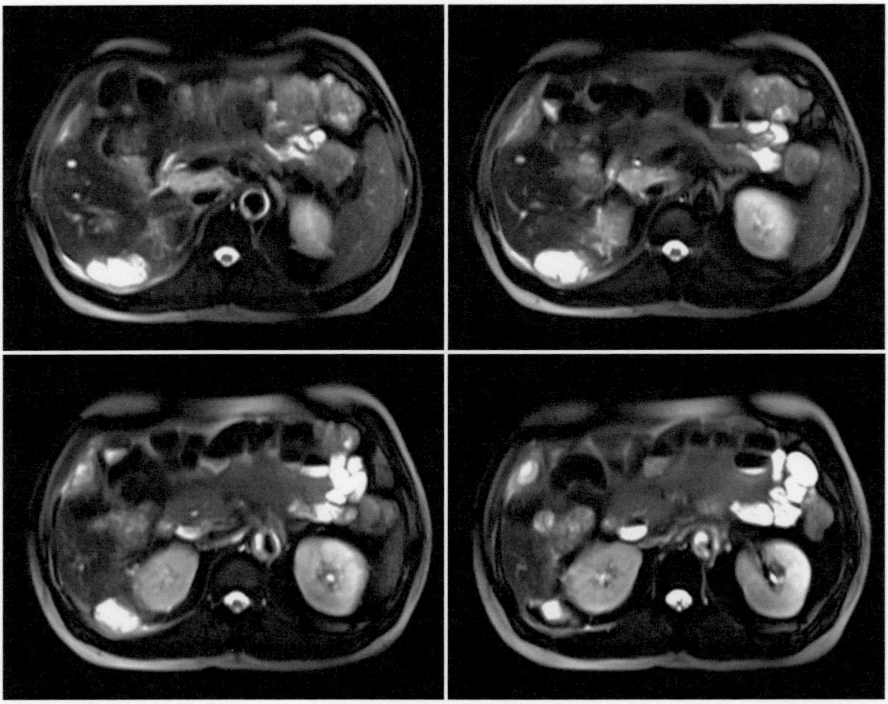

Fig. 2.70 On February 1, 2020, MR enhancement of liver: Round-like long T1 and long T2 signal shadow, about 12 mm, clear boundary, arterial phase edge enhancement, venous phase, and delayed phase filling enhancement were seen in liver IV segment; multiple flaky long T1 and slightly long T2 signal shadow, fuzzy boundary, about 52 × 44 mm, high signal on DWI, irregular edge enhancement, and honeycomb shape were seen after enhancement; and abnormal enhancement foci were found in adjacent peritoneum after enhancement. It was similar to that of January 16, 2020

Considering the pus culture results of *E. coli* in another hospital, results of drug sensitivity, and previous medication history, we gave the patient anti-infective treatment consisting of piperacillin–tazobactam, metronidazole, and amikacin. After the anti-infective treatment, the peak temperature gradually decreased, and although there were still several temperature rises during the period, they were mainly low-to-moderate fever. The temperature began to stabilize on January 29, and the liver MR enhancement was reexamined on February 1 (see Fig. 2.70). It was similar to that of January 16, 2020.

On February 3, the patient had a fever again without any obvious inducement, and the peak value increased gradually. On February 7, the patient had a fever twice, and the highest temperature reached 39.1 °C (see Fig. 2.71).

On February 8, cefoperazone–sulbactam 3 g q8h for antibacterial treatment was used, and the peak temperature and frequency of fever were both lower than before. On February 10, the results of the upper abdominal enhanced CT returned (see

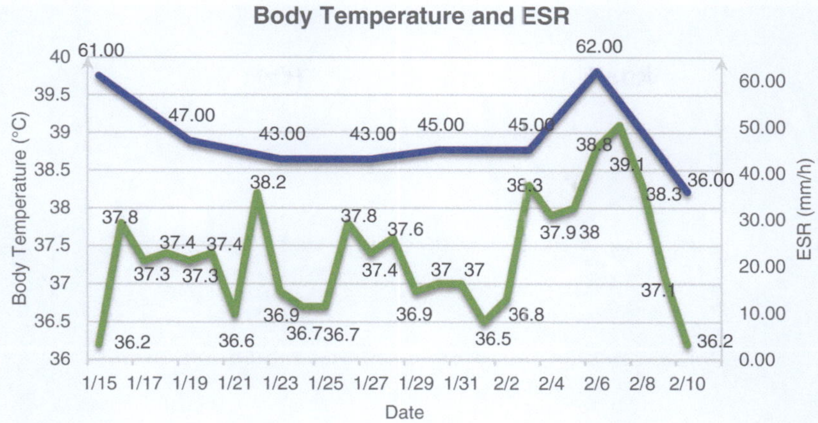

Fig. 2.71 From admission to February 10, the trend of peak body temperature and erythrocyte sedimentation rate was basically the same

Fig. 2.72). After consulting with the general surgery department, it was suggested that after the application of sulbactam, the abdominal CT should be reexamined to observe the size of the lesion and the body temperature. If the effect of medical treatment was not good, drainage of the abscess could be considered. Fever did not recur after continuing with the anti-infective treatment with cefoperazone–sulbactam. However, the abdominal MRI examination on March 3 showed no significant improvement compared with the previous lesions (see Fig. 2.73). During the period of repeated ultrasound examination, there was no significant reduction of the lesions (see Table 2.8) either.

The core idea of this part is completely correct and in line with clinical logic - the typical manifestation of effective anti-infection treatment for liver abscess is reduction in body temperature + shrinkage of the lesion. However, the patient's normal body temperature for 3 weeks but no change in the size of the lesion - this situation where the changes in body temperature and lesion size are not synchronized does indeed not conform to the conventional expectations for effective anti-infection treatment of liver abscess. This leads to the judgment of be alert for other special factors, and the logical chain is complete and in line with medical common sense. As expected, the professor of surgery directly considered that the gallbladder was dysfunctional and gallstones had fallen into the liver, resulting in an abscess and delayed healing. On March 5, after the patient was transferred to the general surgery department, he underwent a special segmental hepatectomy, cholecystectomy, and liver abscess incision and drainage under general anesthesia. During the operation, there was a hard mass in the liver III and IVB segments, about 4 cm in diameter, and a hard mass in the liver and kidney crypt, about 4 cm in diameter. After incision, a large amount of pus gushed out from the mass, and several hard objects similar to gallstones were seen in the mass. The abscess cavity was fully opened. Most of the hard masses in segments III and IVB of the liver were removed, and a large amount of pus and necrotic tissue were also seen in the mass (see Fig. 2.74). On March 12,

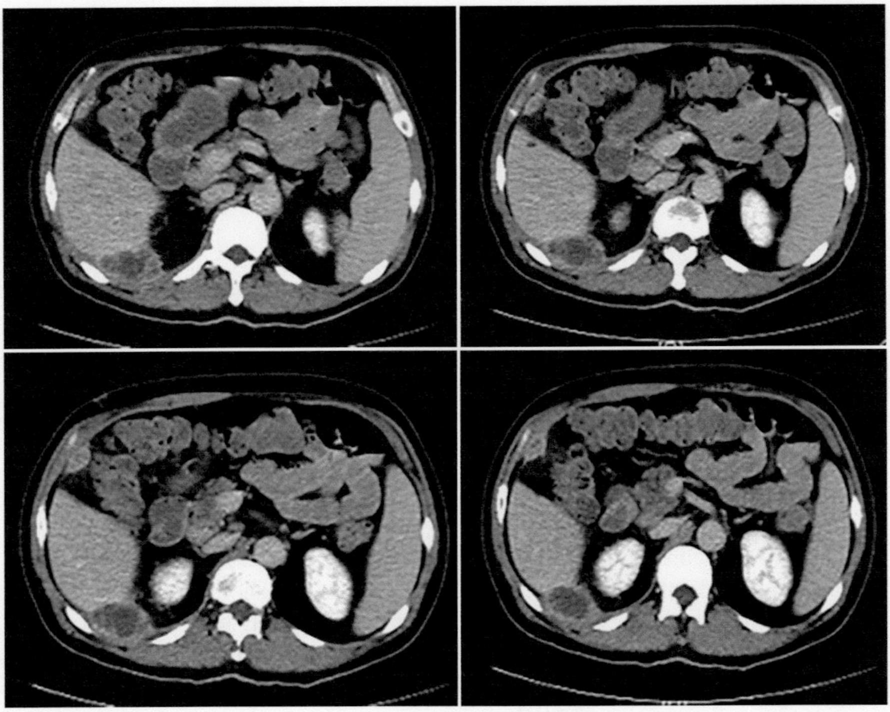

Fig. 2.72 On February 10, 2020, CT enhancement of the upper abdomen showed that the right liver had leaf-like low density, the size was about 6.4 × 34.2 cm, and the CT value was about 38 hu. During the arterial phase of the enhanced scan, the lesions showed circular enhancement, with an enhancement halo around and an unclear edge. A mass-like low-density shadow could be seen behind the S6 segment of the liver (an abscess between the liver and the kidney could be formed), and the edge was clear. After enhanced scan, the lesions showed circular enhancement, the CT value was about 19 hu, and the size was about 4.7 × 3.2 cm. A small, round, and slightly low-density shadow was seen in the S4 segment of the liver, which was about 1cm in diameter

postoperative pathology showed that there were many acute and chronic inflammatory cell infiltrations in the liver tissue, accompanied by microabscess formation, and gallstones were seen in the focal area. Combined with the clinical history, it was considered to be a liver abscess and chronic cholecystitis. Immunohistochemical results showed the following: LCA: (scattered +), CD68: (scattered +), CD1a: (−), S100: (−), CK8: (+), HBsAg: (−), GPC-3: (−), and special staining results: pas: (−), acid-fast: (−), and silver (−). The patient continued to be treated with cefoperazone–sulbactam after the operation. Fever occurred after the operation, which was considered to be absorption fever. The patient's temperature continued to be normal from March 13. CT (see Fig. 2.75), and an MRI reexamination after the surgery showed that the lesions were smaller than before. He was discharged from the hospital on April 7. After discharge, he continued to be treated with faropenem 0.1 g

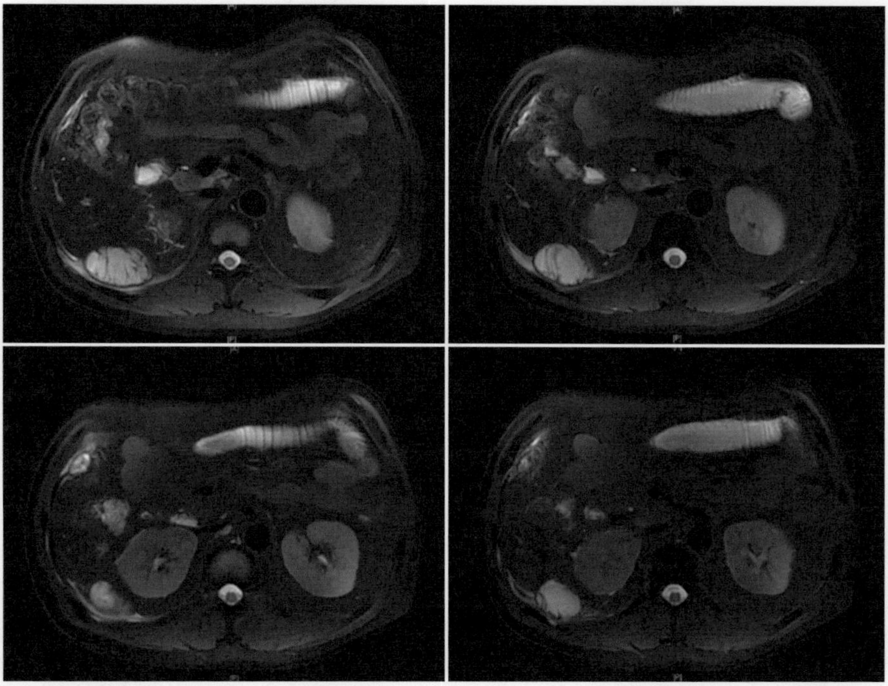

Fig. 2.73 MR enhancement of the upper abdomen on March 3, 2020: round-like long T1 and long T2 signal shadow, about 12 mm, with clear boundary, edge enhancement in arterial phase, filling enhancement in venous phase, and delayed phase and multiple flaky long T1 and slightly long T2 signal shadow, with fuzzy boundary, about 52 × 44 mm in large range, high signal on DWI, and irregular edge enhancement in honeycomb shape after enhancement

TID + levofloxacin 0.5 g QD orally. No fever occurred again. On April 23, the patient's ultrasound at the local hospital showed that the abscess had further reduced.

2.22.4 Discussion

The diagnosis and treatment for liver abscess is a basic skill needed for infectious disease doctors. After finding out the inducement, etiological basis, and predisposing factors of the host and confirming the size and location of the abscess, there is often a clear diagnosis and treatment plan, and most of them can get a good prognosis. However, when the anti-infective treatment effect is not good, we need to consider whether the choice of anti-infective drugs is correct and reasonable; whether there are other factors leading to incomplete disease recovery, such as: 1) Liver cancer that presents with normal body temperature after anti-infective treatment (a manifestation similar to liver abscess); 2) Concomitant liver abscess and liver cancer (i.e., both lesions exist simultaneously); multiple bacterial infections; and

Table 2.8 Comparison of the lesion range of MRI and B-ultrasound

Date	Examination	The left lateral lobe of the liver and near the surface of the liver	Right posterior lobe of the liver and close to the diaphragm	Right posterior lobe of the liver	Near the second porta hepatis	The biggest lesion
01.16	Enhanced MR		52 × 44			12
02.01	Enhanced MR		52 × 44			12
03.03	Enhanced MR		52 × 44			12
01.31	Ultrasound	48 × 37	59 × 47		18 × 17	12
02.12	Ultrasound	66 × 44	76 × 26	16 × 11	15 × 17, 11 × 10	14 × 12
02.18	Ultrasound	57 × 49	53 × 32	15 × 11	32 × 17	14 × 11
02.24	Ultrasound	30 × 32	60 × 48		17 × 16	12
03.02	Ultrasound	33 × 37	76 × 40		17 × 16	12

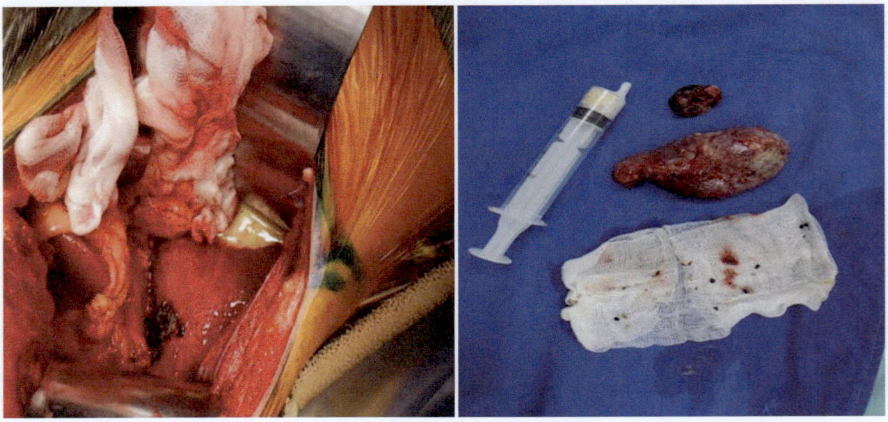

Fig. 2.74 Special segment hepatectomy, cholecystectomy, and incision and drainage of liver abscess under general anesthesia on March 9, 2020

special etiology, which lead to the diagnosis and treatment being not so smooth. In this state, we need to patiently look for the special features of each patient. For example, this patient had multiple liver abscesses after cholecystolithotomy. High-level specialist consultation and cooperation played an important role in the diagnosis and treatment of this patient. At the same time, although we did not find many similar cases in the literature search, from the mechanism point of view, cholecystolithotomy with gallbladder preservation may have led to cholecystolithiasis that could not be completely removed, so it may have been an important inducement of liver abscess associated with biliary factors. Stricter control of indications and contraindications of gallbladder-preserving cholecystolithotomy is needed.

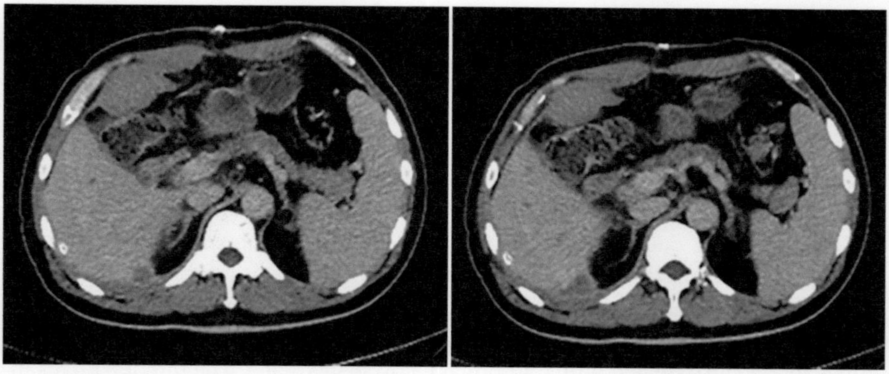

Fig. 2.75 On March 18, CT enhancement of the upper abdomen: postoperative changes of liver, local structural disorder, drainage tube visible. Encapsulated effusion and pneumatosis can be seen in the right abdominal cavity. There were multiple round-like low-density shadows in the residual liver, and no obvious enhancement was found after enhancement, with the maximum of 12 mm

References

1. He ZH, Kou ZQ, Xu AQ. Humanpapillomavirus infection and vaccination. Zhonghuayufangyixuezazhi [Chinesejournalofpreventivemedicine]. 2018; 52(1):106.
2. Sanford JP. The Sanford guide to antimicrobial therapy 2016[M]. 46 th ed. Sperryville: Antimicrobial Therapy Inc.; 2016. p. 114–5.BE
3. Zhang SY, Chen YX. Progress in diagnosis and treatment of pyogenic Iiver abscess [J]. J Clin Hepatol. 2018; 34(7):1577–80. (in Chinese).
4. Luo CQ, Luo F, Progress in diagnosis and treatment of bacterial hepatic abscess [J]. World Latest Med Information (Electronic Version). 2019;19(45):76–7.
5. Yu SL, Weng XH. Antimicrobjal therapy in adult patients with bacterial Iiver abscess [J]. J Pract Hepatol. 2015;18(4):337–9. (in Chinese).
6. Zhang Liangliang, Tuo Hongfang, Wen Junye, et al. A case of liver abscess caused by retained gallbladder stones in the abdominal cavity [J]. Chin J Gen Surg. 2018;33(2):169.

2.23 What Is the Cause of Her Superinfection with Disseminated *Talaromyces marneffei* and *Nontuberculous mycobacteria*?

Zheng Jianming, Lin Siran, Liang Jun, Li Li, Liu Hong, Zhong Wen, Shao Lingyun, and Zhang Wenhong

On November 14, 2016, a 38-year-old woman presented to our institution with intermittent fever, cough, rash, and lymphadenopathy for more than 2 years.

On July 15, 2016, the patient developed a cough with fever, and the temperature was between 37.5 °C and 38.5 °C. On August 12, 2016, chest CT showed chronic inflammation or fibrosis in the lower lobe of bilateral lungs; inflammatory nodules, possibly presented in the upper lobe of the left lung, with pleural thickening, adhesion, and partial calcification on both sides; and a small amount of pericardial effusion. Fiberoptic bronchoscopy showed bronchitis in the right middle and lower lobes and bronchial stenosis in the right middle and lower lobes. Bronchoalveolar lavage fluid smear and culture were negative, but the tuberculin skin test (TST) was positive. Antituberculosis treatment (HRZE) was started on August 17. After that, body temperature, cough, and chest CT were improved. She was discharged from the hospital on September 25 and continued taking oral antituberculosis drugs.

On October 30, 2016, she developed swelling and pain in the right neck, followed by fever, cough, and sore throat. She was then treated with piperacillin and amikacin, and also treated with traditional Chinese medicine. The throat pain disappeared, and the neck mass subsided. However, on November 20, she developed herpes on the face, hard nodules with tenderness on both lower limbs, and painful erythema on both knees. The color ultrasound of superficial lymph nodes suggested the following: "lymph nodes in the right neck were slightly swollen and the lymph nodes in the left neck, bilateral inguinal area and bilateral axillary were visible, no obvious enlarged lymph nodes were found on the bilateral clavicle." The dermatologist considered "pustular psoriasis," and she stopped antituberculosis drugs on November 25. Two days later, the rash gradually subsided, and the body temperature was normal. She was discharged.

On December 10, there was swelling and pain in the right neck, sore throat, fever, joint pain in the lower limbs, and difficulty in walking. On February 11, 2017, there were blisters on her right shoulder and right upper limb, with a white blood cell count of 21.94×10^9/L, neutrophil percentage of 78.5%, CRP of 133 mg/L, and ESR of 10 mm/h. She then experienced repeated clinical visits in the dermatological department and gained previous diagnoses of "Sweet syndrome," "Acute febrile neutrophilic dermatosis," "Herpes zoster," "pustular psoriasis," and "drug hypersensitivity syndrome." She had been given compound glycyrrhizin tablets, acitretin capsules, and methylprednisolone (20 mg qd), and her skin rash subsided.

On June 8, 2017, she developed a cough and chest pain and was diagnosed with pneumonia. She was treated with piperacillin, levofloxacin, cefoperazone, and sulbactam, but the effect was poor. Lymph node biopsy was performed on September 8, and *Nontuberculous mycobacteria* was cultured from the medium for fungi, which was identified as *Mycobacterium chelonae (M. chelonae)/Mycobacterium abscessus (M. abscessus)*. On January 16, 2018, cefoxitin, clarithromycin, and moxifloxacin were given as a triple therapy. On February 7, she stopped the drugs due to the possibility of drug fever, and then clarithromycin, moxifloxacin, and cefoxitin were added in turn. The dosage of cefoxitin was adjusted from 12 g to 8 g, and there was no recurrent fever. After getting discharged on June 15, she continued to take oral clarithromycin and moxifloxacin. The cervical lymph nodes did not get enlarged, and the inguinal lymph nodes shrank. The results of drug sensitivity were as follows: amikacin (sensitive), azithromycin (sensitive), clofazimine (sensitive), moxifloxacin (resistant), clarithromycin (resistant), doxycycline (resistant), and ethambutol (resistant).

On October 23, 2018, she visited a hospital in Beijing and underwent a left cervical lymph node biopsy, which showed a little acute and chronic inflammation of the fibrous tissue. The molecular pathology showed the following: TB-DNA (−), *Mycobacterium* gene detection (−), and special staining results: pas (−) and acid-fast staining (−). Thus, clarithromycin and moxifloxacin were stopped, but the cervical lymph node of the patient progressively enlarged after stopping the drugs. Miliary herpes appeared again on the whole body. On the morning of October 27, the patient suddenly developed right limb weakness and ambiguous speech, fell out of bed, and had a clear mind. After 10 min, symptoms were relieved. After 1 h, the above symptoms appeared again, lasting for about 10 min. Head MRI (plain scan and DWI) suggested cerebral infarction in the left basal ganglia and showed a mass or tumor penetrated through the right parietal bone. Enhanced CT of the head showed that the bone resorption, destruction of the right parietal bone, and the formation of surrounding soft tissue mass, and inflammatory granuloma or tumor lesions were considered (Figs. 2.76 and 2.77). During hospitalization, a cough occurred, and lung CT showed a lower bronchial mass. Pathological biopsy of that mass suggested granulomatous inflammation. Under the microscope, inflammatory necrosis and multinucleated giant cell reaction were found. No epithelioid cells were found. Acid-fast staining showed no acid-fast bacilli. The lower end of the trachea mass was sent for *Mycobacterium* species identification, and the result was negative. For further diagnosis and treatment, the patient was admitted to our department.

2.23.1 Past Medical History

She was a hepatitis B virus carrier, and no antiviral treatment was given.

2.23.2 Physical Examination

On the right side of the neck, along the lateral side of the sternocleidomastoid muscle and supraclavicular fossa, there were two previous surgical scars (10 cm and 7 cm). The whole body was scattered with miliary herpes, with a thick wall, and the top of the herpes was transparent, mainly in both lower limbs and hands (Fig. 2.76). A 4 cm × 4-cm subcutaneous mass could be seen at the top of the right side, which was soft and had a fluctuating feeling when touched, with slight tenderness on the posterolateral wall. Bilateral retroauricular, cervical, submaxillary, submental, and inguinal lymph nodes had a number of broad bean–like and soybean-like enlarged lymph nodes, which were tough in quality, with an acceptable range of motion, and without adhesion to surrounding tissues. There was no redness, swelling, or wave

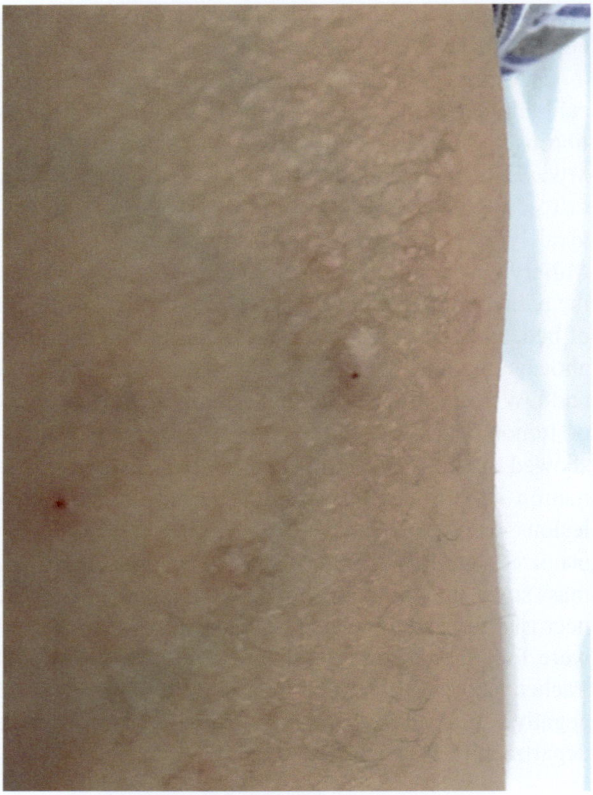

Fig. 2.76 Manifestations of skin rash on the extremities

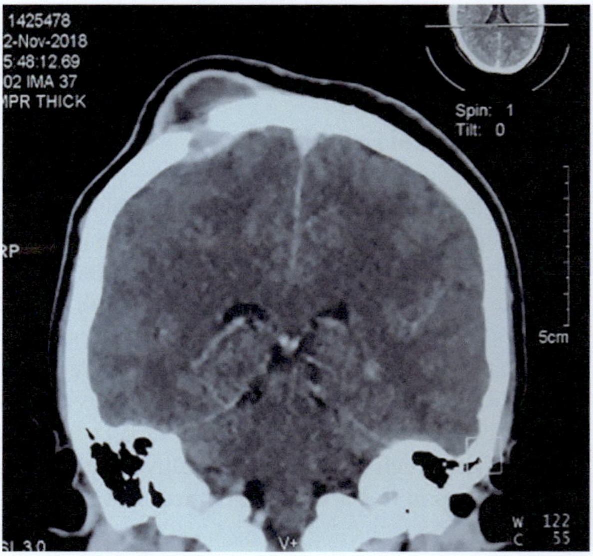

Fig. 2.77 Head CT (November 2, 2018): Bone destruction and resorption of the right parietal bone, with associated formation of a surrounding soft tissue mass. Diagnostic considerations: Is it an inflammatory granuloma? Or a neoplastic lesion?

motion on the surrounding skin. The respiratory sounds of both lungs were clear, and dry or wet rales were not heard. The abdomen was flat, soft, and without any tenderness.

2.23.3 Assessment and Treatment Plan

The culture of the patient's lymph node from the second biopsy showed *Nontuberculous mycobacteria* (NTM) and was identified as a fast-growing *M. chelonae*/*M. abscessus*. After treatment with cefoxitin, clarithromycin, and moxifloxacin in a local hospital, the patient's temperature became normal, and the lymph nodes shrank. Clarithromycin and moxifloxacin were stopped half a month before admission. After stopping the treatment, the cervical lymph nodes of the patient progressively enlarged, and scattered miliary herpes appeared again on the skin of the patient. Her temperature was 37.4–37.8 °C, which was considered a result of the uncontrolled NTM infection caused by the discontinuation of the anti-NTM drug treatment. Therefore, the patient was given anti-infective treatment: imipenem/cilastatin 1 g q8h (November 15–December 13) + amikacin 0.6 g qd (November 15–December 18) + azithromycin 0.5 g qd (November 15). The patient's temperature returned to normal 11 days later (Fig. 2.78). On November 16, after a general surgery consultation, a right neck lymph node biopsy was performed. The pathological report of the lymph node showed suppurative inflammatory fibrosis. After lymphoid tissue culture, *Talaromyces marneffei* was detected. The drug sensitivity test showed that the bacteria were sensitive to amphotericin B, itraconazole, voriconazole, flucytosine, and other drugs. On November 22, the pus of the patient's scalp mass was extracted and put into the *Mycobacterium* blood culture bottle (considering that the patient may have been infected by a special pathogen, the *Mycobacterium* blood culture bottle could cultivate both *Mycobacterium* and fungi). After 12 days, a positive result was reported, and the culture result showed *Talaromyces marneffei* (Figs. 2.79 and 2.80). The patient's lymphadenopathy and scalp mass were caused by a *Talaromyces marneffei* infection. On December 5, itraconazole 250 mg IVGTT (on the first day and on the second day: q12h, and from the third day: qd) was added for antifungal treatment. In the second week after the addition of antifungal drugs, the general condition of the patient improved, and the pain in the wrist joints and the knee joints was relieved. Combined with the above examination results and treatment process, the patient was diagnosed with "disseminated *Nontuberculous mycobacteria* infection and disseminated *Talaromyces marneffei* infection."

Further, the detection of IFN-γ antibody in the peripheral blood showed that the patient's plasma IFN-γ antibody was positive (OD value >4). The patient had "disseminated *Nontuberculous mycobacteria* infection and disseminated *Talaromyces marneffei* infection," and the etiology of the disease was the existence of an autoantibody to IFN-γ, which has been reported to be associated with adult-onset immunodeficiency. The anti-infective treatment was adjusted as follows: azithromycin + cefoxitin against *Nontuberculous mycobacteria* and amphotericin B against

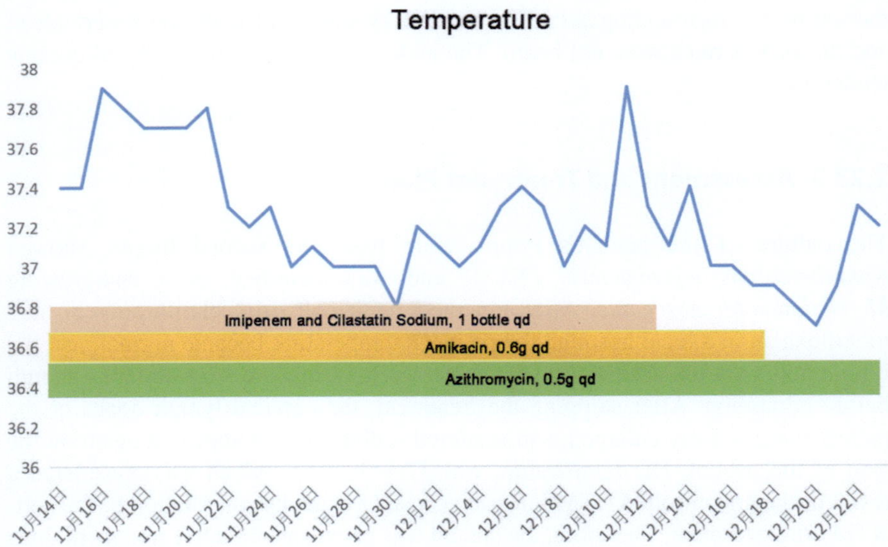

Fig. 2.78 Changes in body temperature during the recovery of anti-NTM drugs after admission

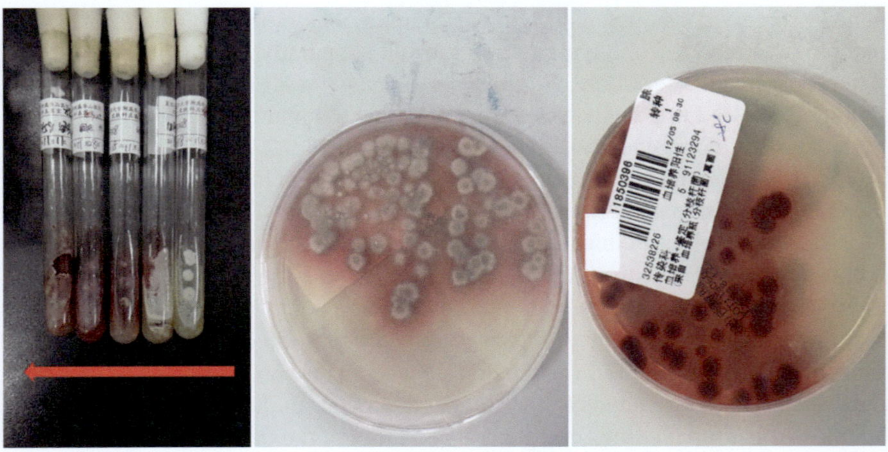

Fig. 2.79 Positive results of lymph node biopsy and head mass pus culture. The red arrow refers to the extension of culture time and the change of strain color. The pathogen of *Talaromyces marneffei* was *Talaromyces* in a 25 °C environment. After 48 h of culture, the colony size was 1–3 mm, and it was gray-white. After 72 h, the colony increased rapidly and turned red. The color of the colony was further deepened, and it was wine-like

Talaromyces marneffei. On December 25, 2018, the patient was transferred back to the local hospital for further treatment. The initial dosage of amphotericin B was 10 mg, increased by 5 mg every day, and maintained at 40 mg. On January 13, 2019, amphotericin B was stopped (the cumulative dosage was 695 mg), and she was given voriconazole 200 mg bid as sequential therapy. The azithromycin + cefoxitin

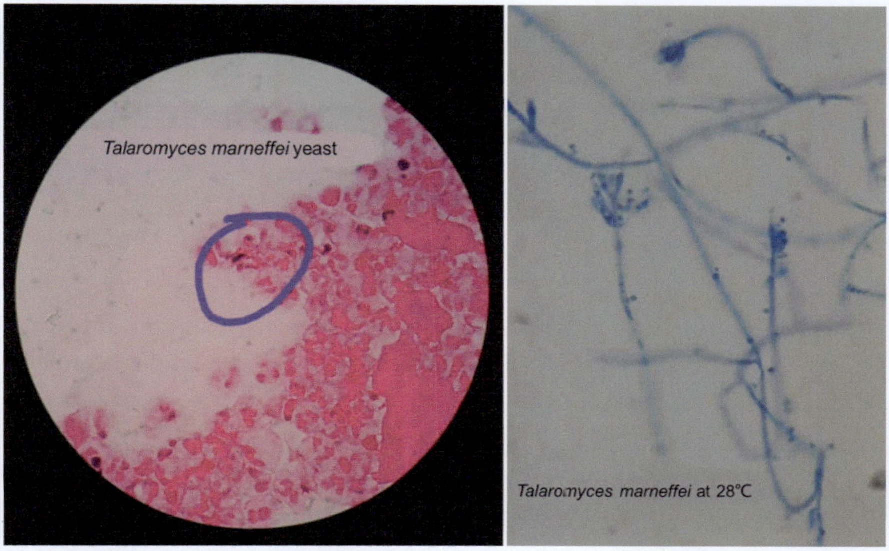

Fig. 2.80 Microscopic morphology of *Talaromyces marneffei*

for anti-NTM treatment was maintained. Her condition gradually improved. Azithromycin and cefoxitin were stopped in April, and itraconazole 20ml bid orally was taken till July 10.

From August to October 2019, the patient had repeated fever with cough and expectoration again, with the highest temperature of 39.7 °C. On October 18, she was admitted to our hospital again. It was considered that the recurrence of NTM could not be excluded. On October 23, she was additionally treated with imipenem/cilastatin 1 g q8h + azithromycin 0.5 g qd for empirical anti-NTM treatment, and on October 24, she underwent a left neck lymph node biopsy. Pathological results showed reactive hyperplasia of lymph tissue, with local fibrous hyperplasia. After treatment, the patient's body temperature gradually dropped to normal, and her cough improved significantly. Considering that the patient's anti-IFN-γ autoantibody was positive, which could lead to cell-mediated immune deficiency and repeated opportunistic bacterial infection, on November 12, the patient was treated with 20 g of immunoglobulin per day for 3 days to block anti-IFN-γ antibody. Anti-IFN-γ antibody titer was measured the next day. However, it was found that the plasma anti-IFN-γ antibody titer had no significant decrease before and after treatment (Table 2.9). On November 13, sputum culture came back *Mycobacterium* positive, and on November 14, blood culture also suggested *Mycobacterium*, which was later identified as *Mycobacterium saskatchewanense*. Considering the patient's serious condition, linezolid 600 mg qd was added to strengthen the anti-NTM treatment on November 20.

The final anti-infective treatment included voriconazole 200 mg bid for antifungal therapy and imipenem/cilastatin 1 g q8h + azithromycin 500 mg qd + linezolid 600 mg qd for anti-NTM treatment. After intravenous treatment for 2 months, the

Table 2.9 Changes of IFN-γ antibody in plasma of patients before and after immunoglobulin pulse therapy

Time	OD value of IFN-γ autoantibody by ELISA
Before immunoglobulin pulse therapy	3.32
One day after immunoglobulin pulse therapy	3.43

patient was discharged on December 24, 2019. At present, the patient is still on oral medication, with her condition stable and leading a normal life. Continuous follow-up is necessary.

2.23.4 Comments

The etiology of the fever of unknown origin for this patient was confirmed as an infection, and the pathogens were NTM and *Talaromyces marneffei*, which were not only rare pathogens but also opportunistic pathogens. We know that patients with opportunistic infections usually have the potential factors of immune deficiency. This patient had a variety of opportunistic infectious pathogens at the same time, and they had disseminated manifestations, which was rare. This required us to develop an anti-infective schedule while carefully looking for the reason for immune deficiency. The patient seemed to have no obvious immune deficiency, so we needed to find out the causes behind the seemingly "normal immunity."

A study published in *The New England Journal of Medicine* in 2012 showed that 81% of patients with disseminated NTM had high titers of anti-interferon-γ autoantibodies. Because IFN-γ is an important cytokine against intracellular pathogens, patients with anti-IFN-γ autoantibodies are prone to infections caused by intracellular parasitic bacteria, including Mycobacterium *(MTB and NTM), Listeria, Salmonella, Histoplasma, Burkholderia pseudomallei,* and *Talaromyces marneffei*, which lead to disseminated infections. In addition, patients with anti-IFN-γ autoantibodies are more likely to have a reactivation of subcutaneous and diffuse varicella zoster. Among the reactive dermatoses associated with the antibody, neutrophilic dermatosis was the most common, followed by erythema nodosum, pustular psoriasis, and rash pustulosis. So far, the reported patients with anti-IFN-γ autoantibodies were previously healthy adults, most of whom were Asian-born. This shows that the distribution of the antibody has a certain regional specificity.

According to the literature, we found a factor rarely recognized in the past: positive anti-IFN-γ autoantibody; the existence of anti-IFN-γ autoantibody in the patient may have been the reason why the patient was infected with a variety of opportunistic infectious pathogens. Infection in patients with immunodeficiency is often difficult to cure, and long-term maintenance treatment is needed to reduce recurrence. There are still many problems to be solved regarding how to correct the immune deficiency. Immunoglobulin was tried to be used to neutralize the autoantibodies in the patient, but the effect was not good. Gene editing or monoclonal antibodies against specific autoantibodies may be the future treatment. But in the absence of an effective way to correct this immune deficiency, the focus of treatment is to carry out the corresponding antibacterial treatment for the existing infection. Maintenance treatment may be a feasible scheme to keep the patient's condition stable.

References

1. Wonekulab P, Wipasa J, Chaiwarith R, et al. Autoantilbody to interferon-gamma associated with adult-onset immunodeficiency innon-HIV individuals in Northemn Thailand. PLoS One. 2013;8(9):e76371.
2. Kampman B, Hemingway C, Stephens A, et al. Acquired predisposition to mycobacterial disease due to autoantibodies to lFN.2gamma.J Clin Invest. 2005;115(9):2480–8.
3. Browne SK. Anticytokine autoantibody-associated immunodeficiency. Anmu Rev lmmunol. 2014;32(1):635–57.
4. Browne SK, Burbelo PD, Chetchotisakd P, et al. Adult-onset immunodeficiency in Thailand and Taiwan. N Engl J Med. 2012;367(8):725–34.
5. Koizumi Y, Sakagami T, Nishiyama N, et al. Rituximab restores lFN-gamma-STAT1 fumction and ameliorates disseminatedmycobacterium avium infection in a patient with anti-interferon-gamma autoantilbody. J Clin Immunol. 2017;37(7):644–9.
6. Chan JF, Lau SK, Yuen KY, et al. Talaromyces (Penicilium) mareffei infection in non-HlV.infected patients. Emerg Microbes Infect. 2016;5(3):e19.
7. Kawila R, Charwarith R, Supparatpinyo K, Clinical and laboratory characteristics of penicilliosis mammeftei among patients witland without HlV infection in Northem Thailand: a retrospective study. BlC Infect Dis. 2013;13:464.
8. Ning C, Lai J, Wei W, et al. Accuracy of rapid diagnosis of Talaromyces mamefei: a systematic review and meta-analysis. PLoS One. 2018;13(4):e195569.
9. Zhu Y M. Ai J W, Xu B, et al. Rapid and precise diagnosis of disseminated T. mamefrei infection assisted by high-throughpusequencing of multifarious specimens in a HlV-negative patient: a case report. BMC Infect Dis. 2018;18(1):379.
10. Kaplan JE, Benson C, Holmes KK, et al. Guidelines for prevention and treatment of opportuistic infections in HIV-infectedadults and adolescents: recommendations fiom CDc, the National Institutes of Health, and the HV Medicine Association of theInfectious Diseases Society of Americal. MMWR Recomm Rep. 2009;58(RR-4):1-207.E1–4.

2.24 Left Atrial Myxoma Complicated with Subacute Bacterial Endocarditis

Chen Mingquan and Huang Yuxian

A 38-year-old male complaining of a two-month history of recurrent fever was admitted to our hospital. He had developed fevers (temperature as high as 39.6 °C), chills, and general malaise without any obvious predisposing causes. The local clinic gave supportive therapy for the presumed common cold, but he showed no improvement. Two weeks later, he visited another hospital, where the blood routine showed WBC of 9.67×10^9/L and neutrophils of 74.81%. Bone marrow examination was normal; multiple blood cultures were negative. The antibiotic therapy consisting of cefmetazole and levofloxacin failed, while ibuprofen was effective for the fever. The patient had thus been taking ibuprofen for three weeks. However, he had suffered from consistent low-grade fevers and continual fatigue in the past two weeks, so he presented to our hospital for further diagnosis and treatment.

During the past two months, he had lost 10 kg. His medical history was notable for hepatitis B virus infection and fatty liver disease.

2.24.1 Physical Examination

The patient had a mildly anemic face. No petechiae or ecchymoses in the mucous membrane of the skin were observed all over the body. No finger clubbing was observed. No lymphadenectasis was palpable in the superficial lymph nodes in the cervix and supraclavicular regions. The breath sounds of both lungs were clear. The heart boundary was not big; the heart rhythm was regular (HR = 100 bpm); the cardiac sound was dull and distant; no murmur or pericardial friction sound was auscultated in each auscultatory valve area, seated or supine. The abdomen was soft, without tenderness or rebound tenderness. The liver and spleen were not palpable under the costal margins; the hepatic region was normal; the hepatic and splenic regions were not sensitive to percussion. No abnormality was observed in the nervous system.

2.24.2 Diagnosis and Treatment Procedure

On his first day of hospitalization, the patient reported hyperpyrexia (as high as 39.6 °C), chills, and tachycardia (HR = 106 bpm). His skin was red and moist without any complaint of pruritus; no lymphadenectasis was palpable in the superficial lymph nodes all over the body; the cardiac sound was dull, without murmur or pericardial friction sound. The blood routine suggested a continuing decrease in hemoglobin. Neither the ultrasound nor the pulmonary CT reported obvious lymphadenectasis. With all of the medications terminated, the patient received mechanical cooling methods. A few hours later, the clinical laboratory reported that the blood culture had yielded gram-positive bacteria. Taking the clinical manifestation and the repeated blood culture tests into consideration, the patient was diagnosed with gram-positive bacteremia.

Gram-positive bacteremia is mostly caused by *Staphylococcus*, *Streptococcus*, and *Enterococcus*. These bacteria normally enter the bloodstream through the skin, oral cavity, respiratory tract, and gastrointestinal tract. Since our patient had anemia and tachycardia, regardless of the body temperature, cardiogenic bacteremia was the most likely. Bacteria with relatively low virulence had to be considered, as he had low-grade fevers during the later course of the disease. After further inquiry, the patient recalled pain in the right dorsal pedis without redness or swelling four months ago, which recovered spontaneously 4–5 days later. Considering the connection between the pain and potential embolism, we conducted echocardiography. The echo reported left atrial and ventricular enlargement, a heterogeneous mobile mass that was consistent with the left atrial myxoma, and aortic root dilation without vegetation. The repeated blood cultures suggested *Streptococcus gordonii*. The diagnosis of left atrial myxoma complicated with subacute bacterial endocarditis was made. *S. gordonii* is an opportunistic pathogen belonging to *Viridans streptococci* (also known as oral *Streptococcus*), which initially colonizes in the periodontal environment. *S. gordonii* can cause bacterial endocarditis. It exhibits resistance to erythromycin and clindamycin but is sensitive to penicillin, cephalosporin, and vancomycin. The busy work, frequent tiredness, and occasional oral ulcer history might assist the bacteria to gain access systemically.

We prescribed vancomycin 1.0 q12h, and the repeated blood culture three days later came out negative. However, the low-grade fever remained, which indicated an inflammatory reaction induced by atrial myxoma. Myxoma-related fever is associated with IL-6 released from the tumor. Liu et al. reported fever as the primary symptom in 29.2% of atrial myxoma patients. The optimal therapy for endocarditis based on atrial myxoma has not been decided. Early diagnosis and surgical intervention can effectively prevent cardiovascular events and death caused by embolus dislodgment and artery thrombosis. While the antibiotic therapy was routinely continued, the cardiothoracic surgical team was consulted. The patient eventually underwent atrial tumor excision.

The coronary artery computed tomography angiography (CTA) and echocardiogram before the surgery confirmed left atrial myxoma and aortic root dilation (39 mm). The patient underwent bicuspid replacement and left atrial myxoma excision. The exploration during the surgery witnessed the myxoma rooted in the inferior part of the atrial septum (size about 5cm × 3cm × 3cm), a thickened mitral valve, and multiple vegetations in the valve. The pathological biopsy revealed left atrial myxoma, complicated with angiogenesis, hemorrhage, and inflammatory cell infiltration, and the chronic inflammation of the mitral valve, complicated with abscess. Our patient became afebrile three days after the surgery. He completed the antibiotic therapy and remained asymptomatic during the four-week follow-up (Fig. 2.81).

2.24.3 Comments

The patient had an underlying left atrial myxoma complicated with endocarditis, and the confusing symptoms delayed a definitive diagnosis for over one month. Apart from meticulous thinking, the combination of blood culture results and echocardiogram findings played a significant role in the diagnosis.

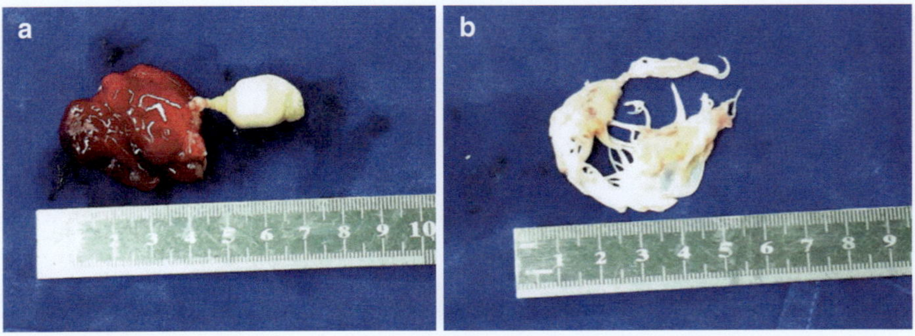

Fig. 2.81 (**a** and **b**) The myxoma specimen from the surgery, sized about 5cm × 3cm × 3cm, rooted in the inferior of the atrial septum; thickened mitral valve; and multiple vegetations

Atrial myxoma is one of the most common primary cardiac benign tumors, typically presenting as the triad of vascular obstruction, embolic disease, and constitutional symptoms. The perplexity of clinical manifestations can predispose to misdiagnosis, the rate of which can be as high as 70%. As far as we are concerned, health care providers lack knowledge of clinical features, and the insensitivity to minor presentations, such as temporary vessel occlusion and embolism, has led to misdiagnosis. In the present case, the history of dorsal pedis pain provided us with an important clue. Clinicians should avoid complete reliance on laboratory testing.

The patient's symptoms started with fever, and empiric antibiotics showed little effect, which predisposed to the likelihood of noninfectious diseases. The febrile changes during the disease progression suggested underlying organic disease, complicated by infections. The blood samples should be sent for repeated cultures before antibiotic administration. If necessary, the antibiotics can be suspended for several days before blood culture, and the sample amount can be mildly increased to obtain a positive yield. The optimal timing for taking a sample is undetermined because of its variability according to the presentations.

Last but not least, the recurrent fever led to the neglect of operating echocardiogram and delayed diagnosis. An echocardiogram is the recommended diagnostic method for endocardial myxoma because it is relatively inexpensive, noninvasive, accessible, and repeatable. The diagnostic sensitivity can reach 98%, significantly reducing the possibility of delayed and wrong diagnosis. When necessary, transesophageal echocardiography can be used to find tumors with a diameter of less than 2 mm.

There is no consensus yet on balancing the advantages and disadvantages of surgical timing in myxoma, complicated by bacterial endocarditis. It is generally believed that surgical treatment should be selected in time, while antibiotic treatment is continued.

References

1. Sabiston D, Spencer F. Surgery of the Chest. New York: A Harcourt Publishers Intenational Company; 2001. p. 2069–85.
2. Liu Hanying, et al. Echocardiographic Diagnosis of Intracardiac Myxoma. Chin J Cardiol. 1984;12(3):204.
3. Lv Lei, et al. Advances in research on the role of interleukin-6 in cardiovascular diseases. J Cardiovasc Rehabil Med. 2009;18(5):510–11.
4. Liu Su, et al. A report of 30 cases of cardiac myxoma. J Cardiopulmon Vasc Dis. 2000;19(3):232.
5. A Case of Right Ventricular Myxoma Complicated by Infective Endocarditis. Youjiang Med J. 2000;5: 811.
6. Collazos J, Martinez E, Mayo J. Spontaneous bacterial peritonitis ceuged by Streptococcus gordonii. J Clin Gaatroenteml. 1999;28:45–6.
7. Dousl CW, Heath J, Hampton KK, et al. Identity of Viridans streptococci isolated from calles of infective endocaditis. J Med Microb. 1993;39:179–82.
8. Guidelines on the prevention, diagnosis, and treatment of infective endocarditis (new version 2009). Eur Heart J. 2009.

Fever of Unknown Origin in Malignant Diseases

3

Li Ning, Chen Shu, Mao Richeng, Zou Mingde, He Fanrong, Wu Ping, Chen Mingquan, Zhang Jiming, Shao Lingyun, Huang Yuxian, Zhang Wenhong, Chen Peidong, Jia Wen, Zheng Jianming, Du Zunguo, Zhang Bingyan, and Jin Jialin

Although the incidence of tumors has been increasing in recent years, due to the rapid development and wide application of imaging diagnostic technology, the percentage of tumor diseases in FUO has continued to decline. The most common malignancies of FUO are lymphoma and leukemia (especially nonlymphocytic leukemia). The most classic solid tumor in FUO is renal cell carcinoma. Fever is related to the necrosis caused by the rapid growth of tumor tissue, the infiltration of tumor cells, the response of human leukocytes to tissue necrosis and other inflammatory stimuli, and the release of endogenous pyrogens from the tumor tissue itself.

1. Lymphoma: 16%–30% of lymphomas have fever as the main symptom or the initial symptom, especially those with deep lesions. Periodic fever is the most characteristic. Pel-Ebstein fever (fever for 3–10 days and no fever in turn) often indicates Hodgkin's disease. Some lymphomas present with cyclic fever and have a long course, up to 3–4 years. Since the disease may have no specific symptoms, and superficial lymph node enlargement may not be obvious, the diagnosis is quite difficult, and some patients can only be confirmed after death by autopsy. The continuous increase in serum lactate dehydrogenase for no other reason may be a clue to the diagnosis (due to the strong metabolism of tumor cells). Noninvasive examinations such as CT, B-mode ultrasound, MRI, PET/CT, etc., are helpful to understand whether there are swollen lymph nodes in the abdominal cavity and retroperitoneum. PET/CT examination has a certain effect on the assessment of the location and nature of lymphoma.

L. Ning · C. Shu · M. Richeng · Z. Mingde · H. Fanrong · W. Ping · C. Mingquan · Z. Jiming · S. Lingyun · H. Yuxian · Z. Wenhong · J. Wen · Z. Jianming · D. Zunguo · Z. Bingyan (✉) · J. Jialin
Department of Infectious Diseases, Huashan Hospital, Fudan University, Shanghai, China

C. Peidong
Department of Infectious Diseases, Jing'an District Central Hospital of Shanghai, Shanghai, China

W. Zhang, X. Weng (eds.), *Fever of Unknown Origin*,
https://doi.org/10.1007/978-981-95-1401-4_3

2. Leukemia: Acute leukemia may be accompanied by fever, and diagnosis is not difficult. It is the preleukemia of nonleukemic leukemia that makes the diagnosis difficult. The peripheral blood picture can be normal, and the bone marrow smear cannot confirm the diagnosis. It is generally believed that fever is the main manifestation of preleukemia in 10%–39%. In addition to fever, there are manifestations such as anemia, purpura, and neutropenia. Fever is more common in the prophase of monocytic leukemia.
3. Liver tumors and other solid tumors: It is well known that liver cancer can cause long-term fever of unknown origin. Primary liver cancer is more common in China. There is no difficulty in general diagnosis in patients with fever, severe right rib pain, hepatomegaly (with nodules), jaundice, ascites and weight loss, etc. clinically. Early diagnosis when fever is the main manifestation is confusing and often accompanied by leukemia-like reactions. Elevated serum AKP is helpful for diagnosis, and qualitative and quantitative tests of alpha-fetoprotein in the blood have diagnostic value, but it must be pointed out that alpha-fetoprotein-negative hepatic cell carcinoma accounts for 10%–15%. Noninvasive examinations such as B-mode ultrasound, CT, MRI, etc., are all helpful for positioning diagnosis. Radionuclide liver scan has a certain diagnostic value. The diagnostic accuracy of selective hepatic angiography is more than 92%, and nodules with a diameter less than 1 cm can also be detected. Others such as kidney tumors, adrenal tumors, nasopharyngeal carcinoma can colon cancer can cause long-term fever. Kidney cancer is very insidious. About 10% of kidney cancer patients have fever as the main manifestation. The body temperature can be as high as 39–40 °C. The fever can be stopped after tumor resection. Such tumor cells can synthesize and release endogenous pyrogens in laboratory, while the tumor cells of kidney cancer patients without fever cannot release endogenous pyrogens. B-mode ultrasound, CT, and selective renal angiography are quite helpful in diagnosis. Colon cancer may penetrate the serosal membrane to form a pericolonic abscess. Both polypoid carcinoma necrosis and abscess formation can cause fever. Solid tumors such as pancreatic cancer, lung cancer, and bone cancer have relatively low fever, and are mostly related to widespread metastasis with tumor necrosis or infection with blocked drainage. Occasionally, benign tumors such as leiomyomas of the stomach, small intestine, and uterus can also cause fever.

In this chapter, we selected 10 classic fever cases that were finally diagnosed as tumors, highlighting the positioning value of PET/CT examination and the diagnostic value of repeated biopsy as well as long-term follow up, hoping to have some inspiration for readers.

3.1 Surgical Removal of Renal Cell Carcinoma with Fever as the First Manifestation, Renal Pathology Indicated Inflammatory Pseudotumor and Second Surgery Proved Clear Cell Carcinoma of Right Kidney

Li Ning

A 52-year-old man was admitted on June 6, 2005 with fever, right-sided lumbago, and had been emaciated for a month. He started fever a month ago with no clear cause, body temperature fluctuated between 37.5 and 38.6 °C with peak temperature at 39 °C, aggravated in the afternoon. Associated symptoms included fatigue, chills, and pain in right waist. He reported no radicular pain, cough, expectoration, sore throat, abdominal pain, diarrhea, frequent or urgent urination, pain with urination, joint swelling, or rash. The patient showed a normal hemogram, ESR of 120 mm/h with negative blood cultures. Immunological indices including ANA, ENA, RF, ANCA, dsDNA, etc., are normal. B-ultrasound, CT scan and MRI examination revealed right renal masses with retroperitoneal lymphadenopathy. On June 9, palliative right nephrectomy was performed and pathologic diagnosis suggested inflammatory pseudotumor (the nidus was composed of large cells with a large number of inflammatory cells infiltration and reactive hyperplasia of fibrous tissue). After consultant with Shanghai Cancer Center, the pathologic diagnosis was approved. After surgery, levels of leukocytes and neutrophils were low, HGB 90 g/L. His body temperature stabilized at 38 °C, given nimesulide treatment, and discharged after temperature fell to normal. However, he was febrile again on July 7. His body temperature rose to around 38.5 °C and aggravated in the afternoon with a band-like sensation of headache in the frontal region. He was treated with ceftriaxone sodium but effect was not good. During the course of disease, he lost 5 kg, but he didn't have recurrent oral ulceration or alopecia. On July 18, he was admitted to our department for further treatment.

3.1.1 Physical Examination on Admission

Temperature, 39 °C; respiratory rate, 30 breaths/min; heart rate, 98 beats/min; blood pressure, 110/70 mmHg. The patient was conscious but listless, slight pallor of palpebral conjunctiva, ecchymosis or petechiae were not found on the skin or mucosa around the whole body. Superficial lymph nodes were impalpable. Both pupils were equal in size and shape and reacted normally to light. Neck was not stiff; no congestion in throat, no hypertrophy of bilateral tonsils. Breath sound of both lungs was clear, and no rales were heard. The patient had normal beats in the precordial region and no expansion of heart border, heart rate 98 beats/min, heart rhythm was normal, pathologic heart murmur was not detected. Abdomen was soft, no tenderness and rebound tenderness, liver and spleen were impalpable at subcostal region, no liver percussion pain, no shifting dullness, percussion pain at right kidney region, both legs were not swollen. Pathologic reflexes were negative.

3.1.2 Treatment Course

Admission routine blood tests: leukocytes, 6.4×10^9/L; erythrocytes, 3.14×10^{12}/L; hemoglobin, 88 g/L; platelet, 1136.4×10^9/L. Routine urine tests: erythrocytes, 6–7/HP. Liver and kidney function, blood glucose, blood lipid and electrolyte were basically normal. Blood cultures were conducted three times when body temperature >38.3 °C, all negative. Immunoglobulin, C3 and C4 were at normal level. Hepatitis markers were all negative, and tumor markers were within the normal range. T, B, and NK cell counts were within the normal range. Immunological indices including ANA and ENA were normal. Surgery pathology results were reviewed again; two coagulated necrotic areas were found in the slice. Tuberculosis infection was most likely and tumor could not be excluded. Antituberculosis treatment started on August 3 with isoniazid, pyrazinamide, ethambutol, and prednisone 30 mg/day. The next day, the body temperature of the patient became normal, ESR decreased moderately, and the retroperitoneal lymphadenopathy was alleviated gradually. The patient was discharged on September 12. Two weeks later, his fatigue and emaciation exaggerated, body temperature fluctuated between 37 and 38 °C, progressive decrease of protein was detected by further tests. On October 12, his body temperature reached 39 °C, and he was admitted once again on October 14. CT scan revealed retroperitoneal lymphadenopathy with massive necrosis of lymph nodes. A laparotomy was performed for lymph node biopsy, and no obvious space-occupying lesion was detected in liver, spleen, or alimentary canal. Near the retroperitoneal lymph node, there were clustered swollen lymph nodes beside the aorta. The pathologic examination was conducted by Shanghai Cancer Center: right renal cell carcinoma, and the renal cell carcinoma metastasized to retroperitoneal lymph nodes, most of which were clear cells.

3.1.3 Comments

The patient had fever, right-sided lumbago, weight loss, and multiple blood cultures were negative, immunological indicators such as ANA, ENA, RF, ANCA, dsDNA, etc., were normal, antibacterial therapy was ineffective, and glucocorticoid therapy was not effective. B-ultrasound, CT, and MRI examinations suggested the right kidney mass and retroperitoneal lymphadenopathy. Palliative right nephrectomy was performed and pathologic diagnosis suggested inflammatory pseudotumor (the nidus was composed of large cells with a large number of inflammatory cells infiltration and reactive hyperplasia of fibrous tissue). Later, due to the progress of disease, a laparotomy was performed for lymph node biopsy, and no obvious space-occupying lesion was detected in liver, spleen, or alimentary canal. Near the retroperitoneal lymph node, there were swollen lymph nodes beside the aorta. The pathologic examination was conducted by Shanghai Cancer Center: right renal cell carcinoma. The renal cell carcinoma metastasized to retroperitoneal lymph nodes, most of which were clear cells. It is consistent with the diagnosis of renal clear cell carcinoma.

Kidney cancer mostly occurs in patients aged 50–70, and the incidence rate is higher in men. The location of the kidney is concealed. When a disease occurs, a change in urine is usually the first manifestation, which is often a signal for the patient to seek medical aid. Hematuria is a common symptom of kidney cancer, but before the appearance of hematuria, the manifestations of kidney cancer can be varied. Sometimes the tumor is very large, with signs of metastasis to lungs and bones; sometimes it can also show no symptoms. In addition to the three typical symptoms, hematuria, low back pain, and lumps, kidney cancer also has many non-urinary extrarenal manifestations, such as fever, anemia, abnormal liver function, hypertension, polycythemia, and hypercalcemia. The most prominent manifestations of this case are fever and increased ALP, which are relatively rare in patients with renal cell carcinoma and are easy to be ignored in clinical practice. In this case, renal imaging showed renal mass, and the patient was still febrile, which aggravated in afternoon, accompanied by weight loss, after palliative surgery. Considering that the secretion of EP by kidney cancer can cause high fever, but generally after kidney cancer resection, the body temperature will decrease. This patient's fever still existed after renal mass resection, and the first histopathological consultation at Shanghai Cancer Center also suggested inflammatory pseudotumor; after reviewing pathology result, two areas of coagulative necrosis were found, so the possibility of kidney cancer is small. Because we cannot exclude the possibility of *Mycobacterium tuberculosis* infection, antituberculosis treatment combined with hormone therapy was conducted. The body temperature returned to normal, but it soon rebounded, and the retroperitoneal lymph nodes appeared swollen and necrosed, which cannot be explained by *Mycobacterium tuberculosis* infection, and finally the retroperitoneal lymph nodes were surgically removed for biopsy, and pathologically confirmed to be renal clear cell carcinoma. In clinical practice, once the histopathological results are not consistent with the clinical manifestations, the initial results should be suspected, because the antituberculosis treatment after the operation was ineffective in this case. The second surgery and pathological examination are necessary, and it is obvious that the clear diagnosis depends on persistence of the clinician.

In recent years, due to the higher attention given to health examinations, the incidence of kidney cancer has increased year after year. According to domestic literature reports from 1995 to 2005, the average detection rate of asymptomatic kidney cancer in our country is about 33%, while for the same period in foreign countries, asymptomatic kidney cancer accounts for about 50%, which means that nearly half of patients have no clinical manifestations and are diagnosed through physical examinations. In the past, the main reason for patients with kidney cancer seeking medical aid was hematuria, low back pain, and abdominal masses (*triad of kidney cancer*). Therefore, before the advent of imaging diagnosis, the diagnosis was often based on *the triad of kidney cancer*. However, due to the continuous development of medical imaging technology in recent years, the average detection rate of asymptomatic kidney cancer has continuously increased. The clinical detection rate of *the triad of kidney cancer* is less than 15%, and they are often patients with terminal cancer. Therefore, *the triad of kidney cancer* has not been used clinically as the main diagnostic evidence for kidney cancer.

Among newly diagnosed kidney cancer patients, about 30% have metastatic kidney cancer, which manifest as hemoptysis, bone pain, pathological fractures, and other symptoms. In addition, because renal cell carcinoma can produce a variety of endocrine hormones, it can cause other discomforts, called the paraneoplastic syndrome of kidney cancer. Paraneoplastic syndrome can manifest as hypertension, anemia, weight loss, cachexia, fever, polycythemia, abnormal liver function, hypercalcemia, hyperglycemia, increased ESR, neuromuscular disease, amyloidosis, galactorrhea, abnormal blood coagulation mechanism, etc. About 10%–40% patients will have paraneoplastic syndrome, so the clinical manifestations of kidney cancer are relatively complicated.

For the diagnosis of kidney cancer, *Chinese Guideline for Renal Cell Carcinoma*, formulated by the Chinese Urological Association, gives advice as follows: First, it recommends necessary laboratory tests include blood urea nitrogen and creatinine due to their indication of the patient's renal function before treatment. In addition, further tests, such as liver function, complete blood count, hemoglobin, blood calcium, blood glucose, erythrocyte sedimentation rate, alkaline phosphatase, and lactate dehydrogenase are recommended, because they are mostly correlated to prognosis factors. Second, it recommends the necessary imaging examinations include abdominal B-ultrasound, chest X-ray, and abdominal CT scan. The latter two are the primary evidence for preoperative staging. Third, it recommends that the selective imaging examinations include abdominal CT scan without contrast, radionuclide renogram or IVU, radionuclide bone scan, chest CT scan, head CT scan, MRI scan, and abdominal MRI scan. These tests are not routine for clinical practice, only used under some specific conditions. For instance, abdominal CT scan without contrast is usually used as reference for the selection of operative incision; radionuclide renogram or IVU is necessary when enhanced CT scan can't be performed and renal function of the contralateral kidney is unknown; radionuclide bone scan is necessary when the patient suffers bone pain, fracture, or elevated alkaline phosphatase. Fourth, some tests may be recommended for patients from wealthy places or in relatively good economic status including renal contrast-enhanced ultrasound, spiral CT scan, MRI, PET, and PET-CT. Fifth, needle biopsy and renal angiogram are not recommended because needle biopsy for kidney cancer has about 17.5% false negative and false positive rate, and needle biopsy brings about 5% complication rate. Thus, needle biopsy is not considered as a preoperative examination for operable patients. Moreover, since the clinical application of CT scan, MRI, and several advanced imaging examinations, renal angiogram as an invasive test is no longer recommended as routine test. For patients who received a partial nephrectomy or have a renal artery embolism, preoperative routine angiography is still necessary, but it will not be taken as a diagnostic basis for kidney cancer though.

Surgical resection is the main treatment for kidney cancer. The effects of radiotherapy, chemotherapy, and immunotherapy are not satisfactory or certain. According to statistics, kidney cancer combined with radiotherapy has no effect on 5-year survival rate.

References

1. Godley PA, Stin Chcombe TE. Renal cell carcinoma[J]. Curr Opin Oncol. 1999;11:213–7.
2. Marshall FF, Taxy JB, Fishman EK, et al. The feasibility of surgical enucleation for renal cell carcinoma[J]. J Urol. 1986;135(2):231–4.

3.2 Fever with Insect Bite Rash for 12 Years

Chen Shu

A 14-year-old female was admitted to hospital because of intermittent fever for more than 12 years. The patient developed chills and fever after mosquito bites at the age of one and a half, and the temperature was between 38 and 40 °C. Physical examination at the local hospital showed "scattered papules on the limbs and oral mucosal herpes, liver was 1.5 cm below the ribs, and spleen was 3 cm below the ribs". The blood routine test showed that WBC was 13×10^9/L. The therapeutic effect is not good with multiple antibiotics. Over the course of the treatment, new rashes such as bleeding spots and herpes appeared successively in the extremities, face, and torso, accompanied by enlargement of bilateral cervical lymph nodes. Peripheral blood smear revealed 15% abnormal lymphocytes, the heterophilic agglutination test was 1:14 (+). Therefore, the patient was considered as infectious mononucleosis (IM). After oral administration of prednisone, the body temperature was normal and the lymph nodes shrunk.

Since then, the patient had a fever about 4–6 h after mosquito bites every summer and autumn, and the body temperature was 38–40 °C. The skin of the bite would successively appear red and swollen, crystal transparent blisters, blisters turn purple and black, skin necrosis, ulcers could reach muscle, the diameter is about 0.5–2 cm, and finally scabbed. About 1 month after the onset of the disease, the body temperature stabilized and the lesions healed. The fever was accompanied by redness, swelling, and pain of superficial lymph nodes and hepatosplenomegaly, and the enlarged spleen could reach the level of navel. Blood routine tests showed that WBC was $4 \sim 7 \times 10^9$/L, of which lymphocytes accounted for 60%–80%. The patient was treated in several hospitals and diagnosed as "low cellular immune function" and "chronic granulomatosis-Job syndrome?" There was no significant improvement with antibiotics, anti-infection, and gamma globulin support. One month before her admission, the patient developed fever again, and the body temperature was between 38 and 40.5 °C, but there were no new rashes. The treatment effects of ceftriaxone, roxithromycin, vancomycin, and tobramycin in local hospitals were not good. And the patient came to our hospital for further treatment.

Since the onset of the disease, the patient had a good appetite and good sleep, no obvious abnormality in stool and urine, and no significant weight loss.

3.2.1 Physical Examination

Body temperature: 37.8 °C, Pulse rate: 120 beats/min, Respiratory rate: 21 beats/min, Blood pressure: 105/65 mmHg. The patient had a clear mind and a thin body. She was normally developed. There was no yellow staining or petechiae on her sclera or skin. 0.3–1 cm scars could be seen on her face and lower limbs, which were concave on the skin. The superficial lymph nodes are not enlarged. The bilateral pupils are equal in size and round, and the light reflex is present. No abnormal secretions were found in the external auditory canal or the nasal cavity. There was no cyanosis on the lips. The pharynx is congested but the tonsils are normal. No ulcer was found in the oral mucosa. The neck was soft and the thyroid was normal. The trachea was in the middle. The chest was symmetrical, with clear breath sounds in both lungs. The apex beat was 0.5 cm outside the left midclavicular line, and the heart dullness area expanded slightly to the lower left. The heart rhythm was regular with no pathological murmur in any valve area. The abdomen was full and hard, only the middle and lower abdomen were soft. The upper liver was in the fourth intercostal space, and the lower liver was 4 cm below the ribs. The spleen was 4 cm below the level of navel and 1 cm beyond the midline of the abdomen, which was hard without tenderness. Shifting dullness (−). There was no edema in the lower limbs. The biceps reflex was present, but the knee reflex was not elicited. Babinski sign (−), Kerning sign (−). The muscle strength of the limbs was normal and the pulse of the dorsalis pedis artery is normal.

3.2.2 The Process of Diagnosis and Treatment

After admission, the patient had a persistent high fever with a body temperature of 39–40 °C and complained of pain in the spleen area. Laboratory examination: the blood routine test showed that WBC increased progressively (12.1–23 × 10^9/L), mainly by lymphocytes (90%–95%). Hb: 70–89.5 g/L. Liver function was abnormal with decreased albumin, and the level of Ig E was 2924 IU/mL. Flow cytometry results of peripheral blood showed that the ratio of CD3, CD4, and CD8 cells decreased significantly. B-ultrasound indicated hepatosplenomegaly. The patient was bitten by a mosquito during a routine examination after admission. Two days later, a blister, about 0.3 cm in diameter, appeared at the bite site. Penicillin was given, but there was no significant improvement in body temperature, so anti-infective treatment was discontinued.

After a discussion of difficult cases, the patient was considered to have an immunodeficiency involving T and B cells, because of a long-term fever and a significant decrease in the proportion of peripheral blood CD3, CD4, and CD8 cells. However, there was no abnormal response to BCG vaccination when the patient was young, so the possibility of primary disease might be small. Bone marrow puncture was required to rule out other diseases.

Bone marrow puncture report showed that the bone marrow nucleated cells proliferated significantly. The ratio of granule red was inverted, and the ratio of granule line was reduced and shifted to the left. Toxic granules and vacuoles could be seen in some granulocytes. The proportion of erythroid was fair, but enucleation disorders and basophilic spots could be seen in some late immature red blood cells. The proportion of lymphocytes on the slice was increased, and the cell bodies varied in size, most of them were large and medium-sized. The cytoplasm was light blue and contained many different thick or thin azurophilic granules. Some were inclusions with round or irregular nuclei. Some had depressions, and the nuclear chromatin was clumpy. Most of the nucleoli were missing, and 1–2 nucleoli could be seen in some cells with binuclear and mitotic phases. Broken cells were more common, and some tissue macrophages could be seen. POX: 96% large granular lymphocytes (−), 4% granular cells were positive. PAS: large granular lymphocytes 58% (−), 7% (+), 25% (++), 10% (+++). Conclusion: Large granular lymphocytic leukemia (LGLL), flow cytometry result of bone marrow cells: CD56+ 50.95%.

Diagnosed as large granular cell leukemia (NK cell type).

After consulting hematologists, CD1348 was prescribed for treatment.

A few days after the diagnosis was confirmed, the patient suddenly defecated a large amount of black stool and vomited coffee-colored liquid. And her skin was not easy to stop bleeding. Coagulation function showed that APTT and PT were significantly prolonged. Secondary disseminated intravascular coagulation (DIC) in large granular cell leukemia was considered. Although she was actively rescued, the patient's condition worsened and died one day later.

3.2.3 Comments

The patient's course of illness was up to 12 years, which is long among the reported cases of fever. The patient has visited the doctor several times during the course for more than 10 years, but they were not able to make a clear diagnosis. The diagnosis of such a long-term unexplained fever is usually very difficult. However, this patient has very clear and specific accompanying symptoms. Ulcerated skin lesions after mosquito bites, accompanied by fever, hepatosplenomegaly and lymph node enlargement are the characteristic manifestations of chronic EB virus infection (CAEBV). The long-term misdiagnosis is related to the lack of understanding of the disease by clinicians.

The patient's rash often has the following characteristics: The disease occurs after a mosquito bite, the skin lesion at the site of the bite might successively be red and swollen, crystal transparent blisters, and blisters turns purple and black, followed by progressive skin necrosis, ulcers occurred and could reached muscle layer, and the diameter is about 0.5–2 cm and then scabbed. This is inconsistent with hydroa vacciniforme (HV). The disease is closely related to chronic Epstein-Barr virus infection, and the high sensitization after mosquito bites is related to NK cells. Chronic EB virus infection (CAEBV) is associated with nasopharyngeal carcinoma and lymphoma. Clinicians should be alert to the possibility of malignant tumors and should do everything possible to identify or exclude the possibility of malignant diseases. Nasopharyngeal examination, bone marrow and lymph node biopsy should be routine. The patient was finally diagnosed as invasive large granulocytic leukemia (NK cell type) by bone marrow examination. Large granulocytic cell leukemia (NK cell type) is a rare cause of fever of unknown reason, because it needs to be diagnosed by pathology. It is currently believed to be closely related to CAEBV and is one kind of chronic EBV lymphoproliferative disease. Secondary DIC may lead to a poor prognosis.

Epstein-Barr virus (EB) virus, belonging to the gamma subfamily of herpesvirus, was first discovered in the Burkitt lymphoma cell line in 1964. Acute EB virus infection can cause infectious mononucleosis (IM). IM is self-limited, and the symptoms alleviate and disappear after a few weeks.

In a few cases, chronic or recurrent IM-like symptoms may occur after EB virus infection. The clinical manifestations include fever, lymphadenopathy and hepatosplenomegaly, etc., and these symptoms could last for more than 6 months, which is called CAEBV. EBV-DNA can be continuously detected in blood samples of such patients.

In the initial research related to Epstein-Barr virus, it is suggested that the target cells of infection are B cells and tonsil epithelial cells, which could lead to a series of lymphoproliferative diseases, such as B cell lymphoma and nasopharyngeal carcinoma. Viruses can promote tumor formation through a variety of mechanisms, including B cell activation, affecting autoimmune function and inactivation of tumor suppressor factors. Recently, more studies have pointed out that Epstein-Barr virus can also infect T cells and NK cells. Similar cases mostly occur in Japan, South Korea, and Native Americans (Mexico, Peru, Central America), but are rare among Caucasians and Black people. In 2008, EBV lymphoproliferative disease (LPD) international classification conference divided it into EBV+ B-LPD and EBV+ T/N-LPD. The latter is equivalent to the T/NK cell subtype of CAEBV, including Hydroa Vacciniforme (HV), HV-like lymphoma, severe mosquito bite allergy (SMBA) and childhood systemic EBV+ T/NK-LPD. Systemic EBV+T/NK-LPD in children is proposed for the first time as an independent disease of mature T/NK cell tumors. The manifestations of T-cell type of CAEBV are usually high fever, lymphadenopathy and hepatosplenomegaly. EB virus-specific antibodies show high titer, and the disease progresses rapidly. NK cell type of CAEBV has high sensitivity to mosquito bites, rashes, high titers of Ig E, and EB virus-specific antibodies are not necessarily elevated.

Hydroa vacciniforme-like Epstein-Barr Virus associated lymphoproliferative disorders was first named in 2000. The rash is similar to HV, but the systemic symptoms are severe and related to Epstein-Barr virus infection. HV is a photosensitive cutaneous disorder of unknown origin first reported by Bazin in 1862. It is characterized by papules, blisters, necrosis and scab in exposed areas such as the face and limbs, which can be relieved spontaneously after puberty. In 1999, Iwatsuki proposed that some children with HV have systemic symptoms such as fever, hepatosplenomegaly, and lymphadenopathy. Such patients are called “severe HV” or “atypical HV”. Epstein-Barr virus infection is closely related to the disease, and severe HV could develop into Epstein-Barr virus-related cutaneous T cell lymphoma.

Poor prognostic factors for EBV + T/NK-LPD patients include: development of lymphoma or leukemia, complications after hematopoietic stem cell transplantation, pancytopenia, infection, DIC, etc.

Researchers have tried a variety of treatments for CAEBV, including antiviral therapy (ribavirin, ganciclovir), immunomodulators (IFN-α, IL-12), chemotherapy (etoposide, hormones), and EBV-positive cytotoxic T cells. Hematopoietic stem cell transplantation is a more effective option, but the long-term effect still needs time to be proven over time.

References

1. Cohen JI. Esptein Barr virus infection[J]. N Engl J Med. 2000;343(7):481–92.
2. Okana M. Haematological associations of epstein-Barr virus infection[J]. Ballieres Best Pract Res Clin Haematol. 2000;13(2):199–214.
3. Merlo A, Turrini R, Dolcetti R, et al. Adoptive cell therapy against EBV-related malignancies: a survey of clinical results[J]. Expert Opin Biol Ther. 2008;8(9):1265–94.
4. Kanegane H, Nomura K, Miyawaki T, et al. Biological aspects of Epstein-Barr virus (EBV)-infected lymphocytes in chronic active EBV infection and asstociated malignancies[J]. Crit Rev Oncol Hematol. 2002;44(3):239–49.

3.3 Pulmonary Sarcoma with Recurrent Chest Pain and Fever Suspected of Pulmonary Embolism

Mao Richeng, Zou Mingde, He Fanrong, Wu Ping, and Chen Mingquan

The patient, a 43-year-old male, was admitted with the chief complaint of recurrent intermittent chest pain and fever for more than 2 months. Two months ago, there was no obvious cause of knife-cut pain on the right back and deep breathing worsened, which was accompanied with continuous dry cough. In addition, there was no hemoptysis, sputum, chest tightness or shortness of breath, no back skin damage, and herpes. He went to the local clinic and improved after receiving a three-day treatment with penicillin. He presented with back pain again and went to the county hospital a week later. The lung CT revealed a lung tumor to be discharged. He was transferred to the outpatient clinic of a tertiary hospital in Shanghai, where pulmonary infection was considered, then he was transferred to the local hospital for 18 days of cephalosporin and levofloxacin anti-infection treatment. The symptoms of chest pain were relieved a little, but he started having a fever of 37.5–38.5 °C. It started at 15:00 in the afternoon and peaked at 21:00. The temperature automatically descended and became normal without sweats and chills in the next morning. One month ago, the patient went to a tertiary hospital in Shanghai again, and was admitted to hospital with the diagnosis of "right lung abnormalities to be examined: lung cancer? pneumonia?" by the outpatient department. Lung mass puncture was performed with the guide of color ultrasound, and routine pathological examination showed that there were a few lymphocytes and epithelial cells without malignant cells. Repeated sputum search for acid-fast bacilli was all negative, but blood test T-SPOT.TB was positive, thus pulmonary tuberculosis infection was not excluded. Although he was transferred to local hospital for anti-tuberculosis treatment for two weeks, chest pain and fever were not improved. At the same time, the antituberculosis treatment was ceased due to his intolerance of excessive gastrointestinal reaction. Now for further diagnosis and treatment, he went to our outpatient department and was admitted to hospital as "the nature of lung shadow to be determined". Since the illness, the patient had malaise, poor appetite, good sleep, normal urine and feces with no significant weight loss. Personal history: smoking history for more than 20 years, 20 cigarettes a day.

3.3.1 Physical Examination

The patient had a temperature of 37.1 °C, a heart rate of 76 beats/min, a respiratory rate of 18 counts/min, a blood pressure of 109/77 mmHg, steady breath, rough breathing sounds in both lungs, no obvious dry or wet rale, and a grade 3/6 systolic murmur in pulmonary valve stethoscope area was heard. Abdomen was soft without tenderness or rebound pain. The liver and spleen were not palpable under the right and left costal margins. There was no edema in both lower limbs.

3.3.2 Process of Diagnosis and Treatment

On admission, laboratory studies revealed the following: leukocytes, 13.86×10^9/L; hemoglobin, 124 g/; neutrophils, 9.64×10^9/L; erythrocyte sedimentation rate, 42 mm/h; carbohydrate antigen 125, 36.87 U/mL; ferritin, 503.9 ng/mL; neuron specific enolase, 32.37 ng/mL; C-reactive protein, 89.9 mg/L. Liver function, kidney function, PCT, DIC were all within normal limits; findings on autoantibody profile (ANA, ENA, dsDNA, ANCA) were unremarkable. Lung CT: multiple patchy high-density shadows could be seen in the lower lobe of the right lung, considering inflammation of the right lung (Fig. 3.1).

The patient was first treated with ceftriaxone 2.0 q12h with moxifloxacin 0.4 qd intravenous for anti-infection therapy, and the body temperature was maintained between 37 and 38 °C. One week after admission, it was suggested that the effect of antibiotics was not obvious. At the same time, the patient complained of repeated chest pain, which was not alleviated after the use of antibiotics, and the lung CT enhanced scan was performed (Fig. 3.2).

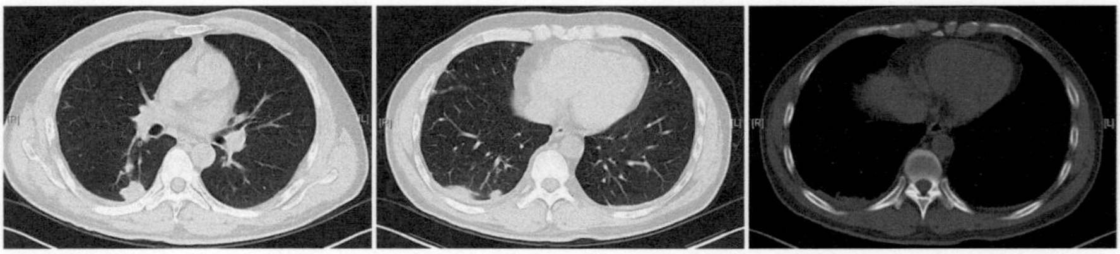

Fig. 3.1 CT scan

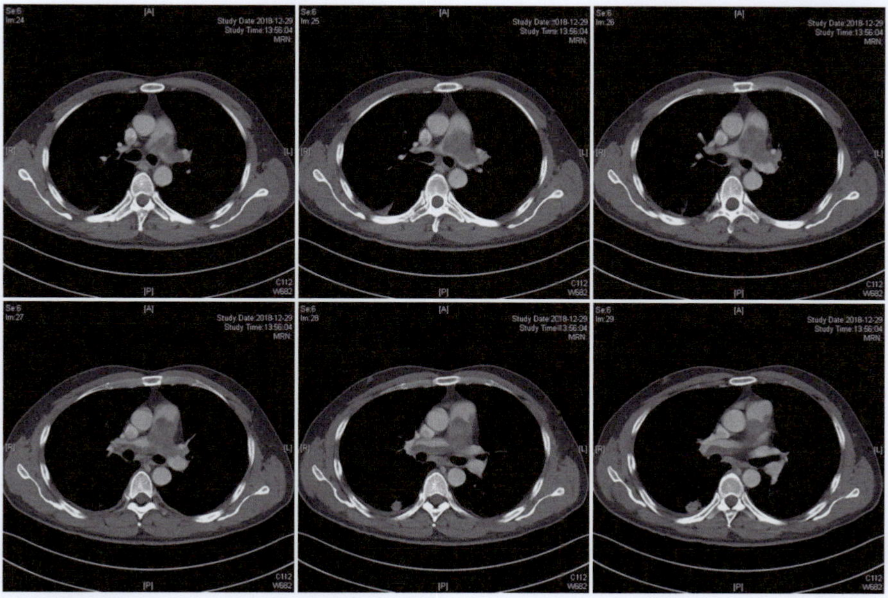

Fig. 3.2 CT scan

Fig. 3.3 PET-CT

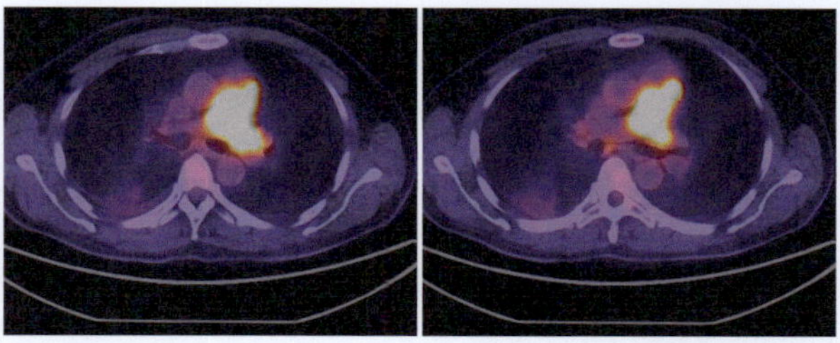

There were no obvious enlarged lymph nodes in the hilum of lung and mediastinum on both sides. The heart didn't dilate. There was no obvious effusion in the bilateral pleural cavity. Patchy low-density shadows could be seen in the right pulmonary artery and branches of the right pulmonary artery, with a CT value of about 33 Hu. The embolisms in the right pulmonary artery and right pulmonary artery branches were badly possible. Please combine with D-dimer, blood oxygen saturation and clinical signs.

Respiratory consultation was performed immediately, considering the possibility of pulmonary embolism and lung shadows. It was suggested that nutrition support for cardiac muscles should be given, and blood routine, liver function, kidney function, DIC, myocardial markers, proBNP and blood gas should be monitored during anticoagulation. After subcutaneous injection of low molecular weight heparin 4100 U for 12 h, blood routine, liver and kidney function, DIC, myocardial markers, proBNP, and analysis of blood gas three times were all normal. However, the patient still complained of repeated chest pain, and PET-CT was performed for further diagnosis (Fig. 3.3). PET-CT: The metabolism of striped FDG in the right and left

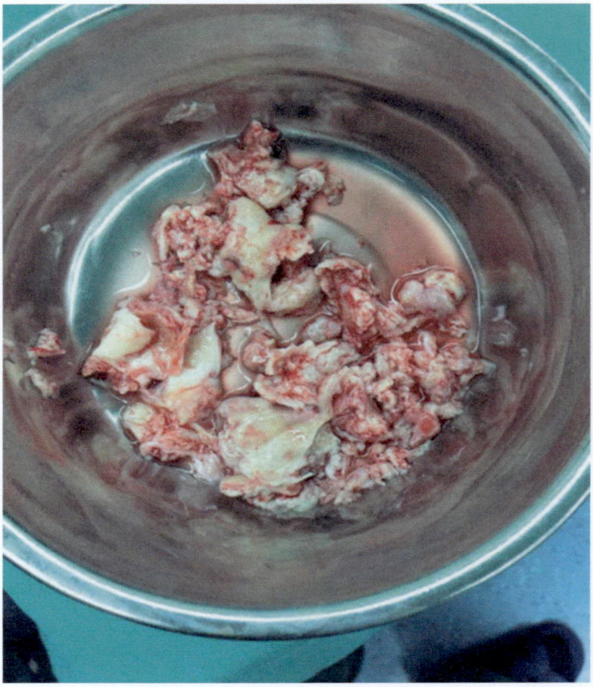

Fig. 3.4 Surgical specimen

pulmonary arteries increased diffusely. The uptake range was about 5.9 cm × 5.1 cm and the maximum value of SUV was 27.9; the shape of heart was enlarged and the metabolism of FDG in the right ventricle increased unevenly, please combine with clinical practice. The metabolism of FDG of the scattered irregular dense shadows in the right lung increased slightly, especially in the right lower lung near the pleura, and the maximum value of SUV was 5.3: considering the possibility of inflammatory proliferative lesions. But the lung biopsy showed no abnormalities.

Cardiothoracic surgery consultation: the patient had repeated chest tightness, chest pain, and anti-infection and antituberculosis treatment were ineffective, and autoantibodies and vasculitis antibody were negative; lung CT suggested pulmonary embolism, while anticoagulation therapy was ineffective; PET-CT showed that the metabolism of striped FDG in right pulmonary artery and left pulmonary artery increased diffusely, considering the possibility of vascular endothelium-derived tumor, thus pulmonary artery biopsy was recommended in the cardiology or interventional department. After contacting the department of cardiology and interventional department, both of them indicated that the risk of pulmonary artery puncture was very high. Later, we contacted the cardiac surgery department of a hospital in Shanghai to perform left and right pulmonary artery endothelium stripping (Fig. 3.4).

Postoperative pathology: pulmonary sarcoma with necrosis. Immunohistochemical results: CK (−), SNA (−), S100 (−), CD31 (vascular+), CAM5.2 (−) ERG (−), Ki67 (40%), HMB45 (−), MelanA (−), MSA (−), PGM1 (histocyte+). At this point, the patient was finally diagnosed as pulmonary sarcoma with necrosis.

3.3.3 Discussion

Pulmonary artery sarcoma is a rare malignant tumor of pulmonary vascular system, originating from pulmonary artery endothelial cells, and C/P-catenin mutations present in the tumor cells. The incidence of PAS is low. Since the first report of PAS in 1923, about 300 cases have been reported at home and abroad, most of which are cases solely, with an incidence rate of 0.001%–0.030%. The age of onset ranges from 2 months to 86 years old, but it is more common at the age of 40–60 years old, and there are more females than males. Clinical manifestations include hemoptysis, weight loss, fever, syncope, dyspnea, cough, and chest pain. Laboratory tests are unremarkable. The imaging examination reveals massive filling defects in the main pulmonary artery and left and right pulmonary arteries; the boundary of the mass is irregular, which could be polypoid or lobulated; PAS grows expansively, hence the proximal end of the lesion protrudes toward the right heart outflow tract, and the affected pulmonary artery is thicker than the pulmonary artery of same grade; the sarcoma invades the pulmonary artery, which may cause "wall erosion sign" and further grow out of the cavity; the sarcoma extends to the pulmonary artery branch, and the hilar vessel presents a "clover" appearance; due to the rich blood supply of tumor tissues, enhanced CT shows tumor enhancement; internal tissues of PAS are prone to necrosis and bleeding, so the enhancement is uneven. Echocardiography, CTPA, MRI, and PET-CT are helpful for diagnosis.

At present, there is a lack of effective treatment for PAS. Recent studies have shown that surgical resection, radiotherapy and chemotherapy are the main treatments for PAS. The surgical methods include pulmonary endarterectomy, pneumonectomy, etc. Complete resection may be the most effective treatment currently. However, the onset of PAS is concealed, and the diagnosis is in a state of progress. The tumor of most patients cannot be completely removed when they see the doctor, and the prognosis is very poor. Chemotherapy and radiotherapy are used for palliative care and patients who have relapsed after surgery, the efficacy of which is still controversial, and there is no standard scheme for PAS. The natural course of untreated PAS is the continuous growth of tumor to form tumor thrombus and superimpose thrombus, resulting in progressive aggravation of pulmonary artery obstruction, and most of the patients die of heart failure.

This case suggests that we need to pay attention to the causes of chest pain when we encounter patients with recurrent fever and chest pain. In addition to thoracic wall disease, cardiovascular disease, respiratory disease, mediastinal disease, subphrenic abscess, liver abscess, and other common diseases, pulmonary vascular diseases such as pulmonary sarcoma should also be considered.

Pulmonary artery sarcoma is known as the tumor with the shortest survival time, with an average survival time of 6 weeks without surgery, which can be extended by 12–18 months after surgical treatment. This kind of tumor has the characteristics of high mortality, high metastasis rate, and high misdiagnosis rate. The Cleveland Center in the United States once made statistics that 50% of the 391 patients were found by autopsy and 30% were misdiagnosed as other benign lesions. Only 20% of the patients were diagnosed before death or operation.

The patient also went to many hospitals, and the final diagnosis was confirmed by postoperative pathology. The lung CT of the patient revealed multiple patchy high-density shadows in the lower lobe of the right lung, which may be pulmonary sarcoma with intrapulmonary metastasis. Although the patient underwent complete surgical resection, the prognosis was still poor in view of the high degree of malignancy of the disease. The patient has been engaged in painting for a long time and has been exposed to a large number of chemical toxic substances, which may be a high risk factor for the disease. Clinically, patients with recurrent chest pain, fever and suspected pulmonary embolism need to be excluded from the possibility of "pulmonary artery sarcoma". The CT findings of pulmonary sarcoma have certain characteristics: the filling defect of the proximal pulmonary artery occupies the whole lumen; the proximal end of the intraluminal lesion protrudes to the right cardiac outflow tract; the involved pulmonary artery is thicker than that of the same grade pulmonary artery; enhanced CT shows inhomogeneous enhancement; the above features are different from pulmonary thromboembolism. In addition, MRI and PET-CT are helpful in differentiating diagnosis.

References

1. Pu X, Song M. Clinical and radiological features of pulmonary artery sarcoma: a report of nine cases. Clin Respir J. 2018;12(5):1820–9.
2. Wei N, Lanyan Z. Advances in the diagnosis and treatment of pulmonary artery sarcoma. Int J Respir. 2017;37(11):863–7.

3.4 Non-Langerhans Histiocytosis Erdheim-Chester Disease Diagnosed by Biopsy

Chen Mingquan and Zhang Jiming

A 28-year-old male was admitted to the hospital on April 23, 2010 due to blurred vision for more than 1 year, with fever and pain in the lower limbs for more than 10 months.

The patient developed blurred vision since October 2009 and was diagnosed as Koyanagi-Harada disease by a local hospital. His blurred vision recovered after he was treated with oral prednisone for two months, and the glucocorticoids was stopped without reduction process.

Two weeks after prednisone was stopped, the patient began to have consistent low fever with the highest temperature of 38.5 °C. The fever started in the afternoon with chills and subsided spontaneously at night. The patient developed severe pain in the front of both lower limbs and it was too painful to squat. He also developed the symptoms of occasional cough with a little clear phlegm accompanied by intermittent headache. He denied symptoms of chest pain, chest tightness, abdominal pain, or diarrhea.

On February 19, 2010, He went to the local hospital, and blood routine test showed white blood cell count of 10.10×10^9/L and neutrophil percentage of 77.8%. Chest radiographs showed increased and thickened lung texture. No abnormalities were found from cranial CT. He was diagnosed as "bronchial infection" and prescribed with azithromycin. However, the symptoms didn't relieve.

On February 28, 2010, he was transferred to another hospital. On physical examination, multiple superficial enlarged lymph nodes were palpable. Laboratory studies revealed a white blood cell level of 7.23×10^9/L, a neutrophil percentage level of 82.7%, a C-reactive protein level of 96.5 mg/L. ANA, PPD, and blood culture were all negative. His chest radiograph showed a patchy shadow in the left lower lobe, while chest CT showed no obvious abnormality. A left neck lymph node biopsy was conducted and the pathology showed "reactive hyperplasia". The local hospital also considered the patient as "bronchial infection". After he was prescribed cefoperazone-sulbactam and vancomycin, the symptoms of cough and expectoration improved, but fever remained. The patient asked for discharge one week later. He had fever consistently, and his temperature would return to normal after taking nimesulide and then rose again the next night.

One week later, the patient was admitted to the hospital again because of consistent fevers. His bone marrow culture was positive for *Staphylococcus hominis* twice during the hospitalization, and the bone marrow smear showed no obvious abnormalities. Lower extremity MRI showed abnormal signal foci in the bilateral tibia, fibula, and medullary cavity. He was diagnosed with "bilateral tibia and fibula osteomyelitis" and treated with norvancomycin for three days. After that, his body temperature returned to normal.

However, the patient developed fever again in the next few days, which implied the four-day antibiotic therapy of vancomycin was ineffective. Local physicians changed the antibiotics to rifampicin, teicoplanin, linezolid, and clindamycin, but his body temperature was still not controlled and gradually rose to 39.2 °C. At the same time, his lower limb pain failed to relieve. The repeated blood culture results remained negative.

The patient was then transferred to our hospital on April 13, 2010. The autoimmune antibodies, HLA-B27, and serum tumor markers were all negative. The bone scintigraphy showed systemically increased radiation in large joints. Rheumatic and orthopedic diseases were excluded after consultation with physicians from the department of rheumatology and orthopedics. Bone marrow infection was still suspected based on previous bone marrow culture and lower limbs MRI abnormalities.

However, vancomycin and rifampicin were both ineffective during the course, and repeated bone marrow culture showed no bacterial growth. We considered the previous bone marrow culture as contaminated and stopped the use of antibiotics. Xinhuang tablets were prescribed to symptomatically relieve fever. Abnormalities of the joint lesion were considered as "reactive arthritis" for lacking evidence of infection. Symptomatic antipyretic and pain relief therapy was given, and the patient was told to follow-up regularly in outpatient clinics. However, he continued to have fevers after discharge and developed intermittent headaches and both lower limb pain. He took Xinhuang tablets regularly and nimesulide intermittently for antipyretic and pain relief according to the doctor's advice.

During the course, he went to local hospitals several times to consult the possibility of rheumatic disease, but the results were all negative. The patient also sought Chinese medicine for help, but the effect was not satisfying. At the end of September, the patient's right frontal, temporal, and occipital constant pain worsened, which could be relieved by nimesulide. From October 10–15, the patient was hospitalized in a provincial pulmonary hospital, where sputum smear and lumbar puncture were conducted. The smear showed acid-fast bacilli negative, and cerebrospinal fluid examination showed white blood cells of 15×10^6/L, glucose of 2.68 mmol/L, and protein of 0.35 g/L. The CSF culture of bacteria and cryptococcus were negative, and chest CT showed bronchial infection in both lungs. Cranial MRI revealed punctate long T1 long T2 signals in the pons and bilateral mastoid inflammation. The patient was admitted into our hospital again for further diagnosis and treatment. During the course of the illness, the patient had a good mental state, poor appetite, and slumber, with normal defecation and urination. He had lost 5 kg in weight.

3.4.1 Personal History

He worked as a painter for 10 years, often in contact with chemicals such as xylene.

3.4.2 Physical Examination

On physical examination, scattered ring-shaped erythema were found behind the left ear, back, and both lower limbs, with clear borders, covered with a few scabs. Hypopigmented spots were found scattered on both sides of the anterior tibial skin. Multiple finger/toe nail plates were thickened, deformed, and presented to be yellow-white. Multiple lymph nodes were palpable on both sides of the cervical, supraclavicular, trochlear, axillary, and inguinal region. The larger lymph node is tough with a diameter of 10 mm and good mobility. The spleen can be reached one finger under the ribs with a medium texture. The bilateral anterior tibial tenderness is obvious. Muscle power, pathological signs of the nervous system were normal, as was the remainder of the examination.

The patient was negative for jaundice, with no deformities of head, normal facial features, and soft neck. His trachea is in the middle, and thyroid gland is not enlarged, with normal breath movements and clear breath sounds. No obvious dry and wet rales were present. The heart rate was 78 beats per minute, with normal sinus heart rhythm and no pathological cardiac murmurs. The abdomen is flat and soft, with no tenderness, rebound pain and normal bowel sounds of four times per minute. No percussion pain is presented in liver and kidney area. The spleen can be reached under the ribs one finger with a medium texture, comparing with unreachable liver. The bilateral anterior tibial tenderness is obvious. There is no deformity in the limbs and spine. Muscle power, muscle tension was normal, as was the remainder of pathological signs of the nervous system.

3.4.3 Presentation of Cases

After admission, he was treated with linezolid for two weeks. His temperature was not controlled, and the bone pain still severe. Since repeated blood cultures were negative, we stopped the antibiotic treatment and increased methylprednisolone to 40 mg intravenously per day. The body temperature dropped to a lower grade, but the lower extremities' pain worsened and, he couldn't bear any weight.

Further examination found no obvious evidence of fungal infection with low titers of peripheral blood G test, and negative GM and T-SPOT test. Reexamination of MRI confirmed abnormal signals in the bone marrow cavity of the tibia, which implied the possibility of bone marrow infiltration, such as the infiltration of hematology diseases. The whole-body bone scintigraphy showed symmetrically abnormal increased radioactivity of shoulder joints, elbow joints, hip joints, knee joints, and ankle joints on both sides. In order to clarify the scope and nature of lesions, PET-CT examinations were conducted to show: (1) Multiple abnormal FDG metabolism increase in the whole-body bone marrow and a slight increase in anterior inferior mediastinal lymph nodes, which most likely implied malignant disease, so puncture biopsy is recommended; (2) the pancreatic FDG metabolism slightly diffusely increased, considering the possibility of inflammatory lesions; (3) mild left maxillary sinusitis; (4) hepatosplenomegaly; and (5) the metabolism of FDG in the left adrenal gland is slightly increased.

Bone marrow biopsy showed that it was infiltrated by malignant cells derived from histiocytes. Pathological biopsy of tibial bone showed that there were sheets of foam-like cells in the tissues showing lipid granuloma-like changes. Combined with medical history and imaging, it was diagnosed as Erdheim-Chester Disease (ECD). In consideration of the ineffectiveness of diagnostic antibiotic therapy and increased steroids therapy, infectious diseases and connective tissue diseases can possibly be ruled out. In order to make the definite diagnosis, bone marrow pathological immunohistochemistry was performed, suggesting: S-100 (−), CD1a (−), CD68 (+), CD138 (small amount +), K (−), KP-1 (−), Lys (+), Ki67 (10%+), CD21 (−), and it was in line with ECD performance. At this point, the patient was diagnosed with ECD. It is believed that the patient's endocrine and nervous system may also be involved based on the clinical and pathological characteristics of ECD. So pituitary MRI was performed, showing full pituitary gland and bilateral retrobulbar diffuse nodular abnormal signal, which can be consistent with granulomatous lesions. ECD diagnosis is also supported.

The patient started receiving interferon combined with glucocorticoid therapy after the diagnosis was confirmed. Unfortunately, he died of severe lung infection and pancytopenia 7 months later.

3.4.4 Pathological Discussion

ECD is a rare non-Langerhans histiocytosis of unknown cell origin. So far, no more than 240 cases have been reported worldwide, predisposing ECD to misdiagnosis. ECD mainly occurs in the middle-aged and elderly, and the average age of onset is 54 years old (21–77 years old) without gender difference. The disease involves a wide range of regions, and the most common site is long bone (32%). 50% of patients have other tissue infiltrations, including skin, retroorbital and periorbital tissue, hypothalamus-pituitary axis, heart, kidney, central nervous system, retroperitoneal cavity, liver, spleen, skeletal muscle, and adrenal gland. Rare cases report the infiltration of breast, thyroid, and testicles.

The diagnosis of ECD depends on the tissue biopsy, imaging, and clinical manifestations. Tissue biopsy is the golden standard for diagnosis. Typical histological findings could be concluded as: HE staining shows a large number of tissue cells rich in foam-like lipids or eosinophilic cytoplasm; immunostaining is characterized by CD68 (+), CD1a (−), Smur100 (+/−); absence of Birbeck particles under the electron microscope. The typical diseases that need to be differentiated are Langerhans histiocytosis (LCH), histiocytosis X, The typical diseases that need to be differentiated are Langerhans cell histiocytosis (LCH), including its historical subtypes such as Hand-Schüller-Christian disease. The diagnosis is based on the immunological markers on the surface of the cell membrane.

The treatment of ECD is still controversial because of the rare incidence and insufficient observational data. The methods of treatment include corticosteroids, cyclosporine, interferon, leukemia chemotherapeutic drugs, surgical resection, radiotherapy, etc. The prognosis of this disease is mainly related to organs involved, worse than that of LCH. Respiratory distress, extensive pulmonary fibrosis, and heart failure are the main causes of death. The 3-year survival rate is 50%, and there is yet no report of self-remission.

The clinical course of our ECD patient lasted for more than a year. The main manifestations were blurred vision, fever, and pain in both lower extremities. Twice bone marrow cultures performed at the local hospital were positive for coagulase-negative staphylococci, and MRI of the lower limbs was suspected to be bilateral tibiofibular osteomyelitis. Long bone osteomyelitis is commonly considered as a complication of staphylococcal bloodstream infection, so it made the diagnosis go through a detour. However, the ineffective antibiotic treatment and negative blood culture reexamination helped broaden our horizon. A tibia biopsy should be done as soon as possible to clarify the diagnosis, which worked as an important step to clarify the diagnosis. It must be mentioned that ECD is a rare disease, so other

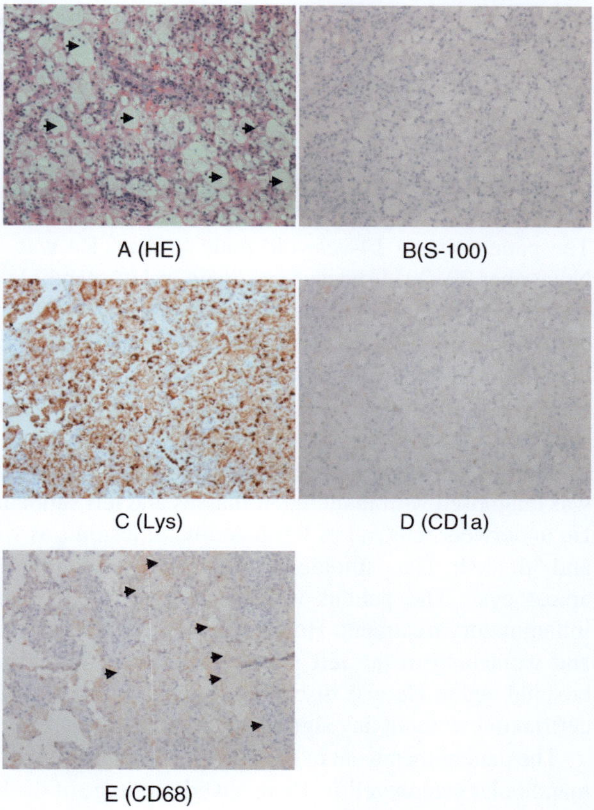

Fig. 3.5 Histopathology of tibia bone. (**a**) HE staining shows a large number of vacuolar cells, full of lipids, and a small amount of lymphocyte infiltration. (**b**) monoclonal antibody enzyme-labeled S-100 negative; (**c**) monoclonal antibody enzyme-labeled Lys negative; (**d**) The monoclonal antibody is negative for CD1a; (**e**) The monoclonal antibody is positive for CD68

common diseases must be excluded before consideration of ECD in the differential diagnosis of long-term fevers. Histopathology and immunohistochemical examination are the important keys to the final answer (Fig. 3.5).

References

1. Devouassoux G, Lantuejoul S, Chatelain P, et al. Erdheim Chester disease: a primary macrophage cell disorder. Am J Respir Crit Care Med. 1998;157:650–3.
2. Park JW, Chung CU, Shin JY, et al. Erdheim-Chester disease with hepatitis, glomerulonephritis, aplastic anemia and lung involvement. Tuberc Respir Dis. 2009;67:345–50.
3. Martinez R. Erdheim-Chester disease: MR of intraaxial and extraaxial brain stem lesions. AJNR Am J Neuroradiol. 1995;16:1787–90.
4. Kong P M, Pinheiro L, Kaw G, et al. Erdheim-Chester disease: a rare cause of interstitial lung disease. Singapore Med J. 2007;48(2):e57–9.
5. Jeon l, Lee SS, Lee MK. Chemotherapy and Interferon- a treatment of Erdheim-Chester disease. Pediatr Blood Cancer. 2010;55:745–7.

3.5 Langerhans Cell Histiocytosis Presenting Fever with Lytic Bone Lesions of the Mandible and Right Femur, Which Had Been Suspected of Chronic Osteomyelitis for More Than 2 Years

Shao Lingyun, Huang Yuxian, and Zhang Wenhong

The patient was a 14-year-old male student. He was admitted to our hospital on November 29, 2011, because of "pain in left mandible for 10 months, followed by fever for 16 months, and pain in right thigh for 15 months."

In September 2009, the patient was admitted to a local hospital for pain in left mandible. He received root canal therapy, anti-infective therapy (mainly cephalosporins and metronidazole), symptomatic treatment and glucocorticoids (no detail available), and his symptoms were partially relieved.

The patient was admitted to a local hospital for treatment on March 25, 2010, and was diagnosed with mandibular masses and left submandibular infection (Fig. 3.6). He underwent removal of left mandibular lesions, as well as extraction of 4th, 5th, and 6th teeth. The pathological results suggested inflammatory cell infiltration and apical cyst. The patient was discharged as the pain was relieved after anti-inflammatory treatment. However, two days after discharge, the pain was recurrent and worsening in the left lower posterior teeth, and the patient was admitted to hospital again. He was discharged against medical advice after being treated with ceftriaxone without any significant improvement.

The patient then went to a hospital in Shanghai twice and was diagnosed with left mandibular osteomyelitis. He received curettage of the left mandibular lesion (April

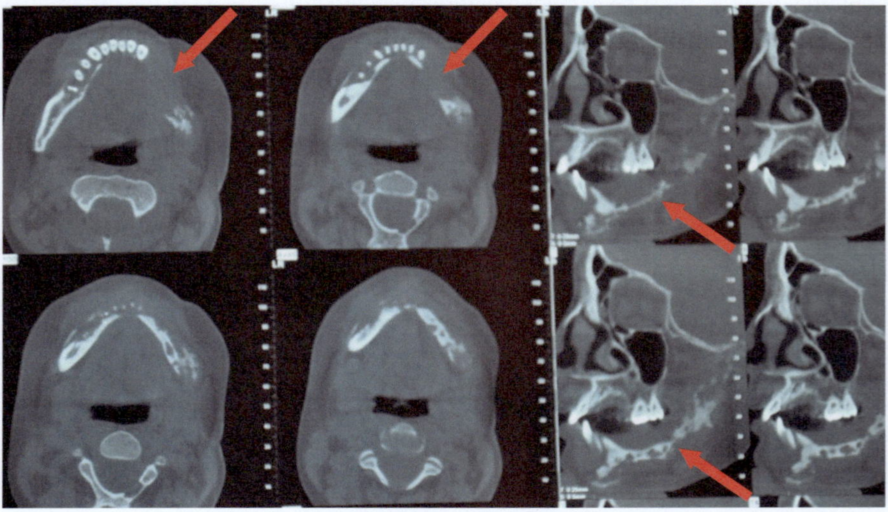

Fig. 3.6 Section from a CT on March 25, 2010, showed the low-density shadow in the left mandibular alveolar bone (arrow)

21, 2010) and curettage of the left mandibular ramus osteomyelitis (June 23, 2010). The pathological results demonstrated fibrous cyst wall-like tissue in left mandibular, with infection and multinucleated giant cell infiltration, no lining epithelium, and focal osteomyelitis and irregular bone edge absorption. The diagnosis was osteomyelitis (left mandible). Symptoms were relieved after antibiotics and glucocorticoids treatment. However, one week after discharge, he developed stiffness of the buccal mucosa of the left jaw, swelling and pain of the gums with fever of 39.6 °C, accompanying by occasional chills, without obvious sweating. Pathology of mucosal biopsy showed inflammation. Intermittent antibiotics and dexamethasone could relieve the symptoms temporarily.

At the end of July 2010, the patient developed sudden severe pain in the right thigh without obvious trigger, which was persistent, accompanied by a fever of about 38.0 °C and a maximum temperature of 39 °C, with occasional chills and without obvious sweating. The body temperature would decrease after administration of antipyretic drugs, but would soon rise again. Subsequently, the patient visited a hospital in Suzhou, where an MRI examination showed that the anterior cortex of the right femur had abnormally low density with a little periosteal reaction. He was still diagnosed with osteomyelitis and was treated with meropenem, rifampicin, and azithromycin, but the pain and fever were not relieved significantly. Symptomatic treatment with indomethacin suppository and analgesics were administered.

From September 2010 to June 2011, the patient went to a hospital in Wuxi for 4 times and was still diagnosed with osteomyelitis (mandible, lower end of right femur). Facial artery and right femoral artery catheterization were performed to give 12-day meropenem therapy through catheterization 5 times, and systemic anti-infective therapy with meropenem and rifampicin was given at the same time. However, the patient's symptoms continued to recur, and the range of pain in thigh expanded. The leg pain and fever were completely improved with the first four intramedullary injections, but the leg pain and fever persisted after the fifth intramedullary injection. During this period, a biopsy for the lytic bone lesions of the right femur was performed on September 21, 2010 in the orthopedics department of the hospital. Pathology of right femur lesions showed broken bone tissue with fibrosis and vascular hyperplasia, and infiltration of lymph node cells, plasma cells, and neutrophils in the focal area. After being discharged from the hospital in Wuxi in June 2011, he returned to the local hospital and continued intravenous antibiotics (penicillin, ceftriaxone, etc.), but the effect was still not good.

In September 2011, he was hospitalized in the orthopedics department of a hospital in Shanghai and was diagnosed with "right femoral chronic hematogenous osteomyelitis, postoperative mandibular osteomyelitis." During the hospitalization, his laboratory tests showed that the blood bacterium and fungus cultures were all negative, autoantibodies were negative as well, and CRP was 214.00 mg/L, ESR was over 140 mm/h, serum 1,3-beta-D-glucan test (October 12, 2011) was 120 pg/mL. In repeated complete blood count tests, anemia was suggested, with basically normal white blood cells and neutrophils.

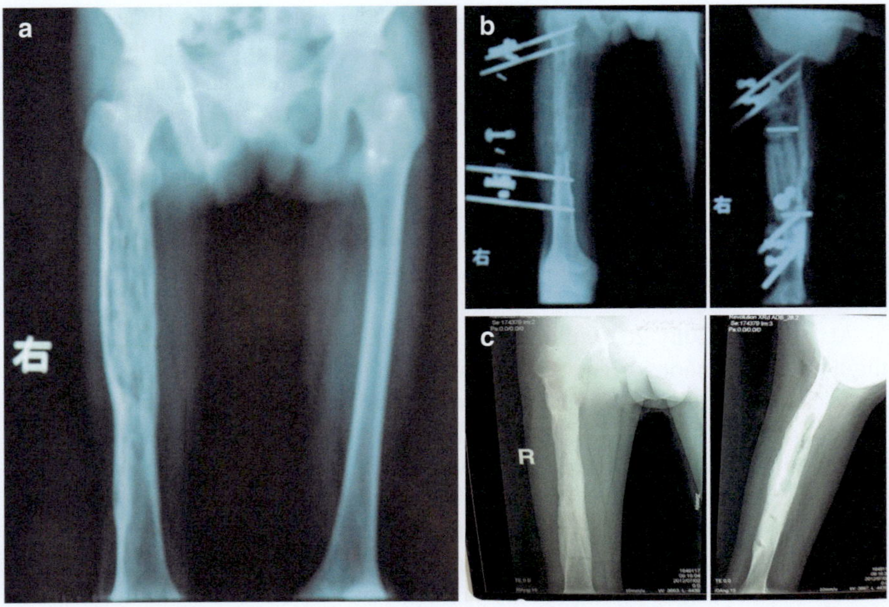

Fig. 3.7 X-ray of the patient's femur. (**a**) Before surgery, in a hospital in Shanghai, in September 2011; (**b**) After surgery, in a hospital in Shanghai, in September 2011; (**c**) After chemotherapy, in July 2012

On September 27, 2011, debridement of right bone femoral osteomyelitis and antibiotic artificial bone implantation and external fixation with external fixation surgeries were performed (Fig. 3.7a, b). Culture of tissues obtained from operation showed *Campylobacter coli*, without any yeast-like fungi. Pain in bones were relieved after anti-infective treatment, but fever still persisted. He was transferred to pediatric department for further treatment and was given a variety of antibiotic and antifungal medications (penicillin, cefoperazone-sulbactam, vancomycin, fluconazole, imipenem, clarithromycin), and antipyretic analgesics for symptomatic treatment. The patient's temperature still wasn't reduced, so the family members required to discharge and took treatment in the local hospital. Though antibiotics (ceftriaxone, penicillin, ornidazole) was continued in the local hospital, the fever still persisted at around 38 °C, with a peak of 39.6 °C, mainly in the afternoon, accompanied by occasional chills. During the period of illness, the patient had pain in right gingival, and there was no rash in skin and mucous, no pain in joint, no oral ulcers, no cough, sputum, abdominal pain, and diarrhea. Antibiotics were withdrawn for 1 week before admission to our hospital for further diagnosis and treatment.

3.5.1 Past Medical History

The patient was diagnosed with acute leukemia at the local hospital at 18 months and was given chemotherapy (vincristine, daunorubicin). The treatment was maintained until the patient was 6 years old. The patient had breast development on both sides at about 8 years old, without obvious pain or discharge. In the past 1 year, the skin pigment changed at the ends of the hands and feet without itching.

3.5.2 General Physical Examination

The patient was conscious, fair in general conditions, and weighing about 30 kg. His left cheek was sunken, and there were pigmentation changes on the tips of the fingers and right toes. Both breasts were developed, without tenderness or discharge. Abdomen was soft, without any tenderness or rebound tenderness. Liver and spleen were not palpable under the ribs. The right lower limb had undergone steel plate fixation, with well-healed wounds. No swelling of the lower limbs.

3.5.3 Management

The patient was given Xinhuang tablets (a tablet with NSAIDs and herbs) after admission. His body temperature gradually decreased, but there was still intermittent low fever (maximum at 37.7 °C). Tumor markers, CD3, CD4, CD8 counts, thyroid function and growth hormone were within normal range. Serum immunofixation electrophoresis, Coomb's test, hepatitis markers, anti-HIV, RPR and serum 1,3-beta-D-glucan test and cryptococcus latex agglutination test were all negative. There was no bacterium in the culture of blood. Emission computed tomography of bones showed that the mandible and right femur had abnormally increased radioactivity (Fig. 3.8).

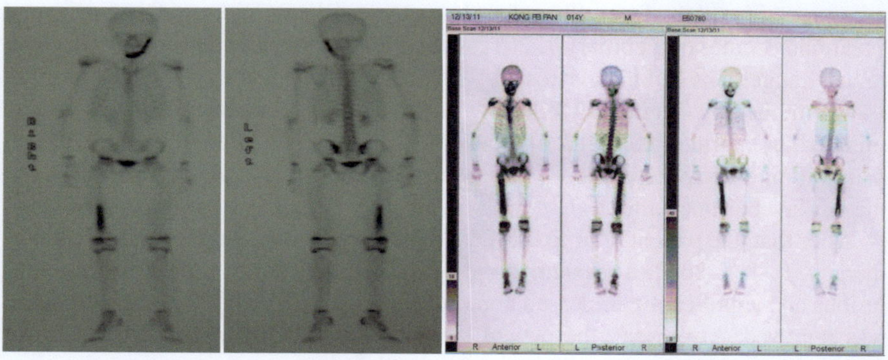

Fig. 3.8 The results of the patient's emission computed tomography of bones. Top picture: conducted in a hospital in Suzhou, in August 2010, suggesting increased radioactivity in the left mandible and right femur; bottom picture: conducted in our hospital, in December 2011, suggesting increased radioactivity in the left mandible and right femur

In view of the complexity of the patient's condition, after completing clinical assessment, the Department of Infectious Diseases held a consultation attended by experts in orthopedics, maxillofacial surgery, and hematology. The experts in the Department of Infectious Diseases believed that the patient had fever and lytic bone lesions for up to 2 years, during which the degree of anti-infective treatment had been literally remarkable, however, the effect was poor, and the disease had been slowly progressing. Therefore, although the pathological diagnosis had been "osteomyelitis", the clinical course could exclude "chronic osteomyelitis". Doctors should not insist upon various antibacterial drugs, instead, consultation with experts in relevant departments should be made to make a clear diagnosis.

Experts of maxillofacial surgery and orthopedics unanimously denied the diagnosis of osteomyelitis, based on their decades of clinical experience. Thus, on February 1, 2012, experts conducted detailed discussions and reviewed the pathological slices obtained from multiple biopsies and operations at the Shanghai Intractable Blood Disease Diagnosis and Treatment Center. The expert group decided that "Langerhans cell histiocytosis" should be considered first, based on the patient's symptoms, signs, bone marrow biopsy, bone marrow smears and other examinations. Pathologists suggested to review the pathological slices repeatedly to determine the diagnosis of "Langerhans Cell histiocytosis" pathologically. S-100, CDla and Langerhans cell (LC) enzymatic examinations should also be performed, if necessary, as well as strategies including seeking Birbeck particles under electron microscope and looking for Langerhans cells in bone marrow puncture. Consequently, the patient was transferred to the Department of Hematology in our hospital on February 2, 2012 for further evaluation and treatment.

After transferring to the Department of Hematology, a repeated bone marrow puncture was conducted (bone marrow slide number: 12–78M1): the bone marrow was actively proliferating, mainly from erythroid and megakaryocytic systems. There was left shift of granule line, some with degeneration. There were obvious mononuclear macrophages and plasma cells on the slice, and a small number of abnormal lymphocytes. No evidence of lymphoma was found. Based on the patient's clinical manifestations and results of radiological examinations, and considering the opinions of experts from Shanghai Intractable Blood Disease Diagnosis and Treatment Center on February 1, 2012, the patient's clinical diagnosis was deemed to be "Langerhans cell histiocytosis".

Chemotherapy (regimen: VLB 8 mg d1 + methylprednisolone 40 mg d1–8) was initiated on February 10, 2012. The patient's body temperature returned to normal, pain in bones disappeared, tooth looseness was relieved, and the buccal mucosa of the left jaw became softer.

After that, the patient returned to the local hospital to finish the course of chemotherapy. In July 2012, a reexamination of the femoral X-ray showed right femur lesions and significantly increased bone substance (Fig. 3.7c). The external fixation was removed. At present, the patient has returned to school, without discomfort such as fever and bone pain, and can perform activities such as running and climbing.

3.5.4 Comments

Langerhans cell histiocytosis (LCH), which was formerly called histiocytosis X, is a group of diseases with the main pathological characteristics of the abnormal proliferation of Langerhans cells for unknown reasons. It has a great variety of clinical manifestations, for example, it only presents as isolated painless bone lesions in mild cases, while it extensively involves multiple organ systems accompanied by fever, anemia and weight loss in severe cases.

The incidence of this disease is estimated to be 1 in 200,000–1 in 2,000,000, and it mainly occurs in infants and children, of which the majority are male patients. In 1987, the International Histiocyte Society established the three-level diagnostic criteria: (1) Presumptive diagnosis: only based on histopathological results with the identification of mononuclear histiocytes in high-power view or oil immersion lens view under optical microscope. (2) Diagnosis: add two or more of the following four indicators on the basis of morphological findings under optical microscope: positive ATPase, positive S-100 protein, positive α-D-mannase, and positive arachis hypogaea lectin. (3) Definitive diagnosis: presence of Birbeck granules on electronic microscopy and/or positive CD1a monoclonal antibody on the basis of morphological findings under optical microscope.

At present, the treatment of LCH is mainly based on the organ involvement, the site of involvement and number of lesions. Treatment options include topical chemotherapy or curettage surgery for patients with single system LCH, and systemic chemotherapy for patients with multisystem LCH. The prognosis of LCH is closely related to the age of onset, the number of involved organs and the impairment of organ function. Generally speaking, the prognosis of bone involvement is better than that of extraosseous tissues, that of solitary bone lesion is better than multiple bone lesions, and that of multisystem LCH is the worst.

In this case, the patient had fever and lytic bone lesions of the mandible and right femur for more than 2 years, and the pathological diagnosis was osteomyelitis, so the initial diagnosis of osteomyelitis was reasonable. However, after more than two years of treatment with dozens of antibiotics and antifungals, even topical antibiotic treatment and debridement of the right femur, it still did not get any better, subsequently the left mandible disappeared and the left cheek was deformed.

It was obviously an overreliance on pathological diagnosis and a false obsession with the power of antibiotics, which was a very common mistake among clinical practitioners. Despite that, the pathological evidence is significant in making definitive diagnosis, and only when the clinicians actively communicated with the pathologists and made profound introspection over the previous diagnosis, which was prompted by the ineffectiveness of anti-infective and surgical treatments, an accurate and proper diagnosis was finally made.

References

1. Henter JI, Elinder G, Soder O, et al. Histiocytosis syndromes in children. Writing Group of the Histiocyte Society. Lancet. 1987;1(8526):208–9.
2. Abla O, Egeler RM, Weitzman S, et al. Langerhans cell histiocytosis: current concepts and treatment. Cancer Treat Rev. 2010;36:354–9.
3. Yuanjun L, Huilin N, Jinsheng T, et al. Clinical analysis of 42 cases of Langerhans cell histiocytosis in children. J Clin Dermatol. 2011;40:348–9.
4. Jingshi W, Zhao W, Mei X, et al. Three cases of Langerhans cell histiocytosis with a literature review. J Clin Exp Med. 2011;10:895–7.

3.6 T Cell Lymphoma of the Small Intestine with Fever as the Initial Symptom

Shao Lingyun, Huang Yuxian, and Zhang Wenhong

A 40-year-old male construction project manager was admitted to the hospital on January 11, 2012 with a 2-month history of repeated fever and chills. Two days after a tonsillectomy on October 1, 2011, the patient developed fever (temperature as high as 38.3 °C), accompanied by chills and pharynx pain, without any other accompanying symptoms. The patient was successively treated with cefuroxime, metronidazole, and amoxicillin-potassium clavulanate, etc., and the temperature was basically controlled half a month later. However, at the end of November 2011, fever accompanied by sore throat and chills occurred again, with the highest temperature of 39.9 °C, and treatment with amoxicillin and levofloxacin showed no obvious effect. On December 19, the patient visited the doctor of the outpatient clinic in our hospital, and the blood culture showed coagulase-negative staphylococcus. After oral administration of cefixime, the body temperature decreased and fluctuated between 37 and 38.5 °C. On January 6, 2012, reexamination of blood culture still showed coagulase-negative staphylococcus, and the body temperature rose again above 39 °C, then he was admitted to hospital.

3.6.1 Physical Examination at Admission

Clear mind, good spirit, and skin and sclera without yellow stain. The superficial supraclavicular lymph nodes were not enlarged. The respiration movements of both sides were normal and symmetrical. The respiration sounds of both lungs were clear, and no obvious rhonchi and moist rales were heard. Heart rate: 90 beats/min. The heart rhythm was normal; no pathological murmur was heard in each valvular area. The abdomen was soft, no tenderness and rebound pain. Liver subcostal not reached, spleen subcostal 2 fingers, medium quality, no tenderness. Normal limb movement, no edema in both lower limbs, symmetrical knee reflex, (++), pathological signs (−).

3.6.2 Auxiliary Examination

Blood routine: WBC: 3.64×10^9/L, N: 47.5%, L: 40.1%, RBC: 3.47×10^{12}/L, HB: 98 g/L, platelet: 142×10^9/L. Abdominal B-ultrasonography showed no obvious abnormalities in liver, gallbladder, and pancreas, while spleen was enlarged (140 × 46 mm). The patient defecated blood and stool 3 times on the day of admission, with a total amount of about 300 mL. No discomfort such as hematemesis, dizziness or cold sweat was found. Check feces OB: 3+. Endoscopy showed gastric sinusitis (hyperemic exudative type, moderate) and polypoid hyperplasia in the gastric fundus. Colonoscopy showed no organic lesions in the entire colorectal mucosa.

3.6.3 The Process of Diagnosis and Treatment

After admission, "coagulase-negative staphylococcal septicemia" was considered and anti-infective treatment was given with vancomycin + fosfomycin, but the effect was not good. The patient still had fever with chills and shivers.

Coagulase-negative staphylococci are the normal flora of human skin and mucous membranes. They are generally not disease-causing and mainly cause nosocomial infections. A blood culture with coagulase-negative staphylococcus positive is generally difficult to distinguish whether it is a contaminating bacterium or a real bloodstream infection. A Swiss study found that 65% of 654 positive blood samples were false positives. Multi-factor analysis showed that fever or hypothermia, tachycardia, shortness of breath, leukocytosis or decrease, and central venous catheters were independent risk factors for coagulase negative staphylococci infection. If three symptoms are met at the same time, the probability of coagulase-negative staphylococcal bloodstream infection increases to 72.3%. Coagulase-negative staphylococci, whether they are contaminated bacteria or pathogenic bacteria, have no significant difference in sensitivity to penicillin, oxacillin, gentamicin, ciprofloxacin, vancomycin, and other drugs. Although this patient had a fever after tonsillectomy and was positive for coagulase-negative staphylococci in blood culture, it may be a pathogen, but the treatment for coagulase-negative staphylococci did not relieve the fever. Therefore, the patient's blood culture results could be caused by pollution. Combined with the patient's repeated fever, tonsillitis, and splenomegaly, further examinations were recommended to rule out hematological disease.

Blood routine showed a progressive decrease in WBC and Hb. Blood routine on January 18: WBC: 1.39×10^9/L, N: 56.8%, Hb: 90 g/L, platelet: 156×10^9/L. Bone penetration on January 19 showed hyperplastic bone marrow with more plasma cells, a small number of atypical lymphocytes (2%) and phagocytes (1%).

The patient had fever, tonsillitis, and splenomegaly. If the diagnosis was hematological tumor, does it originate from the tonsils? However, the pathological sections of tonsils from other hospitals were reviewed, and no malignant cells were found. Further lymphocyte immunolabeling did not find malignant lymphocytes. Thus, tumors originating in the tonsils were excluded.

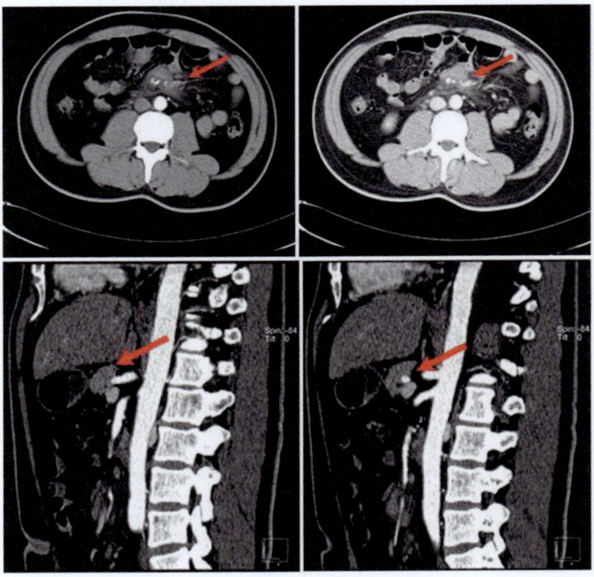

Fig. 3.9 Contrast-enhanced CT of the patient's abdomen. The arrow shows a large area of mixed density at the mesenteric root

The patient further received upper abdominal enhanced CT (Fig. 3.9), suggesting a large mixed density in the mesenteric root, and the possibility of inflammation need to be excluded clinically. After reviewing the abdominal CT film with the radiologist, we consider that group 3 (distal jejunum) and group 4 (proximal ileum) small intestinal lesions are present, accompanied by chronic perforation and local encapsulation. Urgent abdominal supine position plain film showed a small amount of local intestinal gas and no change in intestinal perforation was indicated. There was no obvious abnormality in CTA/CTV of mesenteric vessels. Gastroenterologists considered the cause of bleeding in the lower gastrointestinal tract as uninvestigated, possibly Crohn's disease. On January 21, the patient was given a liquid diet, an anti-infective treatment with tyronen and wenkexin, anti-inflammatory treatment with methylprednisolone, supplemented by parenteral nutrition support treatment, and the patient's body temperature was basically controlled. On January 29, no obvious abnormalities were observed in capsule endoscopy, and the possibility of intestinal inflammatory lesions and perforation was basically excluded. Therefore, it is considered that the large mixed masses in the mesenteric root may be mesenteric lymph nodes. On February 1, PET-CT indicated increased FDG metabolism in enlarged mesenteric lymph nodes and adjacent intestinal tract (the maximum SUV value was 13.5), suggesting the possibility of malignant lesions.

The patient was then transferred to general surgery for laparoscopic mesentery lymph node biopsy on February 3. Intraoperative exploration found that in the middle of the small intestine, there was an inflammatory adhesion between a part of the intestinal wall and the mesentery, and multiple enlarged lymph nodes in the adjacent mesentery were observed and fused with each other, about 6 × 6 cm in size. A lymph node with a diameter of about 2.5 cm was cut off at first, and the adhesion was separated. It was found that there was a perforation of about 1.5 cm in the intestinal wall, and the surrounding intestinal wall was stiff. Therefore, an open approach was decided to disentangle the perforated intestine, remove the intestinal segment with a diameter of about 6 cm, and perform an end-to-end intestinal anastomosis. Postoperative pathological diagnosis: (1) non-Hodgkin lymphoma (mesenteric lymph node), T-cell type, combined with histological morphology and enzymatic labelling results, was first considered as an enteric T-cell lymphoma, type II; (2) Perforation of the small intestine. There is abnormal T lymphocyte infiltration in the surrounding tissue. The patient was diagnosed with enteropathic T-cell lymphoma and was transferred to the hematology department for chemotherapy. However, the patient progressed and died of multiple organ failure on October 12, 2012.

3.6.4 Comments

The main types of intestinal lymphoma are mucosa-associated lymphoid tissue (MALT) lymphoma and enteropathic type T-cell lymphoma (ETCL). ETCL is a type of extranodal T cell lymphoma that accounts for 34% of intestinal lymphomas. It is more common in middle-aged and older men. The typical cases often have a history of cereal protein allergy and celiac disease. However, celiac disease is rare in Asian patients, and the patient in this case has no history of celiac disease. Tumors often occur in the ileocecal part of the small intestine and the ascending colon, but rarely occur in the transverse colon and stomach. Ulcerative colitis and perforation may occur, and ulcerative colitis diagnosed in the past is mostly this disease. Fever, anemia, chronic abdominal pain, diarrhea, weight loss, acute intestinal perforation or chronic multiple intestinal ulcers, repeated bleeding, etc. are the most common in the clinical practice, and can be complicated with the decrease of red blood cells and white blood cells, and thrombocytopenia, hepatosplenomegaly, and occasionally systemic edema have been reported. The clinical process is relatively dangerous and the prognosis is very poor. People often die from repeated gastrointestinal bleeding, perforation, sepsis or tumor recurrence, and metastasis within 1 week to 6 months after diagnosis. Half of the patients could not complete the chemotherapy, and most of the patients relapsed in 1–6 months. Because of the complex and diverse clinical manifestations of ETCL, it is easy to cause misdiagnosis or missed diagnosis.

Some studies have shown that ^{18}F-FDG PET/CT imaging in 35 patients with fever of unknown origin is helpful for clinical diagnosis of 37% of patients, with a positive predictive value of 87% and a negative predictive value of 95%. A study of 48 patients with suspected local infection or inflammatory fever showed that PET imaging was helpful in the clinical diagnosis of 65% of the patients, with a positive predictive value of 95% and a negative predictive value of 100%. The SUVmax of malignant lesions was significantly higher than that of benign lesions. Further analysis showed that 119 of the 144 patients with fever were found to have at least one abnormal radioactive concentration on ^{18}F-FDG PET/CT whole-body imaging, with a detection rate of 82.6%. The sensitivity, specificity, accuracy, positive predictive value, and negative predictive value of PET/CT in the diagnosis of benign and malignant lesions were 97.6% (40/41), 86.5% (77/89), 90.0% (117/130), 76.9%

(40/52), and 98.7% (77/78), respectively. Therefore, whole-body ^{18}F-FDG PET/CT imaging is considered to be an important adjunct diagnostic tool in the diagnosis of long-term fever of unknown origin, helping to provide early location of the primary lesion, and helping to locate and further follow up.

References

1. Elzi L, Babouee B, Vögeli N, Laffer R, Dangel M, Frei R, Battegay M, Widmer AF. How to discriminate contamination from bloodstream infection due to coagulase-negative staphylococci: a prospective study with 654 patients. Clin Microbiol Infect. 2012;18(9):E355–61.
2. Rahkonen M, Luttinen S, Koskela M, Hautala T. True bacteremias caused by coagulase negative Staphylococcus are difficult to distinguish from blood culture contaminants. Eur J Clin Microbiol Infect Dis. 2012;31(10):2639–44.
3. Hui W, Yuexian Z, Xiuli X, Yingchun X, Minjun C. Clinical significance of coagulase-negative staphylococci in blood cultures. Chin J Antimicrob Chemother. 2001;1(2):79–83.
4. Bleeker-Rovers CP, De Kleijn EM, Corstens FH, et al. Clinical value of FDG PET in patients with fever of unknown origin and patients suspected of focal infection of inflammation. Eur J Nucl Med Mol Imaging. 2004;31:37–9.
5. Fengchun H, Yongchang L, Jun Z, et al. The value of 18F-FDG PET imaging in screening for lymphoma in patients with fever of unknown origin. Chin J Nucl Med. 2004;24:11–3.
6. Binqing Z, Yongxue Z, Tao W, et al. Diagnostic value of 18F-FDG PET/CT in fever of unknown origin. Radiol Pract. 2010;25:694–6.
7. Haina G, Xiqun H, Xuming L, et al. Clinical analysis of enteropathy-associated T-cell lymphoma (a report of 5 cases). Gastroenterology. 2005;10:212–6.
8. Huali L, Jing S, Chaofu W. Clinicopathological analysis of enteropathy-associated T-cell lymphoma. J Bengbu Med Coll. 2012;37:650–2.

3.7 Anaplastic Large Cell Lymphoma with Skin Lesions as the First Manifestation

Chen Peidong, Jia Wen, Shao Lingyun, and Zhang Wenhong

A 48-year-old male patient, who worked as a bricklayer and often contact with building materials such as marble, was admitted to the hospital on December 30, 2014, because "the left groin mass was found for more than 4 months and accompanied by fever for more than 2 months." At the beginning of 2014, the patient developed a red maculopapule (about 1 cm in diameter) on the inner side of the left thigh, which was tender and hard with a palpable subcutaneous nodule， but not taken seriously. Later the nodule gradually enlarged. In April, the patient took roxithromycin on his own for one week and the nodule began to shrink and then gradually disappeared. In June, similar skin lesions and subcutaneous nodules appeared above the right knee and behind the left thigh, and gradually enlarged. After consulting a local dermatologist in July, the skin lesions were treated with topical medicine. The lesion behind the right thigh improved, but the other lesion remained enlarging and subsequently ruptured. Biopsy was recommended after debridement. On August 27, the patient went to a hospital in Shanghai for skin biopsy. The results showed that "surface squamous epithelium was obviously hyperplasia with hyperkeratosis, and some areas were ruptured with inflammatory granulation tissue formation." Soon the patient's lesion behind the left thigh improved on its own, meanwhile a subcutaneous nodule appeared above the left groin. However, the patient did not continue to follow up at that time.

Subsequently, the nodule in the left groin of the patient gradually enlarged. The patient began to present with fever on October 18, and the peak body temperature gradually increased, reaching a maximum of 39.8 °C, so he was admitted to a local hospital. Physical examination revealed a mass in the left lower abdomen and groin, and CT enhancement showed "a mass near the iliac artery and the left pelvic wall presented with the density of soft tissue" (Fig. 3.10). The blood routine revealed a white blood cell count of 14.9×10^9/L with the percentages of neutrophils was 77.04%, and a platelet count of 538×10^9/L. Liver function showed that ALT 46 U/L, AST 95 U/L, LDH 251 U/L. The level of C-reaction protein (CRP) was elevated (41.4 mg/L). Therefore, the patient was given ceftazidime, azithromycin, piperacillin, cefoperazone-tazobactam, ornidazole successively, but no obvious improvement was seen.

On November 1, the patient went to a hospital in Shanghai for further treatment. A blood routine revealed a white blood cell count of 19.37×10^9/L, with Neutrophils % of 79.1%, and a platelet count of 543×10^9/L. The erythrocyte sedimentation rate (ESR) was 92 mm/h and the CRP was 155 mg/L. T-SPOT.TB was negative. He was admitted to another hospital in Shanghai on November 6. On November 20, the enhanced pelvic MRI showed that "the left side of the pelvic cavity may have an abscess involving the lower part of the left ureter" (Fig. 3.11). Considering "pelvic abscess", vancomycin, fosfomycin, amikacin, amoxicillin-clavulanic acid, moxifloxacin, azithromycin, and rifampicin were given successively, but the effect was still not satisfactory. On November 21, puncture and imprint cytologic examination of the groin mass was performed and the results showed malignant tumor cells on

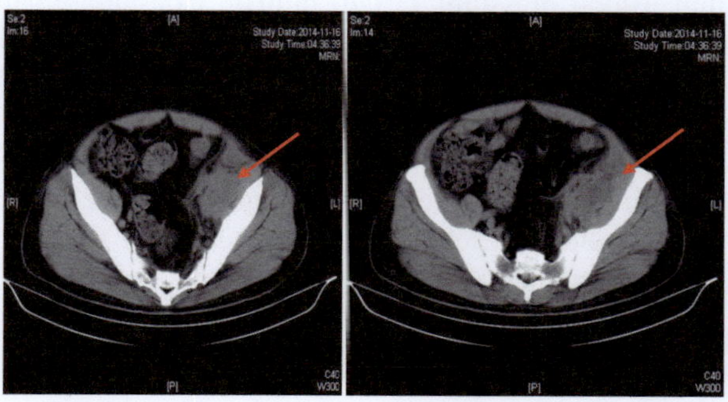

Fig. 3.10 CT scan image of the patient's lower abdomen, showing the soft tissue density shadow next to the iliac artery in the left pelvic wall

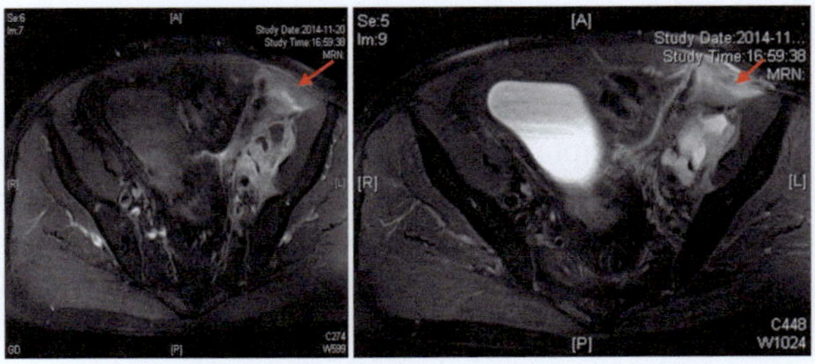

Fig. 3.11 MR enhanced image of the patient's pelvic cavity, showing the uneven density of soft tissue on the left side of the pelvis, with a cyst inside

November 24. The needle biopsy was performed on the same day and the results showed that "fibrous lesions, infiltrating the rhabdomyomus, consider the possibility of invasive fibromatosis." A PET/CT examination was performed on November 26, and the results showed that the soft tissue mass of the left pelvic wall was seen, involving the left ureter, left psoas major, and left iliac muscle, with the highest SUV of 21.0. The boundary with the surrounding tissue is not clear.

Therefore, the patient was admitted to the General Surgery Department of our hospital on December 3, and the operation was performed on December 9. During the operation, a 15 × 10 cm pelvic tumor was seen, which was hard and fixed with unclear borders and local involvement of the sigmoid mesocolon. Because of the surrounding iliac artery, the tumor was unable to be resected, so the abdomen was closed after a biopsy. The pathology examination showed "fatty fibrous tissue with abundant muscular blood vessels. Hemangioma considered", and the report after pathology consultation was "mainly fibrous tissue, accompanied by collagen degeneration, a small amount of inflammatory cell infiltration in the interstitium. Tumorous lesion or fibrous mass caused by inflammation cannot be excluded." He was discharged from hospital to continue medical treatment. As the patient still had fever, and his left groin was painful with a white blood cell count of 31.6×10^9/L, Neutrophil % of 92.54%, a platelet count of 611×10^9/L, he was admitted to our department on December 30.

3.7.1 Physical Examination

Body temperature: 38.4 °C, Pulse rate: 92 beats/min, Respiratory rate: 22 beats/min, Blood pressure: 115/70 mmHg. Conscious, painful face. The conjunctiva was obviously hyperemic. Cardiopulmonary auscultation found no abnormality. Surgical scar which was about 10 cm in length could be seen on the lower abdomen. Scattered pigmentation spots could be seen on both thighs. There was a huge mass, about 15 cm × 6 cm in size, in the left lower abdomen and left groin, which was hard, fixed, and tender with unclear borders. Some broad bean-sized lymph nodes could be reached in the groin, and the remaining superficial lymph nodes were not swollen.

3.7.2 The Process of Diagnosis and Treatment

The complete inspection after admission to the hospital was as follows: blood routine showed a white blood cell count of 34.56 × 10^9/L, with neutrophils 91.00%, hemoglobin of 113.00 g/L, a platelet count of 522.00 × 10^9/L. The ESR was 70.00 mm/h, the CRP was 296.00 mg/L and the ferritin was higher than 1500.0 μg/L. The tumor markers tests showed CA125 was 157.80 U/mL, CA199 was 61.96 U/mL and CA50 was 51.90 U/mL. Liver function showed albumin was 24.00 g/L, globulin was 39.00 g/L, and LDH was 142.00 U/L. Abdominal B-ultrasound revealed left hydronephrosis, left renal parenchymal mass (hamartoma), parenchymal mass next to the left iliac vessels; fatty liver. Superficial lymph node B-ultrasound showed left supraclavicular (13 × 8 mm) and groin (19 × 11 mm) lymph nodes were enlarged.

Due to the patient's persistent hematologic abnormalities, PET/CT reports and other related examinations, hematologic diseases were considered, then bone marrow puncture was performed on December 31. After the bone marrow puncture, methylprednisolone 60 mg/d was given to control inflammation. The patient's fever significantly improved, but the pain remained without NSAIDs. The bone marrow puncture report on January 6, 2015 stated that some naive white blood cells and their mitotic types that cannot be classified, and clusters of fibroblast-like cells were seen. After consulting a hematologist, malignant tumor involving the bone marrow might be considered, among which lymphoma was the most likely, and another biopsy was recommended. Therefore, he was transferred to the Department of Hematology on January 12, 2015. After evaluating the condition, he was given a needle biopsy guided by B-ultrasound. The pathology revealed anaplastic large cell lymphoma. Until now, the patient was finally definitely diagnosed. After CHOP chemotherapy was given, his symptoms improved significantly with his body temperature returned to normal, and the left groin mass shrank significantly.

3.7.3 Comments

Primary systemic anaplastic large cell lymphoma (ALCL) is a type of T-cell lymphoma, accounting for about 2% of all non-Hodgkin lymphoma (NHL), with characteristic chromosomal translocations: t (2,5), TCR gene rearrangement positive. The most common characteristic immunophenotypes are CD30positive, EMA (Epithelial Cell Membrane Antigen) positive. ALCL can be divided into two groups according to whether ALK (Anaplastic Lymphoma Kinase) is expressed or not. ALK-positive groups mostly consist of young men. The prognosis is fairly good with a 5-year survival rate of 70%–90%. ALK-negative group consist more of elderly men, with poor efficacy and short survival lifetime. The main clinical manifestations of the disease include fever, lymphadenopathy, bone marrow or gastrointestinal tract involvement, elevated LDH levels, and skin invasion. Usually, the treatment is the classic CHOP regimen chemotherapy.

The skin lesions of the patient at the beginning of the disease may be another group of related diseases, called CD30+ skin lymphoproliferative diseases, which include lymphoma-like papulosis and primary cutaneous anaplastic large cell lymphoma. ALK is negative in this group of diseases. Lymphoma-like papulosis is mainly manifested as red papules and nodules, which are chronic and may have spontaneous ulcers. They usually heal on their own within 8 weeks, leaving pigmentation, but new lesions may continue to appear. The course of the disease ranges from 3 months to 40 years, and about 10%–20% could progress to primary cutaneous anaplastic large cell lymphoma. The latter disease is more common in older men, and the skin lesions are usually limited, with solid, purple-red lesions, which tend to have ulcers (50%) or spontaneously disappear (25%). The prognosis is good with the 5-year survival rate greater than 90%. Approximately 30% patients progress to extracutaneous lymphoma. It is speculated that this patient may suffer from this group of disease at first and progress to systemic anaplastic large cell lymphoma subsequently.

The patient's first needle biopsy suggested the possibility of invasive fibromatosis, which is an unexplained fibroblastic tumor-like mass that originated in the muscle fascia, also known as ligamentoid tumor. It is benign in pathologic manifestation, but exhibits malignant behavior such as invasive growth. Invasive fibromatosis is most common in the shoulder girdle, thigh, and buttocks of young people. It will not metastasize. Surgical treatment is the first choice but complete resection is required, because it is easy to relapse after surgery. Taking the patient's entire diagnosis and treatment process into consideration, it is possible that the lymphoma cells were not obtained in the first biopsy, but the proliferating tissue around the lymphoma that was stimulated by it was obtained.

For patients with long-term fever, painless lymphadenopathy, and abnormal blood routine, lymphoma is a type of disease that requires high suspicion. Although bone puncture and PET/CT cannot be used as basis for definite diagnosis, they have important suggestive value in the diagnosis. In addition to assessing the extent of involvement, PET/CT can also help to select the site for biopsy and increase the positive rate.

The skin manifestations of anaplastic large cell lymphoma have a certain degree of peculiarities, and some skin lesions can even heal on their own, which can easily mislead clinical judgments and requires special attention. For patients with suspected lymphoma whose malignant cells cannot be seen on the biopsy, if other clinical evidence still leads to lymphoma, it is necessary to insist on repeated biopsy. Because lymphoma needs to be diagnosed and classified by pathology findings to guide subsequent treatment. If the disease indicated by the pathological results does not match the clinical manifestations, the pathological report should not be over trusted. Because the pathological report largely depends on the sample taken, but there is a possibility that the most suitable sample may not be obtained.

References

1. Inghirami G, Pileri SA; European T-Cell Lymphoma Study Group. Anaplastic large-cell lymphoma. Semin Diagn Pathol. 2011;28(3):190–201.
2. Willemze R, Meijer CJ. Primary cutaneous CD30-positive lymphoproliferative disorders. Hematol Oncol Clin North Am. 2003;17(6):1319–32.
3. Dongjie M, Zhiyong Z, Danqing L. Advances in the diagnosis and treatment of desmoid tumors. Beijing Med. 2015;37(3):272–5.

3.8 Fever and Lymph Node Enlargement with Abnormal Elevation of Globulin for 10 months

Zheng Jianming and Zhang Jiming

A 29-year-old male patient was admitted to the hospital on April 7, 2016 with a 10-month history of fever with lymph node enlargement.

The patient had obvious night sweating before the Spring Festival in 2015. Several enlarged lymph nodes of the size of mung beans were found in the right neck and groin, with smooth edges, soft texture, no tenderness, and movable. The patient lost 10 kg in a month, without fever, fatigue, nausea, vomiting, headache, dizziness, and other discomfort symptoms, no diagnosis and treatment. In late June 2015, the patient had a fever of 38.5 °C without other discomfort symptoms. The patient received antipyretic needles at the local hospital (specific details are unknown), and his temperature returned to normal that day. During the latter half of the month, the patient developed mild fatigue, self-measured body temperature every day, low fever appeared in the afternoon, and the axillary temperature was 37.3–37.5 °C, and the fever could be relieved spontaneously in the evening, without other discomfort symptoms. In early July 2015, a routine blood test was conducted in a hospital in Henan Province, with a white blood cell count of 19.46×10^9/L, N% 70%, neutrophil count 13.63×10^9/L, lymphocytes 22.3%, monocytes %: 7.1%, hemoglobin 110 g/L, and platelet count of 523×10^9/L. Erythrocyte sedimentation rate (ESR) 100 mm/h, anti-streptococcal lysin "O" (ASO) 575 IU/mL, C-reactive protein (CRP) 30.3 mg/mL, PCT 0.24 ng/mL. Liver function was slightly abnormal, ALT 69 U/L, ALP 221 U/L, GGT 76 U/L, and globulin 48.3 g/L. HBV and HCV markers were negative, and anti-HIV markers were negative. Ultrasonography showed multiple hypoechoic masses in the anterior, posterior and inguinal areas of bilateral neck (consider: enlarged lymph nodes?). Bone penetration indicated myeloid hyperplasia and increased granulation. The blood routine returned to normal range at the end of July. In August, he went to a hospital in Henan Province. Ultrasound examination showed splenomegaly (length 123 mm, thickness 33 mm), and no obvious enlarged lymph nodes were observed in the retroperitoneum. T-SPOT.TB on August 28 was positive (ESAT-6 > 60, CFP10 > 26). An ultrasound on September 25 revealed bilateral cervical lymph nodes (partial structural abnormality) and bilateral inguinal lymph nodes (partial structural abnormality on the right side). Lymphatic tuberculosis was diagnosed at the local hospital, and an oral tetra-antituberculosis treatment was given: rifampicin 0.45 g qd, isoniazid 0.3 g qd, pyrazinamide tablets 0.5 g bid, and ethambutol 0.75 g qd. After two months of treatment, he did not respond well, he still had a low afternoon fever. In November, cervical lymph nodes were punctured in another hospital in Henan province. Microscopically, proliferative lymphocytes were observed, but no cancer cells were found. Routine blood examination showed WBC count 6.21×10^9/L, hemoglobin 120 g/L, neutrophils 59%, lymphocytes 31.5%, platelet count 318×10^9/L, ESR 105 mm/h. Examination of liver function included ALT 40 U/L, ALP 166 U/L, and globulin 56.2 g/L. Examination of ultrasound revealed bilateral anterior cervical and groin hypoechoic masses (consider enlarged lymph nodes?). Chest CT and ultrasound showed no abnormality. After fiberoptic bronchoscopy, acid-fast bacilli were not found on the bronchial brushing tablets, but lymphatic tuberculosis was still considered at the local hospital. Isoniazid was stopped in the above-mentioned tetra-antituberculosis, and isoniazid plus aminosalicylate compound preparation was added orally at 1 g qd, and the remaining three drugs were taken continuously. However, the patient still had a low afternoon fever and no discomfort symptoms. On February 2, 2016, the above quadruple anti-tuberculosis treatment was stopped, and he went to another hospital in Henan Province to check the liver function, which showed globulin 57.1 g/L, IgG 39.14 g/L, IgA 496 g/L. The urine heavy chain and light chain were negative, but multiple myeloma was considered. There was no difference in bone scanning. The bone penetration indicated that the proliferation of nucleated cells in bone marrow was obviously active, and the granulocytes accounted for 52% and erythrocytes accounted for 26%. Megakaryocytes are more common, and platelets are more common in scattered clusters. At this time, the peak fever temperature in the afternoon rose to 38.8–39.0 °C, and the fever spontaneously subsided to 37.3 °C in the evening, and 37.5 °C in the next morning, without any discomfort. In consideration of mixed connective tissue disease, a hospital in Henan Province was given prednisone 10 mg qd orally and *Tripterygium wilfordii* polyglycosides 30 mg tid orally. But the patient still had a fever. Routine blood examination in March showed normal range of white blood cells, hemoglobin 108 g/L, liver function examination showed ALT 131 U/L, globulin 59 g/L, negative autoimmune antibodies, and negative blood culture. B-ultrasonography suggested liver ptosis and splenomegaly (43 mm thick). Chest CT showed multiple slightly larger lymph nodes in both axilla and splenomegaly. Prednisone and *Tripterygium wilfordii* polyglycosides were stopped. Examination in April showed globulin 72.2 g/L, IgG 93.9 g/L, Procalcitonin (PCT) was normal, and EBV DNA was negative. Mycobacterium infection was still considered, and amikacin, azithromycin and levofloxacin were given intravenous as anti-infective therapy. But the patient still had fever. On March 24, solstice was performed in a hospital in Shanghai for right inguinal lymph node puncture, and the result suggested that there were a large number of lymphocytes, prone to reactive lymph node hyperplasia. At present, the patient still starts to have fever in the afternoon, the peak value of temperature is between 38.8 and 39.2 °C, and the fever can be reduced to 37.3–38.3 °C at night, without any other discomfort. He has been admitted to our hospital for further treatment.

Since the onset of the disease, the patient has a normal mind, normal diet, normal sleep, normal urine and feces, and significant weight loss of 10 kg.

3.8.1 Physical Examination at Admission

T 39.2 °C, P 90 times/min, R 20 times/min, BP 109/64 mmHg, height 170 cm, weight 60 kg.

Clear mind, normal development, poor nutrition, precisely answering the questions, automatic posture, physical examination cooperation, walk into the ward, no abnormality observed in the skin and mucosa of the whole body, and no liver palm. Systemic superficial lymph nodes were enlarged: several enlarged lymph nodes of different sizes were palpable in the bilateral neck, armpit and groin. They were soft, with reasonable mobility, without adhesion, local redness and swelling, tenderness, and fistula scar. No subcutaneous bleeding spots, no rash observed. No skull deformity, soft neck without resistance, no angry jugular vein expansion, trachea in the middle, thyroid enlargement. The chest was symmetrical without deformity, the sternum was not tender, the breathing sound of both lungs was clear, and no rhonchi and moist rales were heard. The heart rate was 90 beats/min, the rhythm was uniform, the abdomen was soft, there was no tenderness in the whole abdomen, no muscle tension and rebound pain, no touch in the liver, spleen and costal area, no percussion pain in the liver and kidney, and bowel sounds were 5 times/min. No abnormality was observed in anus and external genitalia, no deformity in spine and limbs, and no edema in both lower limbs. The muscle strength was normal, the muscle tension was normal, the physiological reflex was normal, and the pathological reflex was not elicited.

3.8.2 Auxiliary Examination

Blood routine: white blood cell counts 7.75×10^9/L, red blood cell counts 3.53×10^{12}/L, hemoglobin: 87 g/L, platelet count: 511×10^9/L, reticulocyte: 1.6%↑, eosinophilic red blood cell: 44×10^6/L↓.

Urine routine and fecal routine, occult blood: negative.

Biochemistry: Alanine aminotransferase 80 U/L↑, aspartic aminotransferase 54 U/L↑, total bilirubin 5 μmol/L, binding bilirubin 2.90 μmol/L, total bile acid 6 μmol/L, alkaline phosphatase 431 U/L↑, γ-glutamyltransferase 96 U/L↑, albumin 24 g/L↓, globulin 74 g/L↑, creatine kinase 24 U/L↓, creatine kinase isoenzyme MB 15 U/L, lactate dehydrogenase 173 U/L, cholesterol 2.32 mmol/L↓, triglyceride 0.62 mmol/L, High density lipoprotein cholesterol 0.38 mmol/L↓.

C-reactive protein 170 mg/L↑, anti-streptococcal lysin "O" 400 IU/mL↑, procalcitonin 0.14 ng/mL↑, ferritin 601.2 ng/mL↑.

There was no significant abnormality in tumor markers.

24 h urinary protein: 1.18 g/24 h↑, urinary β2 microglobulin: 0.72 mg/L↑.

Six subjects of lymphocyte subsets CD: CD3+: 68.51%, CD4+: 35.76%, CD8+: 30.58%, NK+: 10.96%, CD19+: 19.59%↑.

Blood immunoglobulin G 53.3 g/L↑, blood immunoglobulin A 5.77 g/L↑, blood immunoglobulin M 2.23 g/L, blood immunoglobulin E > 2856 ng/mL↑, immunoglobulin G4:4.91 g/L↑, κ-light chain 10.5 g/L↑, λ-light chain 8.23 g/L↑, β2 microglobulin 2.81 mg/L↑, serum and urine immunofixation electrophoresis: negative.

Autoantibody: Anti-nuclear antibody: 1:100, positive +, karyotype: granules, dsDNA: negative, nucleosome antibody: negative, ENA profile: negative, anticardiolipin antibody: negative, complement C3 fragment: 1.86 g/L↑, complement C4: 0.258 g/L, rheumatoid factor <11.40 IU/mL, HLA-B27: negative.

Epstein-Barr virus capsid IgA: negative, Epstein-Barr virus capsid IgG: positive, Epstein-Barr virus capsid IgM: negative. Qualitative test for cytomegalovirus DNA: negative.

T-SPOT. TB: positive, negative control well: 0, antigen A (ESAT-6) well: >30, antigen B (CFP-10) well: 9, positive control well: normal.

Qualitative test of Cryptococcus sera latex was negative, HIV antibody was negative, RPR antibody and TP antibody were negative.

Hepatitis B virus surface antigen: negative, hepatitis B virus surface antibody: positive, hepatitis B virus E antigen: negative, hepatitis B virus core antibody: positive, hepatitis C virus antibody: negative.

Blood culture: no bacterial growth.

Electrocardiogram, chest radiograph and echocardiography showed no obvious abnormality.

PET-CT: bilateral neck and clavicular lymph nodes, mediastinum and bilateral axillary lymph nodes, retroperitoneal lymph nodes, bilateral iliac vascular and pelvic lymph nodes, and bilateral inguinal lymph nodes, with increased FDG metabolism, which is considered to be highly inflammatory and proliferative lesions.

Bone marrow smear, flow cytometry, and bone marrow biopsy: no obvious abnormalities.

3.8.3 The Process of Diagnosis and Treatment

The patient had fever for several months, accompanied by lymph node enlargement and significantly increased blood immunoglobulin. After admission, the serum immunoglobulin reached as high as 74 g/L. Multiple myeloma was suspected in another hospital, but neither bone puncture nor lymph node puncture found tumor cells.

Although the patient was T-SPOT.TB positive, it was ineffective after regular anti-tuberculosis, lymph node pathology did not support the diagnosis of tuberculosis, and other etiological tests were negative, so the evidence of infectious disease was insufficient. The positive significance of 1:100 anti-nuclear antibody in autoantibodies is not significant, and there is no manifestation of multi-system involvement. The quantitative increase of 24-h urinary protein is feasible for further searching for evidence of renal puncture. However, such high level of globulin caused by autoimmune diseases is also a rare manifestation. There is no pathologic evidence for neoplastic disease, and the patient's lymph node enlargement with abnormal globulin should be noted for the possibility of multiple myeloma and lymphoma. In addition to lymphoma, common atypical lymph node hyperplasia should be considered, along with infectious diseases (such as EBV infection, CMV infection and cat scratch disease, etc.), and autoimmune diseases (SLE and rheumatoid arthritis, etc.). Excluding these diseases, the diseases that cause benign enlargement of the lymph nodes also include Castleman's disease, Rosai-Dorfman's disease, and histiocytic necrotizing lymphadenitis (Kikuchi's disease).

The patient had undergone bone puncture and lymph node puncture twice each without definite diagnosis. Immunofixation electrophoresis showed no monoclonal globulin, and no bone destruction was observed, which did not meet the manifestations of multiple myeloma. Myeloma could be excluded according to bone marrow smear and biopsy. With both lymph node enlargement and such a marked increase in polyclonal globulin, several diseases should be considered, such as Castleman's disease, T-cell large granule lymphocytic leukemia, and vascular immunoblastic T-cell lymphoma. Other lymphomas, such as lymphoplasma cell lymphoma, splenic marginal zone lymphoma, and mucosal associated lymphoid tissue type extranodal marginal zone B-cell lymphoma, may be accompanied by elevated immunoglobulin because they originate from post-germinal center B cells.

Lymph node biopsy was performed again to confirm the diagnosis. In order to improve the positive rate of diagnosis, an axillary lymph node with the highest SUV value as seen in PET-CT was selected specially. Results of pathological findings showed that axillary lymph nodes showed vascular hyperplasia with a large number of plasma cell infiltration in the interfollicular area, which was confirmed as polyclonal by enzyme labeling. Combined with clinical and test results, it was consistent with the multicentric Castleman disease, plasma cell type.

The patient was transferred to the hematology department for further treatment and received chemotherapy on April 28: cyclophosphamide 0.4 g D1 + vindixine 1 mg D1 + dexamethasone 20 mg D1 + thalidomide 300 mg D1–7.

After treatment, the patient's condition was stable and he went to the hematology department for reexamination regularly.

3.8.4 Comment

Castleman's disease is an atypical lymphoproliferative disorder of unknown origin, first reported by Castleman in 1956, also known as giant lymph node hyperplasia or angiolymphatic follicular tissue hyperplasia. Pathologically, they are divided into clear vascular type, plasma cell type, and mixed type according to histological characteristics. Clinically, the enlarged lymph nodes can be divided into focal type and multicenter type according to their distribution. Multicentric Castleman's disease is a rare, mostly plasma cell type, characterized by multi-site lymph node enlargement, obvious systemic symptoms such as fever and hepatosplenomegaly, increased immunoglobulin, decreased albumin, and anemia. The etiology and pathogenesis of

Castleman's disease are unknown. Human herpesvirus type 8 infection and abnormal secretion of interleukin 6 are involved in development of the disease. There is currently no effective treatment for multicentric plasma cell Castleman disease. Treatment methods include single-agent chemotherapy, combination chemotherapy, antiviral therapy, and targeted therapy for IL-6 and CD20, with mixed reports on therapeutic efficacy. Some patients may progress to malignant lymphoma, and follow-up should be done closely.

Unexplained fever with lymph nodes enlargement can be a clinical manifestation of a range of diseases. If the key point of lymph node enlargement with significantly elevated polyclonal globulin can be grasped in this case, the differential diagnosis can be greatly narrowed to diseases such as Castleman's disease, T-cell large-granulocytic lymphocytic leukemia and lymphoma. For patients with negative bone penetration and lymph node pathology, where hematological disease is highly suspected, repeated lymph node biopsy may be necessary.

References

1. Armitage JO. Approach to the patient with lymphadenopathy and splenomegaly. In: Cecil medicine. 24th ed. [M] 2012. p. 1107–8.
2. Gang A, Lihui S, Shuhua Y, et al. Case 190: rash, fever, anemia, multiple lymphadenopathy, plasmacytosis, and polyclonal hypergammaglobulinemia. Chin Med J. 2009;89(40):2871–3.

3.9 Pathologically Manifested as Autoimmune Hepatitis, But NK/T-Cell Lymphoma Was a Final Diagnosis After Splenectomy

Zheng Jianming, Du Zunguo, and Chen Shu

A 34-year-old female was admitted to the hospital for liver biopsy on October 10, 2016, because of repeated fever with abnormal liver function for more than 1 year. She started to develop fever in early October 2015 without obvious incentive. The fever was low-grade in the afternoon, about 37.7 °C, and would turn to a normal level on its own. Also, she experienced nausea and vomiting of stomach content, but denied obvious chills, abdominal pain, diarrhea, acid reflux, and belching. Fever was accompanied by headache. Occasionally, she had dizziness and tinnitus, but denied external auditory canal pus, nasal congestion, runny nose, sore throat, sore gums, cough, sputum, chest tightness, chest pain, palpitations, frequent urination, urgency, painful urination, skin rash, joints swelling and pain, mouth ulcers, skin rashes, hair loss, and other discomforts.

She was admitted to a hospital in Anhui Province. Blood routine tests showed a leukocyte count of 1.39×10^9/L, a hemoglobin count of 109 g/L, and a platelet count of 58×10^9/L. Biochemical examination yielded the following: Alanine transaminase (ALT), 64 U/L; blood amylase, 145 U/L; lipase, 156 U/L. Electrocardiogram and chest radiograph showed no obvious abnormalities, while abdominal ultrasound showed chronic cholecystitis and bone marrow cytology revealed proliferative bone marrow. The diagnosis was "(1) pancytopenia: infectious? (2) acute gastroenteritis". Symptomatic treatment was applied to resist infection, protect stomach and raise blood cells (the specific medication is unknown). Symptoms such as fever, nausea, and vomiting were relieved, and the leukocytes rose to 3.22 × 10^9/L. She was discharged from the hospital. However, the above-mentioned symptoms reappeared and no obvious abnormality was seen after gastroscopy, but the blood test showed that the leukocyte was 2.0 × 10^9/L. Orally-taken leucogen and subcutaneously injections to raise the leukocyte (specifically unknown) was applied, but the leukocyte was still between 2 × 10^9/L and 3 × 10^9/L. Body temperature was normal at times, and sometimes was at low-grade fever level.

Her fever reappeared in early February 2016. The body temperature was about 38 °C mainly in the afternoon. The fever could be normal on its own. Nausea and vomiting of the stomach contents still presented. Gastritis, liver function abnormality (unexplained), and leukocyte disorder (granulocytopenia) was considered. She was treated with esomeprazole, polyene phosphatidylcholine, magnesium isoglycyrrhizinate and other drugs, then changed to glycyrrhizic acid diamine capsule orally. Oral diyushengbai tablets (a traditional Chinese medicine for improving white blood cells) and leucogen were used to raise leukocytes. Her body temperature returned to normal, nausea and vomiting also eased. However, her leukocytes were still between 1.84 and 3.16 × 10^9/L, neutrophils fluctuate between 33.30% and 86.41%, ALT fluctuated between 114 and 139 U/L, and aspartate transaminase (AST) fluctuated between 64 and 127 U/L. However, after 3 months, the patient developed fever again in the afternoon, and was still accompanied by nausea and vomiting of stomach contents. Except for continued oral administration of diamine glycyrrhizinate capsules and leucogen tablets, no special treatment was given. She came to our outpatient clinic on October 10, 2016, and laboratory tests revealed the following: ANA, 1:100 positive; p-ANCA, positive; ALT, 548 U/L; AST; 538 U/L; alkaline phosphatase, 649 U/L; glutamyl transpeptidase, 182 U/L; total bilirubin, 15.4 mmol/L; globulin IgG, 17.8 g/L. The report of the plasma EBV DNA test was not available. For further diagnosis, she was admitted to the hospital for liver biopsy. Since the illness, the patient has shown normal mental condition, poor appetite, good sleep, normal bowel movements, and significant weight loss about 10 kg.

3.9.1 Admission at Physical Examination

On examination, her body temperature was 37.5 °C, pulse rate was 80 beats/min, breathing rate was 20 breaths/min, blood pressure was 95/65 mm Hg, height was 165 cm and weight was 51 kg. There was no obvious yellowing of the sclera and the skin of the whole body, no palpable swelling of superficial lymph nodes, no liver palms and spider nevi, no distended jugular vein, middle trachea, and no thyroid enlargement. The thorax is symmetrical without deformity, the sternum is not tender, the breath in both lungs were clear, and no dry or wet rales were heard. Heart rate was 80 beats/min with regular rhythm, soft abdomen, no tenderness, no muscle tension, and rebound pain. The liver reached 2 fingers below the ribs, while the spleen reached 6 fingers below the ribs. There was no percussive pain in the liver and kidney area, negative mobile dullness, and bowel sounded 4 times/min. There was no edema in both lower limbs.

3.9.2 Hospital Course

The patient was a young female presented with fever, abnormal liver function, reduced leukocyte counts, elevated globulin, ANA 1:100 positive, and ANCA positive, suggesting connective tissue diseases such as systemic lupus erythematosus (SLE) or autoimmune hepatitis (AIH). Because the patient had no obvious manifestations of involvement of other systems except the liver and hematologic system, and the characteristic autoantibodies of SLE were negative, the diagnosis of SLE was insufficient, and the diagnosis of AIH required liver puncture. The diagnosis of AIH cannot be made without liver biopsy and compatible histological findings (2019 AASLD AIH guidelines). After liver biopsy, the patient was discharged and waiting for pathological report. Pathology report of liver puncture yielded: CH-G4S3 (Ishak F4), IAIHG-SS (Note: American Society of Liver Pathology Autoimmune Hepatitis Score) 5/5, mild fatty liver (Fig. 3.12). Seventeen points can be gotten according to the AIH score of the American Society of Liver Pathology, and can be diagnosed as AIH.

The patient was admitted to the hospital again on November 3, with a body temperature of 40 °C at the time of admission, and a blood routine test with a leukocyte count of 1.28×10^9/L↓, a hemoglobin count of 101 g/L↓, neutrophils 70.3%, lymphocytes 19.5%↓, monocytes 10.2%↑, a platelet count of 90×10^9/L↓, the plasma EBV DNA report of the last time was 2.16×10^6/L. Considering the close relationship between EBV and hematologic system diseases, bone marrow puncture

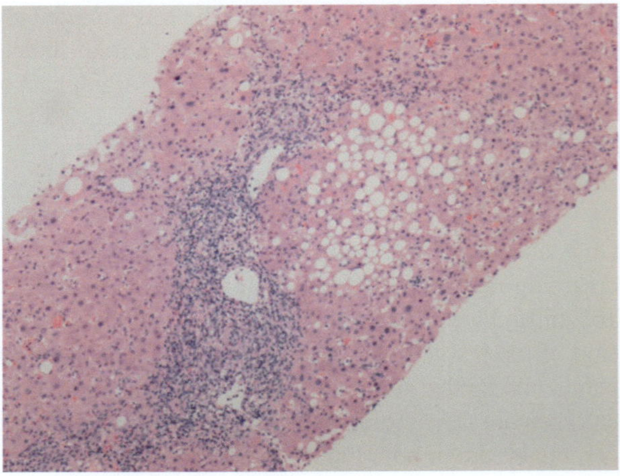

Fig. 3.12 HE 100×, interfacial hepatitis was found

examination and PET/CT examination were performed. Bone marrow smear showed occasional hemophagocytic cells (0.5%), while PET/CT examination revealed splenomegaly, multiple lymph nodes in the right axillary, mesenteric and retroperitoneum, accompanied by increased FDG metabolism, considering hematological tumors. The patient had fever, hepatosplenomegaly, decreased blood cells, increased triglycerides, decreased fibrinogen and increased ferritin, led to the possible diagnosis of hemophagocytic syndrome, although the proportion of bone marrow hemophagocytic cells was less than 2%. No abnormalities of superficial lymph nodes were found in the body examination and PET-CT and peritoneal lymph node biopsy was difficult because of thrombocytopenia. Therefore, on November 5, she was treated with immunoglobulin 20 g qd for 3 days and methylprednisolone 40 mg qd. The patient's body temperature returned to normal, but the platelet count continued to fall. On November 17, the platelet count decreased to 65×10^9/L in the reexamination. On November 18, methylprednisolone was changed to dexamethasone 15 mg qd intravenously. On November 19, the patient had multiple blood stools, ranging from 200 to 300 mL each time. She was treated with fasting, hemostasis, and rehydration, and her condition improved afterwards. The fecal routine and occult blood were normal on November 22. On November 29, the platelet count dropped to 40×10^9/L, and she was treated with 225 mg etoposide intravenously. After that, her hemogram and symptoms improved.

The other results of this patient after she was admitted to the hospital, were a ferritin count of 1302 ng/mL↑, a lactate dehydrogenase count of 596 U/L↑, immunofixation electrophoresis showed no abnormalities, autoantibodies: nRNP/Sm, negative; Sm, negative; SSA, negative; RO-52, negative; SSB, negative; Scl-70, negative; PM-Scl, negative; Jo-1, negative; CENP B, negative; anti-cyclin type I antibody, negative; dsDNA, negative; nucleosome, negative; histone, negative; ribosomal P protein, negative; anticardiolipin antibody, negative; cANCA, negative; pANCA, negative; anti-protease 3 IgG antibody, 2.3 RU/mL; anti-myeloperoxidase IgG antibody <2.0 RU/mL; anti-liver and kidney microsomal antibody, negative; anti-hepatic cytosolic antigen type I antibody, negative; anti-soluble liver/pancreatic antibody, negative; AMA-M2, negative. Since the plasma EBV DNA was positive, further liver immunohistochemistry revealed EBV encoded RNA (EBER) was positive (Fig. 3.13), combined with medical history and this examination: EB virus capsid antibody IgA, negative; EB virus capsid antibody IgM, negative; EB virus capsid Antibody IgG, positive; indicating that with chronic active Epstein-Barr virus infection (CAEBV) combined with EBV hepatitis, and AIH re-scoring less than 15 points, was not enough to diagnose AIH. After the patient was treated with corticoids, the physical examination revealed that the spleen still reached 6 fingers below the ribs, which did not shrink, and the patient's platelets were still low. Therefore, it was recommended to perform splenectomy, which can alleviate the thrombocytopenia caused by hypersplenism and may have new discoveries whether there were specific types of lymphoma.

On December 5, the patient was discharged from the hospital for splenectomy. The postoperative pathology showed tumor cells: CD2 (+), CD3 (+), CD7 (+), CD56 (+), CD43 (+), Ki67 (60%, +), TiA (+), GrB (+), perforin (+), CD20 (−),

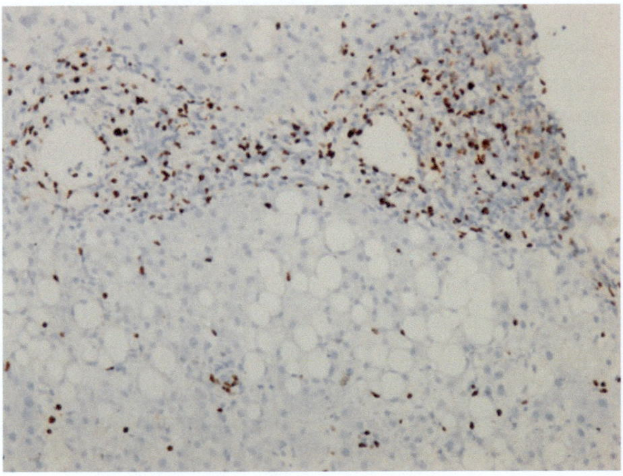

Fig. 3.13 EBER 200×, the brown ones are EBER positive

CD79a (−), CD4 (+), CD8 (+), F8 (+), Gly (−), CD61 (+), MPO (+), CD21 (−), CD23 (−), ALK(−), CD30(−), TDT(−), CyclinD1(−), EBER in situ hybridization was positive, thus NK/T-cell lymphoma was considered. After that, chemotherapy was continued in the Department of Hematology in another hospital, and regular follow-up was conducted there.

3.9.3 Comments

Infectious mononucleosis, caused by acute EBV infection, is a kind of mononuclear-macrophage system proliferative disease, mostly acute and self-limiting, and mainly manifested with irregular fever, lymphadenopathy, sore throat, peripheral blood mononucleosis and abnormal lymphocytes with good prognosis. If EBV is chronic persistent infection, symptoms persist or relapse accompanied by severe complications such as severe hematologic system diseases, interstitial pneumonia and retinitis are called chronic active Epstein-Barr virus (CAEBV) infection [1]. The diagnostic criteria for CAEBV infection are not uniform. The current diagnostic criteria adopted by NIH in the United States are shown in Table 3.1. CAEBV infection can be combined with lymphocyte proliferative diseases such as hemophagocytic syndrome and lymphoma. These diseases can be mutually transformed or exist side by side, and the prognosis is cruel. There is currently no effective treatment for CAEBV infection, and the curative effect of antiviral treatment such as acyclovir or interferon is not clear. The chemotherapy of hemophagocytic syndrome can be applied when combined with hemophagocytic syndrome, and the chemotherapy for lymphoma or leukemia can be applied with the corresponding disease. In recent years, it has been reported that hematopoietic stem cell transplantation can effectively inhibit the viral load and may be an effective measure for the treatment of CAEBV, especially T/NK-cell type CAEBV, which is the basic condition for the

Table 3.1 Diagnostic criteria for CAEBV [1]

Relevant clinical and serological manifestations for more than 6 months	1. Symptoms have continued since the primary EBV infection; 2. Abnormal EBV antibody titer (VCA-IgG ≥1:5120, EA antibody ≥1:640 or EBNA<1:2).
Histological signs of major organ damage	1. Lymphadenitis; 2. Hemophagocytosis; 3. Meningoencephalitis; 4. Persistent hepatitis; 5. Splenomegaly; 6. Interstitial pneumonia; 7. Myelodysplasia; 8. Retinitis
EBV test positive	1. EBV DNA, RNA or antigen test positive in the damaged tissue; 2. EBV DNA test positive in peripheral blood.
It can be diagnosed by meeting at least one of the above items and excluding any immunodeficiency including HIV infection.	

occurrence of EB virus-related T/NK-cell lymphoma. Although the chemotherapy regimen containing L-asparaginase can effectively treat lymphoma, only allogeneic hematopoietic cell transplantation can remove EBV infected cells.

Young women presenting with fever, liver injury and mildly elevated globulin are common in autoimmune diseases. But it should be noted that the diagnosis of autoimmune diseases is often based on the classification of diagnostic criteria. When there are new symptoms that are not consistent with the diagnosis, which is established, it should be reconsidered whether the original diagnosis is correct and whether it is complicated by other diseases. Clinicians also need to distinguish between primary and secondary autoimmune disease. Patients with atypical clinical manifestations and poor response to treatment should be alert to malignant tumors, especially hematological tumors. Even if the disease course is long, clinicians should not easily exclude malignant tumors. This patient is a young woman with elevated ALT, AST and globulin, 1:100 positive ANA and positive pANCA. The pathology of liver puncture was consistent with autoimmune hepatitis, the IAIHG-SS score was 5/5 according to the American Society of Pathology, which can be diagnosed as AIH. However, it should be noted that EBV and non-hepatotropic viruses can cause liver damage, which can be manifested as liver damage similar to AIH pathological changes. The result of plasma EBV DNA was positive. Furthermore, the liver tissue EBER staining positive revealed that it was actually EBV hepatitis caused by CAEBV infection. In the course of treatment, the spleen did not shrink significantly. Considering that EBV has the particularity as a tumor-causing virus and is closely related to hematological malignancies, splenectomy was performed and NK/T-cell lymphoma was finally diagnosed. The diagnosis and treatment process has twists and turns. The complexity of the disease requires doctors to have a broader mind and vision. People still have a long way to go to understand the disease. For patients with unexplained fever and splenomegaly, it is of certain clinical significance to perform splenectomy after carefully excluding other diseases to help confirm the diagnosis.

References

1. Xinhua W, Shu C. Infectious mononucleosis. In: Practical internal medicine. 14th ed. 2013. p. 387–90.
2. Isobe Y, Aritaka N, Setoguchi Y, et al. T/NK-cell type chronic active Epstein-Barr virus disease in adults: an underlying condition for Epstein-Barr virus-associated T/NK-cell lymphoma. J Clin Pathol. 2012;65(3):278–82.
3. Hongying S, Lidan Z, Dong X. Clinical analysis of 24 cases of malignant tumor simulated vasculitis. Chin J Rheumatol. 2015;19(8):534–9.

3.10 The Liver Lesion Resembles Liver Abscess in Imaging, Which Was Later Confirmed by Pathology to Be Liver Sarcomatoid

Zhang Bingyan and Jin Jialin

A 50-year-old female was admitted to the hospital on January 02, 2018 due to repeated fever for more than 2 months. At the beginning of November 2017, the patient started to develop fever with chill without obvious cause. The peak temperature was 40 °C. Body temperature often began to rise in the afternoon and returned to normal after oral antipyretic drugs with sweat. She denied chest tightness, shortness of breath, nausea and vomiting, abdominal pain and bloating, frequent urination, urgency and pain, and joint muscle pain. In December 2017, the patient began to experience cough, accompanied by white sputum, which was easy to cough up. Due to repeated illnesses, she went to the local hospital. And laboratory tests showed a leukocyte count of 22.36×10^9/L, neutrophils of 73.64%, and anti-infectious treatment (detail unknown) was administrated but the symptoms did not improve significantly. Later, she went to a provincial hospital of traditional Chinese medicine and got reexamined: leukocytes, 10.07×10^9/L; neutrophils, 78.9%; hemoglobin, 94 g/L; HBV-DNA, 1.536 × 105 IU/mL; abdominal B-ultrasound showed possible abscesses in right lobe of the liver; abdominal CT showed multiple low-density shadows in the right lobe of the liver, which were abscesses probably; liver cirrhosis; a small amount of ascites and multiple large lymph nodes in the liver hilar. T-SPOT.*TB* test was negative, liver puncture pathology revealed: sliced infarction, regional fibroblasts and small bile duct hyperplasia, with a large number of acute and chronic inflammatory cells infiltration and without liver lobule structure. Teicoplanin, meropenem, and entecavir were administered. Body temperature still fluctuated between 36 and 39.2 °C after medication, and she went to the outpatient clinic of Huashan Hospital. Laboratory tests showed: leukocytes, 7.35×10^9/L; neutrophils, 73.2%; hemoglobin, 80 g/L; chest CT showed small amounts of pleural effusion on both sides, abdominal B-ultrasound showed chronic liver disease, and a substantial mass in the right lobe of the liver. She was admitted to the hospital to receive linezolid 0.6 q12h and cefoperazone/sulbactam 3.0 q12h intravenously for one week, and there was still repeated abnormal body temperature. She was then admitted to our department for further examination and treatment. Since the illness, the patient has good spirit, poor appetite, good sleep, normal bowel movements, and no significant weight loss.

3.10.1 Past History

The patient has a history of hepatitis B for many years. After this onset of fever, she started to take entecavir as antiviral therapy. Liver CT scan suggested cirrhosis.

3.10.2 Physical Examination at Admission

The patient has conscious awareness, eurhythmia, moderate nutrition, cooperative physical examination, mild anemia, no skin rash, no palpable swelling of superficial lymph nodes, no redness of the pharynx, no enlarged tonsils, no tenderness on both breasts and no discharge. Right lower lung breath sounds low, no dry and wet rales, regular heart rhythm, no murmur, soft abdomen, no tenderness, no rebound pain in the whole abdomen. Liver can be reached under the right rib, no palpable spleen under the rib, negative Murphy's sign, no tenderness at Mcburney point, positive percussive pain in the liver area, no percussive pain in the kidneys, non-hyperpopular bowel sounds, and mild edema of both lower limbs.

3.10.3 Hospital Course

After admission, the blood test showed leukocytes, 9.43×10^9/L; neutrophils, 71%; hemoglobin, 75 g/L; erythrocyte sedimentation rate, 30 mm/h; albumin, 26.5 g/L; total bilirubin, 14.9 μmol/L; alanine transaminase, 40 U/L; aspartate transaminase, 76 U/L; alkaline phosphatase, 93 U/L; gamma-glutamyl transpeptidase, 91 U/L; coagulation function showed prothrombin time, 16.3 s; activated partial thromboplastin time, 47.4 s; international normalized ratio, 1.38; D dimer, 1.73; hepatitis B test showed HBeAg negative hepatitis; HBV-DNA, 821 IU/mL, and the markers of HAV, HCV and HEV were all negative. Autoantibodies were 1:320 positive, granular type, and ENA antibody profile were negative; AFP, 23.42 μg/L; CA125, 91.20 U/mL; and other tumor markers were normal. On January 3, PET-CT was performed to further clarify the cause of fever, which indicates that the right lobe of the liver was slightly low-density, with uneven and abnormally increased FDG metabolism. Considering the primary liver lesions, combined with the medical history, infection was first considered; no obvious abnormally increased FDG metabolism was found in other places of the body. There was no abnormal increase in FDG metabolism in the small lymph nodes scattered in the gastric space and retroperitoneum, which led to the consideration of proliferative changes and reactivity changes in spleen and bone marrow.

Therefore, the possibility of liver abscess was still considered (the tumor is not excluded), and linezolid 0.6 q12h and cefoperazone/sulbactam 3.0 q12h were given. On January 2nd, blood culture (1 time) was positive with *Staphylococcus Aureus* growth (oxacillin resistant). Cefoperazone/sulbactam was discontinued and linezolid was still continued. After 4 days of treatment, the patient's temperature peak showed a downward trend. But on January 7, the temperature rose again. Taking into account the possibility of infection by an atypical pathogen in the patient, in order to clarify the etiology, the liver puncture was again guided by B-ultrasound on January 8. During the operation, the mass was punctured twice, but nothing was aspirated. The liver mass tissue was sent out for pathological examination, second-generation sequencing and tissue culture. At this time, the patient's liver-enhanced MRI (Fig. 3.14) on January 11 showed possible cancer of the right anterior lobe of the liver, possible small subcapsular hemangioma of the right lobe of liver and splenomegaly. At this time, the patient's second-generation sequencing and tissue culture both returned negative. Combined with the effect of the treatment, the possibility of liver abscess was considered extremely small at this time.

Liver puncture pathology on January 16 revealed a spindle cell tumor with atypical cells and a large number of lymphocytes and plasma cells infiltration. Combined with the results of enzyme labeling, it was first considered as inflammatory myofibroblastoma. On January 22, liver tumor resection was performed. After that, her body temperature was normal (Fig. 3.15). Postoperative liver pathology suggested (liver) malignant tumors. Combined with morphological findings and enzyme labeling results, the lesion was considered a sarcomatoid carcinoma of epithelial origin. The nontumorous liver tissue showed features of CHB-G3S4 (Chronic Hepatitis B, Inflammation Grade 3, Fibrosis Stage 4).

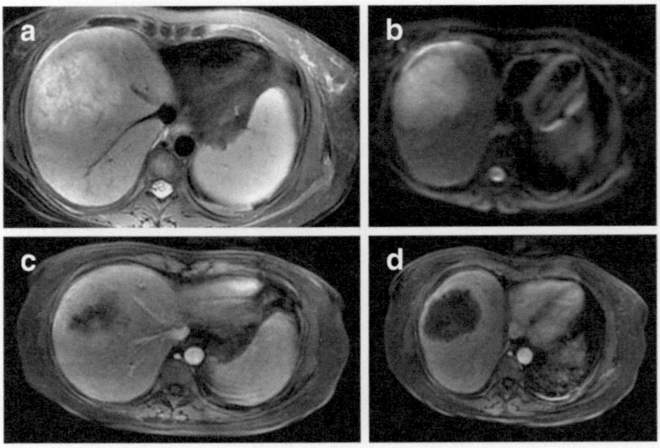

Fig. 3.14 MRI enhancement of the liver: (**a**) Irregular masses can be seen in the anterior lobe of the right lobe of the liver, about 63 × 91 mm in size, showing long T2 signals; (**b**) DWI shows high signals and uneven signals; (**c**) Obviously uneven enhancement around the lesion after enhancement; (**d**) A large area without enhancement in the lesion

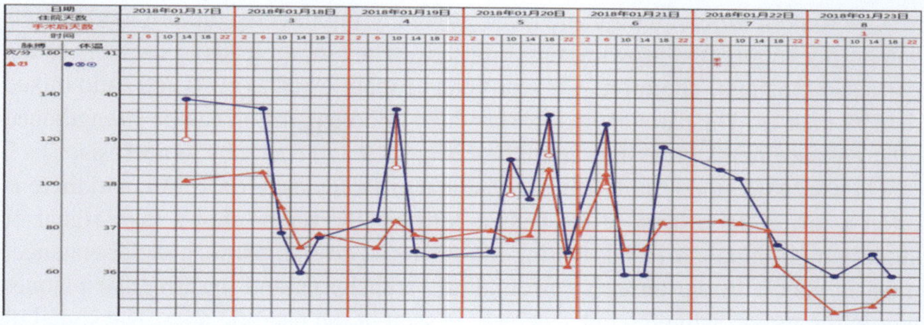

Fig. 3.15 Schematic diagram of the patient's body temperature change: the patient's body temperature dropped to the normal range after the operation

3.10.4 Comments

Hepatosarcomatoid carcinoma was first described by Craig *et al.* in 1989. It is a rare type of malignant tumor that occurs in the liver and has a morphological appearance similar to spindle cell sarcoma, but is actually cancer. It originates from epithelial cells. So far, 29 English cases have been reported on Medline. The disease usually develops in adults between 38 and 76 years old, with an average age of onset of 55.5 years and a male to female ratio of 3:1. Tumors are usually very large, with an average diameter of 12.5 cm, and about 80% of them are >5 cm in diameter when found. In most cases, the clinical manifestations are unspecific, but there may be pain and abdominal distension in the right upper quadrant. Some patients are accompanied by fever, but leukocytes are generally not high or slightly increased, suggesting noninfectious fever, which may be related to sarcoma-like components and ischemia and necrosis of tumor parenchyma. Of the 29 reported cases, 52.7% of patients were HBsAg positive. About half of patients may have elevated AFP, and some of them have elevated CA19–9, CA125 and CEA. Most of the patients had advanced tumors when they were admitted to the hospital. It can invade blood vessels, form thrombus, satellite foci and extra-hepatic manifestations. The most common metastasis places are lungs and lymph nodes, peritoneum, gallbladder, omentum, stomach, mediastinum and adrenal glands. About 60% of patients can relapse in subsequent follow-up. The median survival time is 11.2 months (1.5–30 months), and more than half of the survival time is less than 11.2 months. Therefore, this is a disease with strong aggressiveness, high malignancy, rapid progress, and poor prognosis.

At present, the cause of the disease is unknown, and it may be related to viral infection, hepatic artery embolization chemotherapy, radiotherapy, etc. In recent years, the disease is considered to be of monoclonal origin, and most sarcomatoid carcinomas come from normal liver tissues without cirrhosis. These findings support that tumors arise from pluripotent liver stem cells and then differentiate into tumors with both sarcoma and cancer components.

Due to poor differentiation and rapid growth of tumor cells, tumor blood vessels can hardly supply fast-growing tumor tissues, which often leads to necrosis of the tissues in the mass. Therefore, CT scans can be manifested as cysts and solid mixed density masses. The parenchymal part and the middle partition can be strengthened after enhancement, while the central part is not strengthened due to necrosis.

On liver MRI, the tumor shows low signal or isointensity on T1WI, and there is often a lower signal area in the center. Most of the tumor shows high signal or slightly high signal on T2WI. During the enhanced arterial phase, nodular enhancement is visible in the tumor's surrounding parenchyma and the irregular plaques within the tumor, while no enhancement is seen in the necrotic area. The signal of obvious enhancement in the parenchymal arterial phase around the tumor gradually decrease in the portal vein phase and the delayed phase. On FDG-PET/CT, the characteristics of F-FDG uptake are closely related to the degree of tumor malignancy. High metabolism indicates poor tumor differentiation and high degree of malignancy, which is of great significance in evaluating tumor staging and distant metastasis.

Because the low-density area of the tumor can be seen as a stripe-shaped partition, and there is a little high perfusion around the tumor in the arterial phase. It is often difficult to distinguish atypical liver abscess on CT. However, the low-density CT value is higher than the CT value of liver abscess, and the range of changes is large. There are no ring-shaped low-density around the tumor like hepatic abscess, and there is no increase in leukocytes, which can be used for identification. At the initial stage of the onset of this case, the manifestations were high fever, elevated leukocytes multiple low-density shadows on the abdominal CT. The liver abscess was first considered. However, the patient's multiple abdominal B-ultrasounds outside the hospital showed that the abscess was immature and the puncture was not reached, which is inconsistent with the clinical manifestations of liver abscess. In fact, ultrasound and CT scan can diagnose more than 90% of liver abscess cases, and enhanced CT is better than ultrasound in diagnosing liver abscess. It is reported in literature that MRI enhancement and CT scan have the same diagnostic efficiency. By analyzing the characteristics of liver abscess in the two imaging studies, it is found that CT scan has good practicability in the diagnosis of liver abscess, and can fully understand the location and size of liver abscess and the relationship with the surrounding organs and tissues. CT enhanced scan, especially dynamic enhanced scan, can clearly show the characteristic manifestations of liver abscess in different stages and explain its corresponding pathological changes. However, MRI has high resolution for soft tissues and can better reflect the liquefaction and necrosis of liver tissues than CT. Therefore, combined CT and MRI can significantly improve the diagnostic efficiency of liver abscess.

The current diagnosis of liver sarcomatoid carcinoma mainly depends on pathology and immunohistochemistry. The pathological characteristics of the tumor are both cancer and sarcoma-like biphasic components, often predominantly with sarcoma-like tissue. Immunohistochemical staining shows sarcoma-like component markers, and positive epithelial component markers such as CK, keratin and epithelial membrane antigen (EMA). Surgery is currently the preferred treatment option, supplemented by chemotherapy and radiotherapy when necessary. But because its biological behavior is the same as that of poorly differentiated cancers, it is highly aggressive and often metastases in the early stage of the disease, so most patients undergo recurrence after surgical resection and even liver transplantation. They have poor prognosis and should be followed up closely.

Although abdominal B-ultrasound, liver CT and other imaging methods are efficient in diagnosing liver abscess, in cases where the patient's treatment effect is not good, and repeated liver punctures are found to be unsuccessful in finding the etiology, the possibility of tumors should still be considered and investigation should be carried out carefully. Pathological biopsy is still the gold standard for diagnosis, but liver biopsy is sometimes difficult to make a clear diagnosis due to the small amount of tissue obtained. If necessary, surgical resection can obtain the final diagnosis and play a therapeutic role.

References

1. Li J, Liang P, Zhang D, et al. Primary carcinosarcoma of the liver: imaging features and clinical findings in six cases and a review of the literature. Cancer Imaging. 2018;18(1):7.
2. Li B, Zhang Y, Hou J, et al. Primary liver carcinosarcoma and 18F-FDG PET/CT. Clin Nucl Med. 2016;41(8):e383–5.
3. Xu L, Xiaolin G, Huifan J. A case of liver sarcomatoid carcinoma. Chin J Infect Dis. 2017;35(2):116–7.
4. Peizhong S, Yongqing L, Xingjie L. Diagnosis and treatment of liver sarcomatoid carcinoma. Chin J Gen Surg (Electron Ed). 2016;10(5):378–80.

Fever of Unknown Origin in Noninfectious Inflammatory Diseases

4

Jin Jialin, Chen Mingquan, Yang Feifie, Chen Shu, Huang Yuxian, Bao Suxia, Zheng Jianming, Li Ning, Zhang Jiming, Fan Qingqi, Jia Wen, Shao Lingyun, Zhang Wenhong, Liu Yuanyuan, Qin Yanli, Zhang Shu, Hu Yuekai, Zhang Yanliang, Ruan Qiaoling, Wu Jing, and Wang Xinyu

Fever of unknown origin is sometimes due to various connective tissue diseases/non-infectious inflammatory diseases. The proportion of this group of diseases in FUO has increased in recent years, accounting for about 20%–30%. Common causes include rheumatoid arthritis (RA), systemic lupus erythematosus (SLE), adult-onset Still's disease (AOSD), vasculitis, dermatomyositis/polymyositis (DM/PM), mixed connective tissue disease, etc. Due to the development of sensitive laboratory diagnostic tests (including antinuclear and anti-DNA markers), rheumatic/noninfectious inflammatory are easier to diagnose. The diagnosis is now usually made within 3 weeks. However, the trend of aging results in increasing of the incidence of rare diseases, such as dermatomyositis/polymyositis and temporal arteritis in elderly patients.

Adult-onset Still's disease (adult-onset juvenile rheumatoid arthritis) is one of the most frequent autoimmune diseases resulting in FUO in younger patients. Key clinical features of this disease include an evanescent macular rash, arthralgias, and a sore throat. Patients with AOSD often have high fevers associated with high peripheral white blood cell (WBC) counts, and this combination frequently causes the physician to begin antibiotic therapy for a presumed bacterial infection. However, none of the pathogenic testing is positive and the fever fails to subside after initiation of antibiotics. No specific test is available for AOSD, and other diseases must be carefully excluded before a diagnosis can be made. Serum ferritin levels are

J. Jialin · C. Mingquan · Y. Feifie · C. Shu · H. Yuxian · B. Suxia · Z. Jianming · L. Ning · Z. Jiming · J. Wen · S. Lingyun · Z. Wenhong · L. Yuanyuan · Q. Yanli · Z. Shu · H. Yuekai · Z. Yanliang · R. Qiaoling (✉) · W. Jing · W. Xinyu
Department of Infectious Diseases, Huashan Hospital, Fudan University, Shanghai, China
e-mail: qlruan07@fudan.edu.cn

F. Qingqi
Department of Infectious Diseases, Jing'an District Central Hospital of Shanghai, Shanghai, China

W. Zhang, X. Weng (eds.), *Fever of Unknown Origin*,
https://doi.org/10.1007/978-981-95-1401-4_4

generally markedly elevated, as is the erythrocyte sedimentation rate (ESR). Patients usually respond to glucocorticoid treatment.

SLE is more common in young women, and fever can occur in more than 90% of cases. If the clinical manifestations are typical, the diagnosis is usually not difficult. However, some cases only have fever as the main manifestation and lack the typical rash. When fever is the first symptom, and the rash, bone, joint, heart, kidney, and other system damages are not obvious, it is more likely to be misdiagnosed as an infectious disease.

Reiter syndrome is relatively rare in FUO. Patients present with urethritis and conjunctivitis. Urethritis appears first, which can last for several weeks, and joint symptoms can appear later. Systemic symptoms include fever, diarrhea, and myocarditis. The course of the disease is sometimes 2 months, and years for the elderly.

In elderly patients, polymyalgia rheumatica is the most common autoimmune disorder to cause FUO. This disease results in proximal muscle weakness and a high ESR. Temporal headaches and visual complaints are present, as is temporal arteritis, a vasculitis commonly associated with polymyalgia rheumatica.

Other autoimmune diseases reported to cause FUO include polyarteritis nodosa, subacute thyroiditis, and mixed connective tissue disease. Subacute thyroiditis may present with prolonged fever. On examination, the thyroid is often tender. Serum thyroxine and antithyroid antibodies are elevated, and thyroid iodine uptake rate is decreased in acute phase. Kikuchi's disease, also called histiocytic necrotizing lymphadenitis, has been reported to cause prolonged fever. This self-limiting autoimmune disorder occurs in young Asian females and is associated with generalized lymphadenopathy. Diagnosis is made by lymph node biopsy.

Mixed connective tissue disease is more common in women (about 80%). Symptoms may vary from lupus to scleroderma, or may be cutaneous, but it is difficult to determine which disease it is. Raynaud's phenomenon is particularly prominent (in 90% of patients), which can appear months or years earlier than other symptoms. About 2/3rd of patients with Raynaud's phenomenon have low esophageal peristalsis, diffuse swelling of hands, loss of elasticity, difficulty to pinch, salami like fingers, skin hardening, facial swelling, skin tension and thickening, and poor elasticity. The kidneys may be mildly or not involved. Positive RNP antibody with high potency is one of the characteristics of this disease. It is important to note that symptoms of overlapped connective tissue disease are consistent with the diagnosis of more than two diseases and do not have high titers of RNP antibodies. In the past, MCTD was considered to have a good effect on corticosteroids and a good prognosis, but in recent years, it has been found that the fatality rate in adults is between 4% and 7%. Children are more dangerous, with more heart and kidney involvement than adults, and may have severe thrombocytopenia.

Autoinflammatory diseases should also been included in this category of FUO causes. The term "autoinflammatory" appeared in the pages of Cell in the spring of 1999 to denote an emerging family of clinical disorders characterized by episodes of seemingly unprovoked inflammation without high-titer autoantibodies or antigen-specific T lymphocytes. In contrast, the innate immune system predominates in the pathogenesis of these illnesses. Hereditary recurrent fevers (HRFs) are a group of monogenic autoinflammatory diseases characterized by recurrent bouts of fever and serosal inflammation that are caused by pathogenic variants in genes important for the regulation of innate immunity. Advances in the diagnosis of HRFs have been made owing both to the availability of molecular genetic testing and to the greatly increased clinical awareness of these illnesses.

Most of the HRFs are rare diseases, including familial Mediterranean fever (FMF, gene MEFV, MIM 608107), tumor necrosis factor (TNF) receptor-associated periodic syndrome (TRAPS, gene TNFRSF1A, MIM 191190), and cryopyrin-associated periodic syndrome (CAPS, gene NLRP3, MIM 606416). Patients with HRF often display similar inflammatory symptoms with variable intensity and localization of symptoms, making their clinical diagnosis difficult.

FMF is a hereditary disease characterized by recurrent attacks of fever with peritonitis, pleuritis, arthritis, or erysipelas-like rash. FMF is seen primarily among individuals of Mediterranean ancestry, particularly non-Ashkenazi Jews, Armenians, Arabs, and Turks. TRAPS present with dramatic, sometimes month-long bouts of fever with sterile peritonitis, pleurisy, arthritis, migratory erythema, or periorbital edema. In some cases, renal failure develops due to the deposition of an acute-phase reactant, serum amyloid A (SAA), in the kidneys.

In this chapter, we selected series of non-infectious inflammatory cases in FUO. Through these cases, clinicians will learn the principle of dealing with similar patients.

4.1 Systemic Lupus Erythematosus with Onset of Fever and Chest Pain

Jin Jialin

A 20-year-old woman was admitted to the hospital with chief complaints of fever and left chest pain for 25 days on April 3, 2009.

At the beginning of March, the patient developed traction pain of left chest during deep breathing or posture change without obvious predisposing cause. The pain was not severe and the patient did not pay attention to it. On March 8, the patient developed hyperemia and a few rashes without pruritus on her face, the rash disappeared after applying pearl powder. On March 10, the patient presented with a sudden high fever and a body temperature of 39.2 °C, as well as fatigue and anorexia. No chills, sore throat, or cough was observed. After she received anti-cold medicine and cephalosporins, the body temperature gradually stabilized. On March 16th, she had a fever again and still had chest pain. The blood routine test in local hospital showed Hb of 95 g/L and monocyte of 12.9%, while the other tests were normal. Chest CT scan revealed chronic inflammation of the left upper and lower lung as well as left pleural thickening. The patient was treated with azithromycin and cefradine. The left chest pain gradually eased. The body temperature decreased but then increased again, up to 39.3 °C. After being admitted to a local hospital on March 28, the patient was given levofloxacin and ceftriaxone for anti-infection treatment, but her temperature did not decrease. On the day before admission, the patient developed chills, pale face, and vomiting of stomach contents during intravenous injection of moxifloxacin. The patient was admitted to our department with a diagnosis of "fever of unknown origin" on April 3 for further diagnosis and treatment. Medical history: at the beginning of January 2009, the patient had redness, swelling, and pain in the big toes of both feet, which relieved after about a week of iodophor administration. At the end of January, the patient felt that she could not hold her hands tightly. This symptom improved after activity and did not worsen in the mornings. There was no redness, swelling or pain in the finger joints and other joints. Since the illness, the patient developed fatigue and anorexia, with normal sleep, stool, and urine. Two blood tests before admission were as follows: WBC 1.66×10^9/L, N 80.5%, Hb 90 g/L, PLT 101×10^9/L, and WBC 2.96×10^9/L, N 51.8%, Hb 86 g/L, PLT 101×10^9/L.

4.1.1 Physical Examination on Admission

The general condition was acceptable. The body temperature was 37.4 °C. Her bilateral cheeks and nose skin were congested, and a few petechiae at the intravenous injection site of the left elbow were observed. No rash was seen on the skin of the trunk and limbs. Swollen and clustered lymph nodes can be palpable on the right neck, with moderate hardness and no tenderness. The breathing sounds were clear while some of the lower lungs were low. Her heart rate was regular with 83 beats/min. Abdomen was flat and soft. Liver and spleen were not palpable below the costal margin, and there was no percussion pain in the hepatic region. No edema was noticed in the lower limbs.

4.1.2 The Process of Diagnosis and Treatment

Laboratory examinations after admission were as follows: WBC, 10.83×10^9/L; N, 80.6%; RBC, 3.54×10^{12}/L; HB, 93 g/L; PLT, 129×10^9/L; ANA, 1:3200 positive (homogeneous, granular); SSA/Ro, positive; ds-DNA, positive (quantitative result >250 IU/mL). Complement C3 and C4 were 0.51, <0.06, respectively and both decreased. Urine routine test showed microalbuminuria and quantity of the urinary protein in 24 h was less than 0.05 g. Liver function was normal, and the globulin count was 43 g/L. Thoracic ultrasonography showed no vegetation. Ultrasonography of the abdomen revealed splenomegaly (121 mm × 39 mm), while the liver, gallbladder, pancreas, kidneys, and retroperitoneum were all normal. Ultrasound of superficial lymph nodes showed that there were multiple enlarged lymph nodes with irregular shape from bilateral lower neck to supraclavicle, and several flat lymph nodes with irregular shape in bilateral axillas and groins. Chest CT scan showed inflammation of bilateral lower lobes and a small amount of pleural effusion on both sides. Visual field examination showed decreased visual acuity in the right eye and normal in the left eye. Multiple blood cultures were all negative. As the result, the patient was then diagnosed as "systemic lupus erythematosus".

The patient was treated with methylprednisolone 80 mg/day and her body temperature returned to normal. The dose was reduced to 60 mg/day after 5 days and to 40 mg/day after another 9 days of treatment. Meanwhile, she received oral omeprazole to protect the gastric mucosa and potassium supplementation, calcium supplementation and other treatments. The patient improved during the outpatient follow-up.

4.1.3 Comments

SLE, an inflammatory connective tissue disease, is an autoimmune-mediated disease with unknown etiology. It produces a variety of autoantibodies as its immunological characteristics, and can involve multiple systems and organs such as skin, joints, kidneys, and serous membranes. The clinical manifestations of SLE are complex and diverse. The natural course of the disease is usually manifested as the alternation of aggravation and remission of the disease. SLE is common in young women, and the peak incidence is in the reproductive period of 15–40 years old. The ratio of males to females is 1:7 to 1:9.

The main manifestation in the early stage of this patient is fever and chest pain. Chest CT also showed chronic inflammation of the left upper and lower lung as well as left pleural thickening. Therefore, the initial diagnosis of acute upper respiratory tract infection is established. However, after examination, the decreased white blood cell counts in the peripheral blood, the ANA test with a titer of 1:3200, and the strong positive ds-DNA made it not difficult to obtain the diagnosis of systemic lupus erythematosus (SLE). In fact, her chest pain may be caused by the involvement of the pleura, which is a manifestation of serositis. However, it seems to be special that the patient has no typical rash but enlarged lymph nodes on the neck, splenomegaly in ultrasound image and decreased visual acuity of the right eye. Such manifestations of SLE are not uncommon in clinical practices. SLE is a common disease in fever of unknown origin. The author uses this example as a case to make a detailed description of SLE literature for readers' reference.

References

1. Chinese Rheumatology Association. Chinese guidelines for the diagnosis and treatment of systemic lupus erythematosus. Chin J Rheumatol. 2010;14:342–6.
2. Goldman L, Ausiello D. Cecil medicine. 26th ed. Saunders Elsevier; 2020.
3. Smith PP, Gordon C. Systemic lupus erythematosus: clinical presentations. Autoimmun Rev. 2010;10(1):43–5.

4.2 Rheumatoid Arthritis with Rheumatoid Factor Negative

Chen Mingquan

A 19-year-old man presented to our institution with a 21-month history of recurrent fever with muscle soreness and a 4-month history of joint swelling and pain in July 5, 2006.

At the beginning of November 2004, the patient developed sore throat. During this time, the patient had temperatures as high as 39–40 °C, with associated chills, shivering, and systemic muscle soreness. Fever mostly occurs in the afternoon, and can last several hours to the second half of the night. Body temperature can retreat to normal without obvious sweating. The patient went to the local hospital and checked the blood routine: leukocyte, 10.8×10^9/L; neutrophils, 80%. After 1 week of treatment with cephalosporins for suspected typhoid fever, body temperature dropped to normal. The patient developed similar symptoms again in early December 2004. He visited the local hospital again and the bone marrow examination showed infectious bone marrow imaging. In addition, the patient's blood culture results repeatedly showed negative. Penicillin and cephalosporins were given for 5 days, but the curative effect was not obvious. Therefore, the patient was transferred to another hospital and the leukocyte count showed 10.7×10^9/L. During this hospitalization, the patient treated with clindamycin for 10 days and discharged after returning to normal body temperature. Fifteen days after discharge, the patient had a similar attack again and improved after treatment with penicillin and clindamycin. After that, the patient had fever about every half month with a slight increase in white blood cell count. But the body temperature could be reduced to normal after penicillin, clindamycin, or traditional Chinese medicine treatment.

On March 6, 2005, the patient developed a fever again, accompanied by sore throat and muscle aches. In the right side of the neck, a bean-sized lymph node could be touched, which is soft, with clear boundary, and has no tenderness. The patient was admitted to hospital on March 11, 2005. Laboratory tests are as follows: leukocyte, 18.56×10^9/L; neutrophils, 89.1%; red blood cell count, 3.95×10^{12}/L; hemoglobin, 111 g/L; Platelet, 327×10^9/L; C-reactive protein, 139 mg/L; erythrocyte sedimentation rate, 30 mm/h; Ferritin, 1022 ng/mL. Liver and kidney function was normal. Tumor markers and autoimmunity antibody were negative. Multiple blood cultures and tuberculin test both were negative. The results of bone puncture suggested that hyperplastic bone marrow image and partial degeneration of granulocyte hyperplasia. Epigastric computed tomography was not abnormal. Bone scan revealed that the left side of the fifth lumbar vertebrae was abnormally elevated. Lumbar X filmograph showed L5 was fissured. Type-B ultrasonic showed multiple lymphadenectasis in superficial and retroperitoneal; no obvious abnormality was found in liver, bile, pancreas, and spleen. Because the enlarged lymph nodes were small and deep, no lymph node biopsy was performed. Upon admission, the patient was given clindamycin 0.9 bid and azithromycin 0.5 qd for 6 days for anti-infection. The patient's body temperature dropped to normal without any other discomfort. Review blood routine showed as follows: leukocyte, 12.6×10^9/L; neutrophils, 72%.

The patient requested to be discharged on March 25. There was recurrent fever after discharge and the nature is the same as before. On June 2005, examination results in other hospitals were as follows: C-reactive protein, 61 mm/h; erythrocyte sedimentation rate, 94.6 mg/L. Cytomegalovirus IgG and EB virus IgG both were positive. Rheumatoid factor was negative. On August 2005, the patient underwent a lymph node biopsy on a pulley in other hospitals, the pathological results suggest chronic lymphadenitis. Since 8 September, an intravenous drip of dexamethasone for 3 mg qd for 3 days. Then, change to oral prednisone 2# tid on 12 September and body temperature returned to normal. In January 2006, the patient's hormone dosage was reduced by one tablet every 2–3 weeks. However, fever occurred during each reduction and body temperature was about 37.5 °C. These symptoms can last 2–3 days and relieve themselves–.

In March 2006, the bilateral wrist joint and bilateral knee joint developed redness and pain, especially in the morning. The patient's joints were stiff, which improved after exercise. Subsequently, these symptoms developed to the bilateral ankle joints, bilateral metacarpophalangeal joints, and proximal interphalangeal joints. The symptoms can be relieved after taking Chinese medicine. When the hormone was reduced to prednisone 2.5 mg qd in May 2006, the patient developed a continuous fever with a body temperature between 37.5 and 38 °C and went to a local hospital. During this period, the patient's body temperature returned to normal after hormone addition to prednisone 10 mg qd, plus *Tripterygium wilfordii* polyglycoside 1 tablet tid. Since the onset of the disease, the patient has no headache, nausea and vomiting; no cough or expectoration; no abdominal pain, diarrhea; no low back pain, urinal urgency, frequent urination, or urinal pain; normal defecation and urination. For further treatment, the patient was readmitted to hospital on July 5, 2006.

4.2.1 Physical Examination

The patient had a temperature of 36 °C and no skin rash. On palpation, several lymph nodes in the neck and axilla were palpable. Besides, the lymph nodes are soft, with clear boundaries, and no tenderness. Findings on cardiopulmonary examination were within normal limits. No abdominal tenderness and rebound pain were found, and liver and spleen subcostal were unreached. Limb muscle strength and muscle tension were within normal limits. The bilateral knee joint was slightly red and swollen, with mild tenderness. The metacarpophalangeal joint and interphalangeal joint have obvious swelling and pain, and the movement is slightly limited.

4.2.2 Diagnosis and Treatment

The patient's liver function test is within normal range. Laboratory results were as follows: leukocyte count, 7.06×10^9/L; neutrophils, 55.2%; red blood cell count, 4.73×10^{12}/L, hemoglobin 128 g/L; Platelet, 214×10^9/L; C-reactive protein, 20.7 mg/L; erythrocyte sedimentation rate, 15 mm/h. Rheumatoid factor was negative. Tumor markers and autoimmunity antibody were negative. There was no obvious abnormality in chest radiographs. Hand X-ray showed that the bone of both hands and wrists was not abnormal. B-ultrasound revealed multiple enlarged lymph nodes in bilateral armpit and bilateral groin.

Consult rheumatology for consideration: rheumatoid arthritis, rheumatoid arthritis systemic (Still disease). It is recommended to discontinue the *Tripterygium wilfordii* polyglycosides, decrease the prednisone gradually and increase Methotrexate gradually from 2.5 to 10 mg qw. Give the patient paeoniflorin 0.6, three times a day and folic acid 5 mg, once a day.

The patient's condition was stable and fever, sore throat, swelling, and pain of joints were not found again. Therefore, the patient was discharged from hospital on July 18, 2006. Follow-up for 9 months after discharge, the patient's condition is stable with no recurrence.

4.2.3 Comments

Rheumatoid arthritis (RA) is not a rare disease, mainly involving bone joints, with chronic, symmetrical, poly synovial arthritis, and extraarticular disease as the main clinical manifestations, belong to autoimmune inflammatory disease. The disease often affects the hand joints, wrist joints, foot joints, and other small joints of the extremities, and is characterized by recurrent attacks and symmetrical distribution. Morning stiffness is usually the first symptom. In addition to joint lesions, the systemic manifestations of rheumatoid arthritis can also show fever, fatigue, pericarditis, subcutaneous nodules, pleurisy, arteritis, peripheral neuropathy, and so on. Fever can be of different degrees, mostly low fever or hidden slow onset. Sometimes lymph nodes may be enlarged.

This case has fever, joint redness, stiffness that involve joints of wrist, knee, ankle, metacarpophalangeal, and proximal interphalangeal joints, all bilateral, symmetrical, with obvious morning stiffness, enlarged lymph nodes around the body. Biopsy indicated inflammatory changes, while etiological examinations were consistently negative. The patient's condition relieved after treatment with hormones and immunosuppressants. Although diagnosing rheumatoid arthritis (RA) is usually straightforward, this patient had persistently negative rheumatoid factor (RF) throughout the disease course—making this the main feature of the case, as RF negativity is less common in typical RA. If the rheumatoid factor is more than 1:80, it has great reference value for diagnosis. However, because rheumatoid factors are not specific, they cannot be used as the basis for diagnosis. But they cannot be denied because rheumatoid factor is negative. The diagnosis of rheumatoid arthritis cannot be excluded because rheumatoid factor is negative. Anti-rheumatoid arthritis combined with nuclear antigen antibody (anti-RANA) is important for the diagnosis of rheumatoid arthritis. The positive rate was 95%. However, other types of arthritis can be 20% positive, so the diagnosis still needs to be closely combined with clinical practice. X-ray examination showed that osteoporosis of joint had diagnostic reference value and can be an early change. The occurrence of joint space narrowing, articular surface blur or bone destruction is slightly late, so the diagnosis should be combined with clinical symptoms.

This patient is characterized by long-term fever, sore throat, leukocytosis, and recurrent attacks as the early manifestations and then evolved into bone joint manifestations which is its special. It is suggested that clinicians should follow up for a long time in the case of unclear diagnosis and finally make a definite diagnosis.

References

1. Qingqing W. Diagnosis and treatment of rheumatoid arthritis [J]. Clin Educ Gen Med. 2008;2(6):92–4.
2. Xiuyan Y. Differential diagnosis of arthritis [J]. New Med. 1998;2(29):101–2.
3. Rheumatology Branch of the Chinese Medical Association. Guidelines for the diagnosis and treatment of rheumatoid arthritis [J]. Mod Pract Med. 2004;3(16):184–8.
4. Rheumatology Branch of the Chinese Medical Association. Draft guidelines for the diagnosis and treatment of rheumatoid arthritis [J]. Chin J Rheumatol. 2003;4(7):250–4.

4.3 A 35-Year-Old Female Patient Was Admitted to Our Department Due to Recurrent Fever with Granulocytopenia for 5 Months in December 2018

Yang Feifie, Chen Shu, and Huang Yuxian

Five months before admission, the patient was taking care of a herpetic angina patient and then she developed fever with a body temperature of up to 40 °C, accompanied by chills, headache, sore throat, and muscle and joint aches. She sweated heavily when the fever subsided. She had transient red rashes on the right inner thigh during the first fever and the rashes disappeared the next day. Over the course of disease, she did not have nausea, vomiting, abdominal pain, diarrhea, and jaundice. She took tylenol and her body temperature did not return. She went to the hospital on July 13. The blood routine revealed a low level of both white blood cell and neutrophils. The Coxsackie virus antibody test of her blood was positive. She was given intravenous levofloxacin for 3 days, followed by oral levofloxacin for 8 days, and then her body temperature dropped to normal. After 1 week, she developed fever again and her temperature was up to 37.8 °C. She was admitted to the Department of Hematology of a tertiary hospital in early August. Laboratory studies revealed the following: leukocyte count, 1.7×10^9/L; neutrophil percentage, 12.0%; lymphocytes percentage, 42.2%; monocytes percentage, 44.6%; hemoglobin, 110 g/L; platelet count, 175×10^9/L; C-reactive protein (CRP), 17.4 mg/L; and normal levels of liver functions, kidney functions, and electrolytes. Bone marrow smear showed increased proportion of mature monocytes (7.5%); the presence of immature monocytes (1.5%); moderate quantity of megakaryocytes with platelet function defect. No abnormal primitive or immature cells were seen in bone marrow by flow cytometry. Bone marrow needle biopsy revealed an abnormal proliferation of immature cells, which indicate the possibility of lymphoma. The results of PET/CT revealed the following: (1) Multiple lymph node enlargement in the bilateral clavicle area with SUVmax 2.9 and one swollen lymph node in the right side to be 1.0 × 0.9 cm; (2) Slight liver and spleen enlargement with SUVmax 2.5–2.7. Biopsy of the right cervical lymph node was performed and the pathology showed lymphadenia accompanied by large calcium salt deposition and cholesterol crystal formation. Cephalosporin, penicillin, and low-dose methylprednisolone were administered, and his body temperature dropped to normal. After being discharged from the hospital, her temperature increased repeatedly. She was admitted to the department of hematology three times and underwent bone marrow aspiration plus biopsy every time. The results were the same as before and the cause of neutropenia was unknown. Additional laboratory studies revealed the following: rheumatoid factor, 383.0 IU/mL; antinuclear antibody, 1:160; immunoglobulin G, 3217.0 mg/dL; soluble nucleoprotein antibody, positive; anti-SSA antibody, positive. Then, she was admitted to the department of rheumatology and was considered to be immune overload caused by viral infection. She went to the another hospital on October 25, 2018, and was hospitalized in the Department of Infectious Diseases. She had the following laboratory test results: leukocyte count, 1.6×10^9/L; neutrophil percentage, 0.6%; neutrophils count, 0.0×10^9/L; hemoglobin, 110 g/L; erythrocyte sedimentation rate (ESR), 56 mm/h; CRP, 31.19 mg/L; bone marrow aspiration plus biopsy, the same as before. During this hospitalization the patient still has fever, accompanied by cough and bloody sputum. The results of chest computed tomography (CT) showed small nodules in the upper lobes of both lungs, left lower lung infection with pleural effusion and a small amount of pericardial effusion. She was considered to have pulmonary infection and she was given anti-infection treatment with piperacillin-tazobactam, ribavirin, fluconazole, and moxifloxacin. Her body temperature returned to normal, and the lung infection recovered. One month later, she was discharged from the hospital with oral moxifloxacin and methylprednisolone. However, her fever reappeared 4 days later and returned to normal after 5 days of treatment with methylprednisolone. She went to our department again and stopped methylprednisolone. We asked clinical consultation of the Fudan University Cancer Hospital and their recommendations were as follows: (1) Bone marrow hematopoietic cells proliferate actively with all three lines of hematopoietic cells present, and there are many proliferating lymphocytes. Combined with the immunophenotype of these cells, the diagnosis of lymphoma is insufficient. (2) Lymph node histiocyte proliferative lesions, with large calcium salt deposition and cholesterol crystal formation, which are considered to be reactive hyperplasia. In order to further clarify the cause of repeated fever and lack of granules, she was admitted to our department for hospitalization. During the course of the disease, the patient has good spirits, appetite and sleep, normal bowel movements, and no significant weight loss.

Total thyroidectomy and neck lymph node dissection was performed on her in 2008. The pathology showed papillary thyroid carcinoma. The postoperative recovery was good.

4.3.1 Admission Physical Examination

Body temperature: 36.5 °C, no abnormal skin and mucous membranes all over the body, no liver palms, no swelling of superficial lymph nodes all over the body. There was no yellowing of the skin and sclera. No ecchymosis and rash were seen on the skin and mucous membranes. Scars of thyroid surgery could be seen on the neck. Breath sounds in both lungs were clear with no dry or wet rales heard. The heart rate was 80 beats/min and the rhythm was regular. The abdomen was flat and soft. No tenderness, no muscle tension and rebound pain were found in the whole abdomen. The liver and spleen could not be touched under the ribs. Percussive pain of the liver and both kidneys were negative. Bowel sounds were 3 times/min. There was no abnormality in the anus and external genitalia, no deformity of the spine and limbs, no redness and swelling of the joints, no clubbing, and no edema of the lower limbs. The muscle strength of both limbs was normal, and the pathological reflex was not elicited.

4.3.2 Course of Admission

Complete examinations were conducted. Blood routine: WBC 1.43 × 10^9/L, RBC 3.9 × 10^{12}/L, Hb 97 g/L, N 2/20, L 15/20, M 3/20, PLT 111 × 10^9/L. Lymphocyte subsets: Lymphocyte population 31.42%, CD3+ 78.87%, CD4+ 38.34%, CD8+ 37.01%, NK+ 12.67%, CD19+ 7.19%. Urine routine: Pro 1+, RBC 3801.4/μL, WBC 5.9/μL. Fecal occult blood test: negative. ESR: 40 mm/h. Ferritin: 282.2 ng/mL. Liver and kidney function and blood coagulation function were normal. Serum protein electrophoresis and immunofixation electrophoresis were normal. Tumor markers were normal. Autoantibody: ANA (+), titer 1:3200, particle type; ENA antibody profile: Ro-52 (+), SS-A (+), SS-B (−), cANCA (+), MPO: 5.2 RU/mL, pANCA (−), PR: 32.6 RU/mL. HLA-B27: negative. HBsAg: negative, HCV antibody: negative; EBV DNA, CMV DNA: negative. Blood IgA: 1.41 g/L, blood IgE: <45.12 ng/mL, blood IgG: 24.4 g/L, blood IgM: 1.19 g/L. Repeated blood culture and drug sensitivity tests were all negative.

Ultrasound: total thyroidectomy; lymph nodes were enlarged and considered to be reactive hyperplasia in the left neck (IV), bilateral axillary and bilateral inguinal. The left supraclavicular lymph node needed follow-up. There were no abnormally enlarged lymph nodes on the right neck and clavicle. There was no obvious abnormality in the bilateral parotid glands. Splenomegaly and small cysts of left kidney were found. No obvious abnormalities were found in the liver, gallbladder, pancreas and right kidney. There were no obvious abnormally enlarged lymph nodes around the vessels of the posterior peritoneum. Bone marrow aspiration and biopsy: Bone marrow smear: 16.5% granular lymphocytes can be seen. No obvious abnormalities were found in bone marrow flow cytometry, TCR rearrangement, and chromosome examination. Bone marrow biopsy pathology revealed the follows: more than ten medullary cavities; about 80% were hematopoietic cells; megakaryocytes can be seen; hyperplastic bone marrow; monocyte proliferation was considered according to the morphology and enzyme label; the nucleus had not shifted to the left. Reticular staining (−).

During the course of the disease, the patient had fever, cough and progressive decline in platelets. Chest CT suggested multiple lung inflammation (Fig. 4.1). She was given anti-infection treatment with intravenous imipenem and moxifloxacin, accompanied by intravenous gamma globules of 20 g for 5 days.

Considering the positive results of ANA (1:3200) and SSA, the autoimmune diseases such as Sjogren's syndrome cannot be ruled out, which can cause neutropenia. The labial gland biopsy was also conducted. Then, the patient was given intravenous methylprednisolone 40 mg and oral hydroxychloroquine every day, accompanied by stomach protection, calcium and potassium supplement. The patient's temperature returned to normal, and the count of platelets and white blood cells increased. However, the chest CT showed that the lesions progressed. The result of G test was >1000.00 pg/mL ↑ twice. We considered she had pulmonary fungal infection. Antifungal treatment with micafungin was administered and the other antibiotic were changed to cefoperazone-sulbactam. After that, the patient's white blood cells improved. Chest CT showed absorption in the inflammation site (Fig. 4.2). Labial gland biopsy pathology revealed Infiltration of inflammatory cells dominated by lymphocytes (both >50 foci) and suggested Sjogren's syndrome. Therefore, the patient was diagnosed as Sjogren's syndrome with immune neutropenia and pulmonary infection. She was then discharged from the hospital with oral medications and was followed in the outpatient.

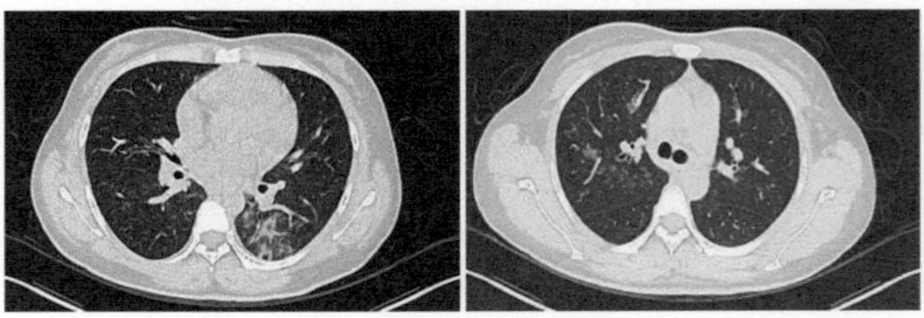

Fig. 4.1 Before anti-infection treatment

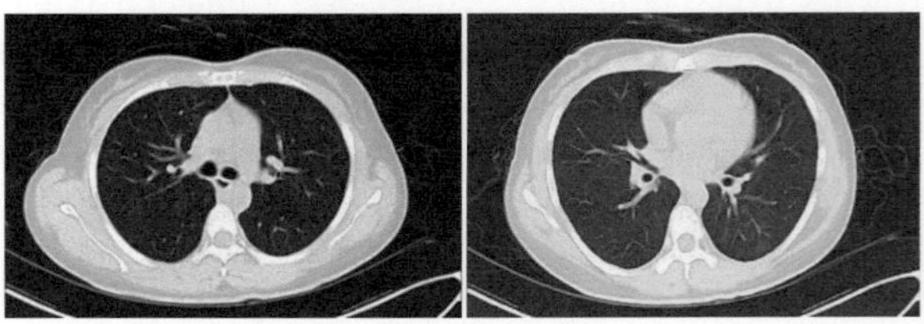

Fig. 4.2 After anti-infection treatment

4.3.3 Comment

Sjogren's syndrome is a chronic inflammatory autoimmune disease, which mainly involves the exocrine glands. In the clinic, about 2/3rd of the patients have systemic disorders in skin, skeletal muscle, liver, or kidney, in addition to dry mouth and dry eyes due to the impaired function of salivary and lacrimal glands. About one-quarter of the patients with Sjogren's syndrome have normocytic anemia. 30% of them have lower counts of white blood cells, and 2% have agranulocytosis.

The patient in this case had a history of close contact with a herpes virus patient at the beginning of the illness. Later, a granulocytic or even agranulocytosis was found. The course of her disease lasted for more than 5 months. The outside hospitals considered hematological tumors. They have done several bone marrow and lymph node examinations several times, but the course of the disease could not be found. In our hospital, the ANA and SSA antibodies were found to be positive. We performed a labial gland biopsy, which finally confirmed the diagnosis. In our case, the symptoms of dry mouth and dry eyes were not obvious, and agranulocytosis was the main clinical manifestation, which affected our diagnosis of the disease. The patient has Sjogren's syndrome with agranulocytosis as the main manifestation. Long-term follow-up is of great importance to detect the occurrence of lymphoma.

4.3.4 Discussion

Immune neutropenia is a group of neutropenia and agranulocytosis diseases mediated by anti-neutrophil antibodies. There are two types of neutrophil surface antigens: one is the antigen shared by neutrophils and other cells, such as HLA; the other is the specific antigen of neutrophils. At present, 10 types of human granulocyte antigens (HNA) have been identified, of which HNA-1 (FcγIIIb receptor) is the most immunogenic glycoprotein on the neutrophil membrane surface. There are four types of immune neutropenia: (1) neonatal alloimmune neutropenia, (2) primary autoimmune neutropenia, (3) secondary autoimmune neutropenia, (4) drug-immune neutropenia. This patient belongs to secondary immune neutropenia, which is the most common autoimmune neutropenia in adults. Neutropenia is often secondary to certain autoimmune diseases such as systemic lupus erythematosus (found in 50% of the cases), rheumatoid arthritis [Felty syndrome (Felty syndrome, a triad of rheumatoid arthritis, splenomegaly, and agranulocytosis)], Sjogren syndrome, immune thyroid disease, thymoma, T-granular lymphocytosis (often accompanied by agranulocytosis), etc. The mechanism of neutropenia can be due to anti-granulocyte antibodies, and cell-mediated destruction or antibodies of granulocyte colony-stimulating factor (G-CSF). In terms of treatment, in addition to therapy of the cause, the key is the prevention and treatment of infections caused by neutropenia. In patients with agranulocytosis, when the body temperature exceeds 38 °C, empirical antibiotic treatment should be given immediately after the risk of infection and drug resistance are evaluated. The principle is to cover the most common and virulent pathogens that can cause serious complications or life-threatening diseases. For high-risk patients, preventive medication is recommended. Fluoroquinolones and sulfamethoxazole/trimethoprim are recommended. Preventive use of third-generation antibiotics is not recommended. It is recommended to start with neutropenia until granulocytes are more than 0.5×10^9/L or obvious evidence of blood cell recovery. In addition, recombinant human G-CSF has been confirmed to have the effect of enhancing neutrophils.

References

1. Guowei L, Xiaoqin W. Immune-related granulocytopenia [J]. Chin J Pract Intern Med. 2006;26(7):487–9.
2. Jianhua F. Research on neutropenia in children [J]. Chin J Contemp Pediatr. 2017;19(4):484–8.
3. Capsoni F, Sarzi-Puttini P, Zanella A. Primary and secondary autoimmune neutropenia [J]. Arthritis Res Ther. 2005;7:208–14.
4. Zhai W, Zhang X, Wei J, et al. A prospective observation study of antibiotic therapy in febrile neutropenia patients with hematological malignances from multiple centers in Northeast China [J]. Int J Infect Dis. 2015;37:97–103.
5. Gafter G, Fraser A, Paul M, et al. Antibiotic prophylaxis for bacterial infections in a febrile neutropenic patient following chemotherapy [J]. Cochrane Database Rev. 2012;1:CD004386.

4.4 Nine-Month History of Fever, Headache and Cerebrospinal Fluid Abnormality: A Rare Case of Neuro-Behçet Syndrome

Bao Suxia, Zheng Jianming, and Chen Shu

A 29-year-old man was admitted for a 9-month history of recurrent fever and headache on June 11, 2014.

He started to have fevers without regular pattern (peaking at 38.3 °C) and severe persistent headache (mainly distending) since September 9, 2013, without nausea, vomiting, chills, sweating or cough. An MRI of the brain performed on September 13, 2013, showed scattered foci of signal abnormalities in the right thalamus and left pons, suggesting intracranial viral infections. He was then treated with antiviral reagents (details unobtainable) and prednisone (10–15 mg po) for about 1 week. But his condition did not improve, and his recurrent headache persisted.

He presented to another hospital on September 23, 2013. Notable laboratory findings were as follows: white blood cell count, 16.4×10^9/L, of which 81.6% were neutrophils; cerebrospinal fluid (CSF) studies on admission showed a pressure of 250 mmH_2O, total cells 250×10^6/L, white blood cells 26×10^6/L, glucose 2.8 mmol/L, Chloride 119 mmol/L, protein 0.59 g/L. He was diagnosed as viral meningitis, antiviral and rehydration treatment was given, and was discharged after his symptoms relief.

After discharged from the hospital, the patient experienced intermittent headaches, which can be relieved by painkiller. He had another episode of fever (temperature ranging from 37.6 to 37.8 °C) 1 month later. His fever was associated with headache and severe night sweating, but he denied cough, expectoration, dyspnea, tightness in chest, abdominal pain or diarrhea. T-SPOT.TB test result from another hospital was positive (antigen A, 10; antigen B:15).

On January 1, 2014, the patient present to our hospital. His CSF studies yielded the following notable results: white blood cells 32 × 10^6/L, multinucleated cells 4/32, mononuclear cells 28/32, Pandy's test ±, glucose 2.4 mmol/L, Chloride 118 mmol/L, protein 590 mg/L. His MRI of the brain (January 16th 2014) showed a widen septum pellucidum filled with CSF, but a normal ventricular system. No abnormal signal shadow in the parenchyma, no midline shift and no abnormal enhancement occurred. A conclusion of the formation of septum pellucidum cavity was concluded. His MRV of the head showed no notable abnormality.

Mannitol dehydration treatment failed to relieve his intermittent headache with fever. A 4-week diagnostic antituberculosis treatment, consist of isoniazid, rifampicin, ethambutol, pyrazinamide and levofloxacin was initiated on January 22th 2014. His CSF studies (performed on February 18, 2014) yielded the following results: white blood cells 172 × 10^6/L, multinucleated cells 35%, mononuclear cells 65%, Pandy's test ±, RBC 5 × 10^6/L, glucose 2.3 mmol/L (blood glucose 7.1 mmol/L), Chloride 120 mmol/L, protein 588 mg/L. His CSF culture was positive for *Acinetobacter lwoffii*.

Therefore, a combination of meropenem and amikacin treatment was given since February 18, 2014. The patient's headache relieved but still was occasionally febrile (temperature peaking at 37.8 °C). The CSF studies performed on February 28th 2014 showed the following results: white blood cells 86 × 10^6/L, multinucleated cells 29/86, mononuclear cells 57/86, Pandy's test ±, glucose 2.3 mmol/L, Chloride 120 mmol/L, protein 477 mg/L.

On March 24th 2014, a follow-up CSF study was performed and showed the following results: white blood cells 50 × 10^6/L, multinucleated cells 40%, mononuclear cells 60%, Pandy's test ±, RBC 70 × 10^6/L, glucose 2.9 mmol/L, Chloride 122 mmol/L, protein 440 mg/L. The patient improved but still had mild headache after a 6-week regimen of meropenem and amikacin. At the time of hospital dismissal, a 1-week regimen of oral levofloxacin and SMZ-TMP was prescribed. He still occasionally had headache with fever (temperature around 37.8 °C). On April 25th 2014, he was admitted to hospital again for repeated CSF studies, which revealed the following results: white blood cells 51 × 10^6/L, multinucleated cells 11/51, mononuclear cells 40/51, Pandy's test ±, glucose 2.3 mmol/L, Chloride 121 mmol/L, protein 639 mg/L. No notable findings were indicated by his MRI of the brain with contrast except for the formation of septum pellucidum cavity.

He was generally well, thus dismissed without further antibiotic therapy. However, after hospital dismissal, he was still occasionally febrile (temperature around 37.5 °C). He denied headache, nausea, vomiting, abdominal pain, diarrhea, cough, dyspnea, tightness in chest. One week ago, he noticed multiple erythema on both feet, which were painful but not itchy. Moreover, 5 days ago, he had another episode of fever of 38 °C with mild headache. After taking two tablets of "Xinhuang tablet", his fever ceased but the erythema did not disappear. The patient presented to our hospital after recurrent episode of fever (temperature of 37.7 °C) and fatigue 3 days ago. He was admitted for presumed central nervous system infection. On admission, he appeared generally well.

4.4.1 Physical Examination

The patient appeared well and conscious. His heart rate was 78 beats/min. Multiple erythema of different sizes, which were slightly elevated in the center, were spotted on both lower extremities. His mucous, abdominal, cardiac, musculoskeletal, and neurologic examinations were without significant abnormality.

4.4.2 Diagnosis and Treatment

On admission, his laboratory studies demonstrated: white blood cell count, 8.25×10^9/L, with 69.9% neutrophils, 21.8% lymphocyte and 0.4% eosinophils; hemoglobin, 137 g/L; platelet count, 267×10^9/L; erythrocyte sedimentation rate, 21 mm/h (elevated); C-reactive protein, 5.13 mg/L; procalcitonin, 0.03 ng/mL; blood IgA 4.4 g/L (elevated), IgG 15.6 g/L, IgM 0.77 g/L, IgE 324 ng/mL (elevated) and IgG4 1.3 g/L; fungal (1,3)-β-D-glucan test <10 pg/mL. T-SPOT.TB and Cryptococcus antigen latex agglutination tests were negative. Studies of liver and renal function, myocardial enzymes, coagulation function, blood lipids and glucose, serum tumor markers, blood lymphocyte subsets, thyroid function, autoantibodies, ferritin, urine and stool, and immunofixation electrophoresis blood test were unremarkable. His chest CT showed no obvious abnormality. The ultrasonography showed liver, gallbladder, pancreas, spleen, kidneys, bilateral ureters, bladder, and bilateral cervical lymph nodes no obvious abnormality, bilateral thyroid nodules (presumed benign). His CSF studies yielded the following results: white blood cells 342×10^6/L, multinucleated cells 28%, mononuclear cells 72%, Pandy's test 1+, glucose 2.3 mmol/L, Chloride 120 mmol/L, protein 731 mg/L (Table 4.1).

His clinical manifestations were mainly fever, headache and recurrent CSF abnormalities, which did not improve after either antiviral, antibiotic or anti-tuberculosis treatment. CSF culture was once positive for *Acinetobacter lwoffii*, however the patient did not improve after treatment with antibiotics according to drug-susceptibility testing. These suggested he might have chronic purulent meningitis, or might be infected with rare pathogens with low virulence, such as fungus, or might have non-Infectious diseases. Central nervous system tumors were unlikely, because of his imaging examination results without notable intracranial or meningeal mass-like lesions, results of multiple CSF studies unrevealing of exfoliated cells and the relatively long 9-month duration of symptoms. A skin biopsy was not performed due to the disappeared skin lesions soon after admission.

Table 4.1 Results of CSF studies

Date	CSF pressure (mmH_2O)	White blood cell (multinucleated cell) ($\times 10^6/L$)	CSF protein (mg/L)	CSF chloride (mmol/L)	CSF glucose (mmol/L)	Blood glucose (mmol/L)	Treatment
2013.9.25	250	26	590	119	2.8		
2014.1.13		32(4/32)	590	118	2.4		Isoniazid + rifampicin + ethambutol + pyrazinamide + levofloxacin
2014.2.18		172(35%)	588	120	2.3	7.1	Meropenem + amikacin
2014.2.28		86(29/86)	477	120	2.3		
2014.3.24		50(40%)	440	122	2.9		
2014.4.25		51(11/51)	639	121	2.3		All medication withdrew
2014.6.12	280	342(28%)	731	120	2.3	6.4	
2014.6.17	>300	234(16%)	686	119	2.6	5.4	
2014.7.7	>300	160(70%)	639	119	2.4	6	Meropenem + linezolid
2014.7.16	260	135(68%)	664	118	2.4	6.7	
2014.7.21	230	134(37%)	591	119	2.3	6.1	Itraconazole
2014.7.29	190	28(2/28)	119	116	2.2	7.6	
2014.8.11	>300	486(71%)	901	121	2.2	7.1	Methylprednisolone 60 mg/day
2014.8.19	230	18(2/18)	386	121	4.2	7	

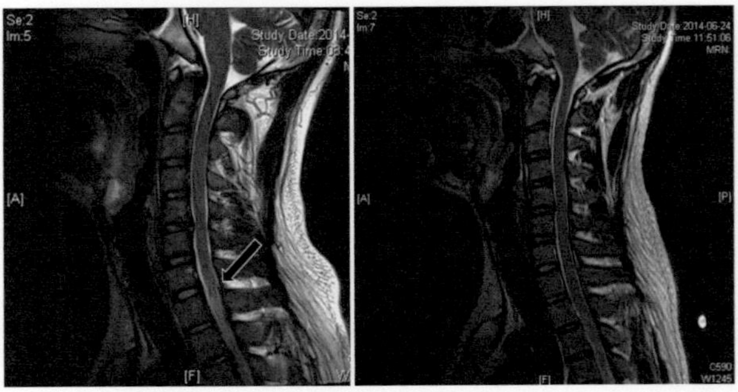

Fig. 4.3 Changes of MRI results of the cervical spine

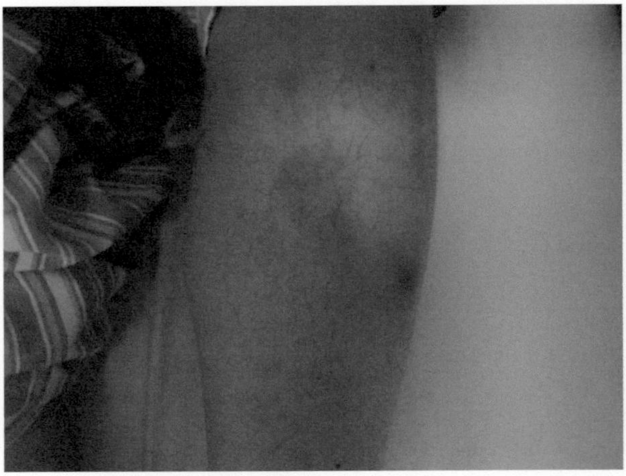

Fig. 4.4 Skin lesions at the site of tibialis anterior

An MRI of the spinal cord (performed on June 17th 2014) revealed cord signal abnormalities at C3-T3 levels and cervical disc herniation at right C5/6 level (Fig. 4.3). His PET/CT indicated: (1) A diffusive decrease of FDG uptake in bilateral cerebellar cortex and an uneven distribution of FDG uptake in bilateral cerebral cortex; (2) An mild increase of bone marrow FDG uptake, presumed reactive changes; (3) Uneven intensity of bilateral thyroid lobes, with scattered calcifications but no marked increase in FDG uptake, presumed benign lesions; Right maxillary sinusitis; Bilateral cervical lymphadenitis; (4) Increased bronchovascular markings; (5) Fatty liver. Based on findings from the MRI of the spinal cord and PET/CT, an MRI of the cervical spine with contrast was performed on June 24, 2014, which revealed signal abnormality in the spinal cord at T3 level (improved comparing to results of MRI on June 17, 2014) and posterior cervical disc herniation at right C5/6 level (Fig. 4.3). Bone puncture was done, but bone marrow smear, flow cytometry, and bone biopsy showed no obvious abnormality.

Abnormal signal was found in spinal cord after admission. However, the cord signal abnormality, along with results of repeated CSF studies improved without any medication treatment. On July 2, 2014, the patient had another episode of fever and developed rash and painful subcutaneous nodules (Fig. 4.4). A skin biopsy was performed, and histological examination revealed a generally normal epidermis, small lymphocytic infiltrations around superficial and deep perivascular in the dermis with several neutrophils present, only a small amount of subcutaneous fat tissue. The immunohistochemistry staining test results was unremarkable for dysplasia. Thereby, any infectious or neoplastic disease should not be considered the cause of this patient. Autoimmune disease is mostly likely cause, but the lack of autoimmune antibodies made it difficult to reach a final diagnosis and precise classification.

Immunosuppressive therapy is the treatment option for autoimmune diseases. However, infection could not be excluded due to his recurrent elevated level of WBC in CSF. A meropenem + linezolid combination regimen and an antifungal regimen of itraconazole were sequentially initiated. Repeated CSF studies showed no improvement, thus excluded infection in this patient. Neurologists, dermatologists and rheumatologists were consulted for the diagnosis of an autoimmune disease affecting both the nervous system and the skin.

Based on results of imaging examinations, the neurologists consider Behçet's disease as the most likely diagnosis, due to the spontaneously resolved parenchymal focus with manifestations indicating vascular involvement. Apart from folliculitis-like rash and erythema nodosum, the dermatologists noticed depigmentation of the scrotum on physical examination, which might be resulting from previous genital ulcerations. The delayed healing of the site of bone marrow biopsy was also noticed and was considered indication of positive pathergy test. Although the patient did not have mouth ulcers in 2014, he reported a history of recurrent painful aphthae several years ago. Histological findings of his skin biopsy were indicative for vasculitis and were also consistent with Behçet's disease. Therefore, a diagnosis of Behçet's disease was established. The rheumatologists agree on the diagnosis and suggested an early admission of glucocorticoid treatment, since the poor prognosis of Neuro-Behçet's disease.

After treatment of 60 mg/day methylprednisolone, the patient's fever, headache, rash and erythema nodosum resolved. His repeated CSF studied performed on August 19th 2014 showed improved results, including a decreased level of white blood cells (18×10^6/L) and normal chemical tests results (Table 4.1). The patient regularly followed up at the department of rheumatology and remained stable thereafter.

4.4.3 Comment

Behçet's disease (BD) is a multisystemic, chronic, vasculitis disease with major manifestations including recurrent aphthae, genital ulcers, eye inflammation and skin lesions. BD can also affect the vascular system, nervous system, gastrointestinal tract, joints, lungs, kidneys, epididymites and other organs. Most patients have good prognosis, except those with ocular, central nervous system or macrovascular involvement.

Interestingly, BD is more prevalent along in the Far East, the Middle East, and the Mediterranean regions, thus also known as the "Silk Route disease". Neuro-BD (NBD) refers to the neurological manifestations of the disease. NBD, with a prevalence ranging from 5% to 50%, can affect multiple systems, but is present in only a few (5%) patients as an initial symptom. Central nervous system (CNS) involvement is more common, and is usually associated with symptoms including headaches, Horner syndrome, pseudobulbar paralysis, epilepsy, aseptic meningitis, papilledema, hemiplegia, aphasia, motor symptoms, paraplegia, and sensory and mental disorders. Peripheral nervous system involvement is less common, and usually present as numbness and weakness of the extremities and peripheral sensory neuropathy. NBD is considered a poor prognostic factor. Brainstem and spinal cord lesions are responsible for the majority of disability and death caused by NBD.

NBD is usually associated with elevated CSF pressure, slightly higher WBC count of CSF. The sensitivity of MRI, revealing the brainstem–thalamic–basal ganglia lesions of hyperintensity signal at the acute phase, can be as high as 96.5% for the diagnosis of NBD. MRI abnormalities of chronic NBD lesions should be carefully differentiated from multiple sclerosis.

NBD should be considered in the differential diagnosis of fever of unknown origin with a relatively long duration. Criteria for the diagnosis of NBD are listed in Table 4.2. In this case, fever, headache and CSF abnormalities are the patient's major manifestations. Symptoms were sometimes alleviated, while sometimes aggravated by empirical treatment including antibiotics, antituberculosis and antifungal regimens. It was so difficult to establish the diagnosis of NBD that eventually it took 9 months. Unusual manifestations are responsible for the delayed diagnosis of this patient. It is even rare to be initially presented with CNS symptoms. Secondly, the skin lesions and recurrent oral ulceration developed at different time points, along with the absence of ocular lesions, add up to the difficulty of diagnosis. Comprehensive and careful analysis of the patient's skin lesions of the 9 months'

Table 4.2 The International Criteria for diagnosis (classification) of Behçet's disease (The ISG criteria, published in 1990, the most widely used)

Sign/symptom	Definition
Recurrent oral ulceration	Minor, major, or herpetiform oral ulcerations, confirmed by a physician or reliable patient report, occurring on at least three separate occasions within a 12-month period
Plus, any 2 of:	
Recurrent genital ulceration	Aphthous ulceration or scarring of the oral or genital mucosa, confirmed by physician examination or reliable patient report.
Eye lesions	Anterior or posterior uveitis, or vitreous cells detected by slit-lamp examination; or retinal vasculitis confirmed by an ophthalmologist or other qualified physician.
Skin lesions	Erythema nodosum or erythema nodosum-like lesions, confirmed by physician examination or reliable patient report; pseudofolliculitis or papulopustular lesions; or acneiform nodules identified by a physician in post-adolescent patients not receiving corticosteroid therapy.
Positive pathergy test	Results interpreted as positive by a physician at 24–48 h post-procedure.

duration, his episode of recurrent aphthae years before and the spontaneously resolved or aggravated symptoms led to the establishment of a diagnosis of BD.

The folliculitis-like rash, erythema nodosum, depigmentation of the scrotum and the delayed healing of the wound are important hints. Manifestations of the nervous system could indicate an overlap of two diseases. However, the improvement of headache, fever and CSF study results after steroid treatment proved that NBD may be the correct diagnosis. The signs and the symptoms might develop at different time points, but they lead to only one diagnosis. Therefore, in order to avoid being one cannot see the wood for the trees, one should always inquiry case history in details, perform physical examination carefully and analyze the evidence comprehensively.

References

1. Rheumatology Branch of the Chinese Medical Association. Guidelines for the diagnosis and treatment of Behçet's disease [J]. Chin J Rheumatol. 2011;15(5):345–7.
2. Silman A. Criteria for diagnosis of Behcet's disease [J]. Lancet. 1990;335(8697):1078–80. https://doi.org/10.1016/0140-6736(90)92643-V.
3. Alibaz-Oner F, Direskeneli H. Update on the diagnosis of Behçet's disease [J/OL]. Diagnostics (Basel). 2022;13(1):41. https://doi.org/10.3390/diagnostics13010041.

4.5 A Rare Adult-Onset Still's Disease Involving Heart Valve with a Tortuous Treatment History

Li Ning and Zhang Jiming

A 19-year-old unmarried female student presented to the department of infectious disease with fever and both hands and lower limbs swollen for more than 20 days on May 13, 2015.

She had enjoyed good health until she went sketching in Huangshan Mountain on April 22, 2015, when she felt chilly with no obvious cause. At that time, her temperature was not measured, while then she soon developed edema on her hands and the back of feet. Then she presented to a hospital in Mountain Huang, founded to be febrile to 39.0 °C, with laboratory studies demonstrating the leukocytosis 16.67×10^9/L, hemoglobin 111 g/L, neutrophil 14.93×10^9/L, platelet 222×10^9/L, CRP, 131.6 mg/L. Considering infectious fever, levofloxacin combined with cefathiamidine was given intravenously for 2 days, while her symptom of fever and edema were not relieved. On April 24, she was transferred to a hospital in Nantong, reexamined blood routine with leukocyte 15.5×10^9/L, hemoglobin 82.2 g/L, neutrophil 12.7×10^9/L, ESR 88 mm/h, ferritin 512.76 g/mL. There was no significant finding in the tests of EB virus antibody, blood plasmodium screening, blood culture, tumor markers, immunoglobulin and complements. Her chest CT showed no obvious abnormality in the chest but with splenomegaly. Abdominal B-ultrasound showed that the echo in the liver area was uniform and dense, and no obvious abnormality was found in the bladder. Superficial lymph node B ultrasound showed bilateral inguinal, bilateral axillary lymph nodes, right neck lymph node enlargement. Her bone marrow smears showed that bone marrow hyperplasia was active, with granulocyte and erythroid accounting for 73.5% and 15.5%, respectively, granulocyte proliferation was active, eosinophils were visible, erythroid proliferation was active, which mainly containing middle late erythroblasts, and mature erythrocytes were different in size, and there were 81 megakaryocytes and platelets. Her bone marrow culture was negative. After admission, she was treated with cefotaxime/sulbactam (4.5 g bid IVGTT). The swelling on both hands and the back of feet subsided obviously, but she was still febrile with the peak temperature of 39.0 °C at night, accompanied with feeling obviously chilly and shivering. Since April 25, levofloxacin was added to strengthen anti-infectious treatment, while she felt chilly, shivering and febrile again at 2 p.m. on that day. She was given dexamethasone 5 mg intravenously and her temperature dropped briefly, but she had fever again the next day, with the peak temperature of 40.2 °C. On April 28, anti-infectious regimen was replaced with teicoplanin, but the patient still had fever, with a peak temperature of 39.2 °C. On May 2, TIENAM® combined with teicoplanin was given but the temperature was still high, so the patient asked to transfer to our department for further diagnosis and treatment. Since the onset of the disease, the patient's mind was ordinary, appetite and sleep were general, urine and stool were normal, and there was no significant weight loss. Current medication: Xinhuang Tablets (1 q.d. po).

4.5.1 Physical Examination on Admission

Temperature 37 °C, pulse 106 bpm, breathing 18 bpm, blood pressure 116/70 mmHg, height 165 cm, weight 51 kg. Clear awareness, one enlarged lymph node with soft texture and good mobility, about 1 cm in diameter, was palpable in the right neck. The breath sounds of both lungs were clear. Heart rate was 106 bpm, with regular rhythm and no murmur; no significant abnormality in abdomen. Nondepressed edema was found on her lower limbs, the back of the right foot near the ankle joint was red and swollen without skin temperature rising.

4.5.2 Hospital Course

After admission, related examinations were conducted. Laboratory studies showed blood routine with white blood cell 4.24×10^9/L, with 55.90% neutrophil and lymphocyte 36.10%, red blood cell 4.03×10^{12}/L, hemoglobin 102 g/L ↓, platelet 115×10^9/L ↓, CRP 88 mg/L ↑, ESR 53 mm/h ↑, procalcitonin 3.27 ng/mL ↑, lactate dehydrogenase 842 U/L ↑. Cell subsets with lymphocyte subsets % 21.78%, $CD3^+$ 82.84% ↑, $CD4^+$ 41.18% ↑, $CD8^+$ 41.78% ↑, NK^+ 9.78%, $CD19^+$ 6.14% ↓, and CD4/

CD8 0.99. Liver function and electrolyte with ALT 59 U/L ↑, AST 135 U/L ↑, albumin 32 g/L ↓, globulin 29 g/L, white globulin ratio 1.10 ↓, bilirubin normal, potassium 3.40 mmol/L ↓, sodium 130 mmol/L ↓, and chlorine 93 mmol/L ↓. Coagulation function with INR 1.13 ↑, Pt 12.30 ↑, APTT 37.60 s ↑, fibrinogen 3.1150 g/L, D-dimer 20.11 ↑, and fibrinogen degradation products 52.10 μg/mL ↑. There was no significant abnormality in TNT, proBNP, glucose metabolism, lipid metabolism, autoantibody, antibody O, rheumatoid factor, blood Cryptococcus latex agglutination test, blood T- SPOT.TB, urine routine, fecal routine and OB.

Completed bone marrow puncture smear showed the number of nucleated cells in bone marrow decreased. Pox staining showed nonabnormal lymphocyte, and NAP staining showed 26% positive and accumulating 40 points. Iron staining showed that external iron without bone marrow granules and internal iron without no erythroblasts. There was no obvious abnormality in abdominal B-ultrasound.

On review of supplementary medical history below, (1) Considering the redness and swelling of the back of the right foot, she was asked carefully whether she was bitten by insects during the sketch in Mountain Huang? (2) With high fever, her toxic blood symptoms were not obvious, which was not characterized like infectious fever. So, the patient was asked if her joints were swollen and painful recently, if she had a sore throat, a rash (ever appeared), recurrent oral ulcers, if her conjunctiva was congested, and if there was a vulvar ulcer, or any other discomforts accompanying? It was learned that the patient did not contact any insect or feel bite during her sketching in Mountain Huang. In addition to the accompanying symptoms in the current medical history, the patient had obvious pharyngeal pain at the initial stage of onset, which was too severe to swallow drinking water. Sometimes there was pain in wrist and ankle joint.

Before the onset of the disease, the patient "went to Mountain Huang for sketching" and had a history of mountain tourism. After regular systemic treatment for Gram-positive and Gram-negative bacteria in other hospitals, the patient's temperature still did not improve. Considering the possibility of atypical pathogen infection, intravenous doxycycline (0.1 g q12h) was given. The patient's temperature soon dropped to normal, and the general situation improved (Fig. 4.5).

After doxycycline treatment, the patient's peak temperature dropped on the second day, then became normal on the third day and maintained for 4 days. On May 20, her temperature began to rise to 38.4 °C (Fig. 4.6). On the premise that

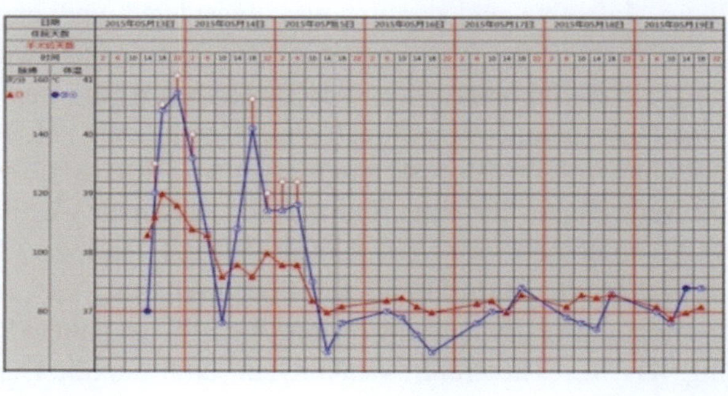

Fig. 4.5 Temperature sheet of the first week after admission (May 13, 2015 to May 19, 2015): the patient's temperature dropped to normal after doxycycline application

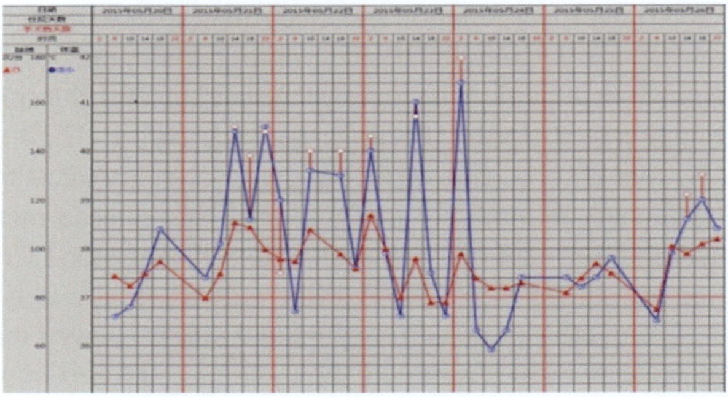

Fig. 4.6 Temperature sheet of the second week after admission (May 20, 2015 to May 26, 2015)

doxycycline seemed to be effective, the temperature appeared to be repeated. Should we consider whether the original treatment direction was correct? Did the process of the disease just enter the intermission which made doxycycline seemed to be effective? Then doxycycline was stopped and the changes of temperature were observed. The patient's temperature remained high at the peak of 41.4 °C. At that time, reexamined blood routine on May 20, 2015, showed white blood cell $11.64 \times 10^9/L$ ↑ with neutrophil % 63.20%, lymphocyte 24.40% and monocyte% 9.90%, red blood cell $3.47 \times 10^{12}/L$ ↓, hemoglobin 87 g/L, platelet $256 \times 10^9/L$. It can be seen that hemoglobin decreased from 102 g/L to 87 g/L 1 week ago. Combined with high fever, chills, leukocytosis and anemia, possibility of infective endocarditis should be considered. In addition, the patient's redness and swelling limiting on the back of the foot, could it be caused by embolus falling off and embolizing blood vessels?

Actively arranged for cardiac ultrasound examination, and then carefully physical examination was done to determine whether there were ecchymoses and petechiae on the skin and mucosa, and reexamined the urine routine to determine whether there was occult blood. Since doxycycline seems to be effective in the treatment of atypical pathogens, doxycycline combined with moxifloxacin were used for anti-infectious treatment.

After treatment of doxycycline combined with moxifloxacin, her temperature suddenly dropped to normal on the second day (May 24). While on the third day, the temperature showed a rising trend (Fig. 4.7). Meanwhile, echocardiography reported rice grain shaped vegetations attaching in the anterior lobe of the mitral valve, mild mitral regurgitation, and a small amount of pericardial effusion. On the evidence of those, infective endocarditis was considered and anti-infectious regimens were adjusted immediately. Doxycycline and moxifloxacin were stopped, and vancomycin (1 g q12h) combined with fosfomycin (8 g q12h) was used to strengthen the anti-infectious treatment for Streptococcus empirically. However, the patient's fever did not improve, and the peak temperature was still 39 °C, even further rising to 39.6 °C on May 28. At that time, the antibiotic regimen was adjusted to vancomycin (1 g q12h) combined with moxifloxacin (0.4 qd). However, the patient's temperature had no obvious downward trend, fever occurred every day, and the peak value continued to rise. In the early morning of June 4, 2015, the patient had a high fever again, reaching 41 °C. Therefore, vancomycin and moxifloxacin were stopped, and the

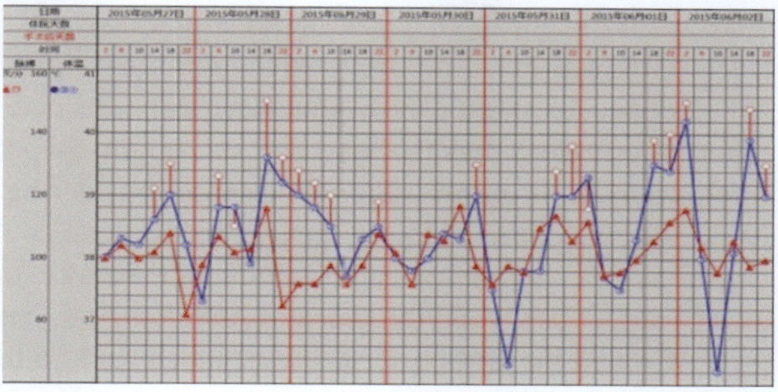

Fig. 4.7 Temperature sheet of the third week after admission (May 27, 2015 to June 2, 2015)

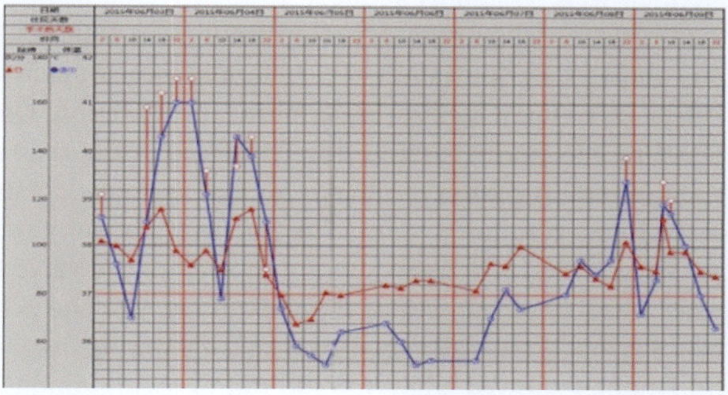

Fig. 4.8 Temperature sheet of the fourth week after admission (June 3, 2015 to June 9, 2015)

anti-infectious regimen was adjusted to doxycycline (0.1 g q12h IVGTT). The next day (June 5) her temperature suddenly dropped to normal (Fig. 4.8), but rose again 3 days later.

The clinical characteristics of the patients are further summarized below. A young female, high fever, sore throat, arthralgia, splenomegaly and lymphadenopathy, high white blood cell count, negative rheumatoid factor and antinuclear antibody, and a long course of treatment without a variety of significantly effective anti-infectious regimens with sensitivity to non-steroidal anti-inflammatory drugs (indomethacin) and corticosteroids. Meanwhile, repeated blood culture in other hospitals and our hospital were all negative. After excluding infectious disease, connective tissue diseases which is more likely adult-onset Still's disease, should be considered. Since adult-onset Still's disease was considered, why did her temperature fall to normal level after application of doxycycline in three times during admission and then rose again after 3–5 days? This phenomenon may be related to doxycycline's immunomodulatory function. It has been reported that doxycycline can regulate the reducing secretion of IL-1 β, IL-12, TNF-α and IL-6 secreted by dendritic cells and inhibit the proliferation of allogeneic T cells stimulated by dendritic cells, which may alleviate the cytokine storm to a certain extent. However, 4 days with dropped temperature after doxycycline monotherapy for the third time, the patient developed fever again on the night of June 8, with a peak of 40 °C and scattered skin rash with pruritus. Dermatology department was urgently asked, considering "allergic dermatitis" after consultation. Doxycycline was stopped and loratadine was given orally. After further discussion, it was still considered that the more likely diagnosis of "adult-onset Still's disease". Therefore, methylprednisolone 40 mg was given intravenously at the same time. Then the patient's temperature dropped to normal level and her rash subsided. On June 11, the patient's echocardiographic results showed a rice grain shaped vegetations attaching the anterior leaflet of mitral valve, which was considering non-infectious vegetations, so the patient continued to use methylprednisolone.

The patient had no fever and the temperature was stable. On June 14, the patient tried to reduce the methylprednisolone to 32 mg qd, but her temperature rebounded (37.9 °C), and the corticosteroids was added back to the original dose. Within one day, her temperature quickly returned to normal. By June 23, the patient's corticosteroids were gradually reduced to methylprednisolone tablets 28 mg qd po, and there was no rebound of her temperature. On June 25, reexamined echocardiography showed the formation of vegetations in the anterior and posterior parts of the mitral valve with slight to mild mitral regurgitation. On June 30, the patient's temperature was normal lasting for 1 week, and she was discharged from hospital in stable condition. After discharge, according to the doctor's advice, methylprednisolone tablets continued to be 28 mg qd and gradually reduced. After regular follow-up, reexamined echocardiography showed mitral valve thickening, multiple miliary vegetations could be seen at the apex of anterior and posterior lobes, the largest one was 3 mm × 4 mm (all organized), and valves opening were not limited, with colorful Doppler showed slight to mild mitral regurgitation. The patient was still taking methylprednisolone, gradually reducing the dosage, normal temperature, and has returned to school.

So far, combined with the patient's symptoms, signs, auxiliary examination, management process, the final diagnosis of adult Still's disease was considered.

4.5.3 Discussion

Still's disease originally refers to juvenile arthritis with systemic onset, but similar diseases can also occur in adults, so it is called adult-onset Still's disease (AOSD). The clinical features are fever, arthralgia and/or arthritis, rash, myalgia, sore throat, lymphadenopathy, increasing of total white blood cell count and neutrophil count, and thrombocytosis, meanwhile severe cases accompany with systemic damage. The predilection age is from 16 to 35 years old, and it can also be seen in the elderly.

There are nonspecific diagnosis criteria of adult-onset Still's disease, while American Cush criteria is recommended mostly, with necessary criteria of fever with temperature over 39 °C, arthralgia or arthritis, rheumatoid factor $<1:80$, antinuclear antibody $<1:100$ and any of the following two items are required, including white blood cell $\geq 15 \times 10^9/L$, rash, pleurisy or pericarditis, and hepatomegaly or splenomegaly or lymphadenectasis. It should be emphasized that adult-onset Still's disease is an exclusive diagnosis, and there is still no specific unified diagnostic criteria. Even after the diagnosis is made, it is still necessary to observe the changes of the condition at any time during the treatment and follow-up.

Multiple organ damage is the characteristic of this disease, while it is easy to be misdiagnosed when only single organ damage manifested. The most common is liver damage, followed by heart damage which can be manifested as arrhythmia, pericarditis, myocarditis, etc. The incidence of pericarditis is relatively high, ranging from 3% to 20%. Myocarditis is relatively rare. But other rheumatic immune diseases involving the heart valve is not rare, it was reported that abnormal echocardiography was found in about 91.7% of patients with diffuse connective tissue disease, while the highest incidence is valve regurgitation caused by valve involvement, as a proportion of 57.8%.

The main reason for the tortuous treatment process of this case is that the mitral valve vegetations were seen by echocardiography for many times, and the patient had high fever, anemia and elevated white blood cells, so it was difficult to ignore the diagnosis of infectious endocarditis. However, the patient's blood culture was negative for many times, and the anti-infectious regimens were ineffective. Although several echocardiographic results showed that there were mitral valve vegetations, the patient was determined to be non-infectious, and the patient's condition was relieved after the application of methylprednisolone.

References

1. Gerfaud-Valentin M, Seve P, Iwaz J, et al. Myocarditis in adult-onset Still disease. Medicine. 2014;93(17):280–9.
2. Carrilho-Ferreira P, Silva D, Silva M d J, et al. Adult-onset Still's disease and cardiac tamponade. Tex Heart Inst J. 2015;42(3):277–80.
3. Yang DH, Chang DM, Lai JH, et al. Etanercept as a rescue agent in patient with adult onset Still's disease complicated with congestive heart failure. Rheumatol Int. 2008;29(1):95–8.
4. Efthimiou P, Paik PK, Bielory L. Diagnosis and management of adult onset Still's disease. Ann Rheum Dis. 2006;65(5):564–72.

4.6 Vascular Macrovascular Vasculitis

Fan Qingqi, Jia Wen, Shao Lingyun, and Zhang Wenhong

A 28-year-old woman, was admitted to the hospital on August 11, 2016 due to "fever for more than 1 month".

In June 2016, the patient started to present with fever. The highest temperature was 39.6 °C, accompanied by neck tenderness and headache, but the headache was not related to temperature, and there was no rash or joint pain. She went to the local hospital on June 23 and checked blood test: WBC 7.15×10^9/L, N 72.3%, Hb 93 g/L, PLT 310×10^9/L, erythrocyte sedimentation rate 120 mm/h, CRP 131.79 mg/L, liver and kidney function: normal, urine routine: normal, ferritin 307.4 ng/mL. A plain lung CT scan revealed a small amount of effusion in the bilateral pleural cavity. After receiving antibiotic therapy (cephalosporin) for 3 days, she still had fever.

She was transferred to a hospital in Jiangsu Province on June 28, and the blood test was similar to before, with CRP of 158 mg/L. Autoantibodies were all negative; EBV-DNA was negative; B-ultrasonography: no abnormalities in liver, gallbladder, pancreas, spleen, and kidney, right thyroid hypoechoic nodules TI-RADS type 2; lumbar puncture showed that cerebrospinal fluid routine and biochemical examination were normal; head MRI scan: no abnormalities; heart ultrasonography: no obvious abnormalities; a small amount of atypical lymphocytes were found by bone marrow puncture. CT showed a small amount of pelvic effusion and pleural effusion on both sides. She was given moxifloxacin for 4 days, but still had fever. After that, the patient was treated with glucocorticoids for 3 days (the specific dose is unknown), and his temperature dropped to normal. However, after stopping the glucocorticoids, she had a fever again and was admitted to our ward on August 11. Since the onset of the disease, the patient's spirit, appetite, sleep, defecation as usual, urination as usual, no significant decrease in physical strength, and no significant weight loss.

4.6.1 Admission Physical Examination

T 38.3 °C, P 98 beats/min, R 18 beats/min, BP 110/70 mmHg (left and right hands), clear mind, no rash on the whole body, pulsation of bilateral temporal arteries, soft neck without resistance, tenderness in anterior neck area. Obviously, the thyroid gland was not palpable bilaterally, the carotid murmur was not obvious, and the lymph nodes were not palpable. Pulmonary examination revealed rough lungs, and no dry or wet rales were heard, cardiac examination revealed the heart rate was 98 bpm with regular rhythm and no murmurs are heard. The abdomen was soft, no tenderness, the liver, spleen, and ribs were not palpable, and the mobile dullness was negative. No swelling of both lower limbs. Meningeal irritation signs were negative, and bilateral pathological signs were not elicited. The muscle strength of the limbs is symmetrical and normal.

4.6.2 Diagnosis and Treatment

Related examinations were completed after admission. Blood routine: white blood cell count, 8.88×10^9/L, Hemoglobin, 85 g/L, Platelets count, 399×10^9/L, neutrophils, 74.0%, RET 1.70%; liver and kidney function: Albumin, 26 g/L, other related checks were normal; blood lipids were normal; coagulation function: PT 15.2 s, FIB 9.0 g/L, D-dimer <0.10 mg/L; ESR, 125 mm/h, CRP, 176 mg/L, ferritin, 456.70 μg/L, LDH, 125 U/L; blood culture: negative; normal thyroid function; thyroid gland Antibody, ANA, ANCA are all negative; urine test: white blood cell 1–3/HP, red blood cell 0/HP, protein negative. After admission, non-specific inflammatory indicators such as CRP and erythrocyte sedimentation rate were significantly increased, and albumin was significantly decreased, suggesting a significant systemic inflammatory response. At the same time, because the patient's neck tenderness was

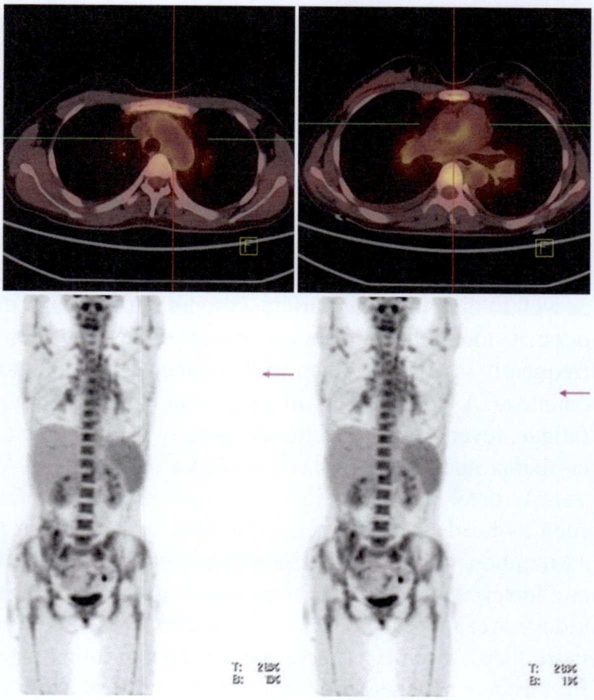

Fig. 4.9 PET/CT image of the patient. It can be seen that the lower part of the bilateral carotid artery, the bilateral subclavian artery, the thoracic aorta, the superior mesenteric artery, and the upper part of the right femoral artery have increased metabolism of FDG

obvious and there was no obvious specific change in thyroid B-ultrasound, ultrasound examination of bilateral carotid arteries was performed. The results showed that the inner diameters of bilateral carotid arteries were diffusely thickened (left 6.3 mm, right 6.4 mm). This important result provided important clues for our diagnosis. In order to quickly and comprehensively assess the patient's pathological changes, we performed a whole-body PET/CT examination on the patient. The results showed that the bilateral lower carotid artery, bilateral subclavian artery, thoracic aorta, superior mesenteric artery, and upper right femoral artery appeared strip-shaped. FDG Metabolism increased signals, with the highest SUV value of 3.2 (Fig. 4.9), combined with medical history, it is considered as an inflammatory lesion.

The PET/CT results of this patient provided an important basis for our diagnosis. This patient, a young woman, had fever with neck and head pain as the main manifestations. Ultrasound of the carotid arteries showed significant internal diameter increase. PET/CT showed increased FDG in many large arteries, suggesting inflammatory lesions. Therefore, after comprehensive analysis, the patient was diagnosed with polyarteritis. Further examination of thoracic aorta MRA and carotid MRA showed no obvious abnormalities, suggesting that the patient has no obvious target organ involvement and the disease is at an early stage. After consultation with the rheumatology department, she was given cyclophosphamide 0.6 intravenous drip, once a month, combined with methylprednisolone 40 mg/day oral treatment, and at the same time given aspirin, atorvastatin antiplatelet and anticoagulant therapy to prevent target organ damage. After treatment, the patient's fever and other symptoms were significantly improved, and the erythrocyte sedimentation rate and CRP quickly fell to normal, and he was discharged from the hospital. After discharge, he was followed up by the rheumatology department for a long time.

4.6.3 Comments

Large vessel vasculitides (LVV) mainly include Takayasu's arteritis (TA) and Giant cell arteritis (GCA). Aortic arteritis often involves the aorta and its main branches, as well as the pulmonary artery, coronary arteries and its branches, causing stenosis or occlusion of the corresponding parts of the blood vessel. The disease occurs more frequently in young women, and it spreads globally, most often in South-east Asian countries. A small number of patients may have symptoms such as general malaise, fatigue, fever, loss of appetite, nausea, sweating, weight loss, myalgia, arthritis, and erythema nodules, which can be acute or insidious. According to different blood vessels involved, symptoms and signs of corresponding organ ischemia appear, such as headache, dizziness, syncope, stroke, vision loss, intermittent fatigue of extremities, weakened or disappeared brachial or femoral artery pulse, neck, upper and lower clavicle areas. There were vascular murmurs in the lower abdomen and kidney area, and the systolic pressure difference between the two upper limbs was more than 10 mmHg. There are no specific laboratory indicators for this disease. Erythrocyte sedimentation rate (ESR) and C reactive protein (CRP) are important indicators that reflect the disease activity of this disease. Imaging examination is a necessary condition for the diagnosis of aortic arteritis. The purpose is to clarify the location and anatomical characteristics of the diseased artery. At present, the commonly used examination methods are: (1) Color Doppler ultrasound; (2) Multi-slice CT angiography or magnetic resonance imaging; (3) Transarterial Digital subtraction angiography (DSA) or selective angiography. With the widespread clinical application of PET/CT, it has significant clinical value in the early diagnosis of arteritis and the judgment of disease activity. In this case, PET/CT showed abnormal FDG metabolism in multiple vascular walls, suggesting inflammatory reactions in the walls, and early diagnosis of arteritis. Takayasu arteritis often has an insidious onset and lacks specificity in clinical manifestations. If the first consulting department is not a rheumatology department or the first consulting doctor lacks relevant experience, the diagnosis will be delayed. The advantages of PET/CT in diagnosing macrovascular vasculitis can assist the diagnosis in the early stage of the disease. However, it is not recommended that all patients with fever under investigation undergo PET/CT examination, and the decision should be based on the patient's clinical manifestations and clues provided by routine examinations. Since macrovascular vasculitis requires glucocorticoids plus immunosuppressive agents and anticoagulation therapy after a clear diagnosis, a rheumatology specialist should be consulted to determine the next treatment and follow-up plan.

References

1. Chinese Medical Association Rheumatology Branch. Guidelines for the diagnosis and treatment of arteritis [J]. Chin J Rheumatol. 2011;15(2):119–20.
2. Lindi J, Hejian Z. Primary vasculitis. In: Chen H, Lin G, Wang JY, editors. Practical internal medicine [M]. 14th ed. Beijing: People's Medical Publishing House; 2013. p. 2640–6.

4.7 Recurrent Fever, Arthralgia, Visual Impairment, Restricted Jaw Movement and Finally Was Diagnosed with Giant Cell Arteritis (GCA)

Fan Qingqi, Jia Wen, Shao Lingyun, and Zhang Wenhong

The patient, a 55-year-old male, was admitted to the hospital on August 18, 2016, for "recurrent fever for more than 2 years."

On March 2014, the patient developed chills and fever with a maximum body temperature of 39 °C under no obvious cause, accompanied by polyarthralgia (shoulder joints, knees, and ankles, etc.) and occipital neck pain, and the arthralgia was migratory. He was sent to local hospital, after more than 10 days of symptomatic anti-inflammatory treatment (detailed information not proved), fever and arthralgia improved. He had no fever for about 4 or 5 months and the same symptoms occurs again in September 2014. After more than 10 days of treatment (the specific plan is unknown), his temperature was normal for 4–5 months. In March 2015, the patient recurred fever, arthralgia and myalgia. He went to a local hospital. The blood test showed that WBC was 8.0×10^9/L, N 64.2%. He was treated with cephalosporin and levofloxacin for anti-infective treatment for more than 1 month, and his temperature dropped back to normal. But 1 month after the drug was withdrawn, the fever appeared again. In September 2015, He was sent to the Department of Hematology of the local hospital and rechecked the complete blood count (CBCs): WBC 11.66×10^9/L, N 72.11%, PLT 301×10^9/L and autoantibodies were all negative. Considering thrombocytosis, he was given ordinary interferon α-2b antiviral treatment for more than 7 months. During this period, the patient had prolonged fever, accompanied by blurry vision, slight loss of vision, and difficulty in opening mouth. He was admitted to our ward on August 19.

The patient had been in good condition with a slightly poor appetite, and had lost 20 kg in weight since the onset of symptoms.

4.7.1 Admission Check

Temperature 38 °C, Pulse 90 beats/min, Respiration 18 beats/min, BP 125/70 mmHg (left upper limb), 140/70 mmHg (right upper limb), conscious, breath sound clear, no icteric sclera, no pale conjunctiva, no tonsils swollen, the trachea is in the middle, and the temporal artery pulsation is normal. There was no goiter, no distention of jugular vein, and there are murmurs in bilateral carotid arteries. Breath sounds in both lungs are rough, no obvious rale and moist rales are heard, and the heart rate is 90 beats/min, the rhythm is regular. The abdomen is soft without tenderness, and liver and spleen were impalpable under the ribs. A pigeon-egg-sized lymph node can be palpated in the right groin area with good mobility and no tenderness. The physiological reflexes of the nervous system are normal, and the pathological reflexes are not elicited.

4.7.2 Diagnosis and Treatment

Relevant examinations had been complete after the patient was admitted to the hospital. CBCs: WBC 10.53×10^9/L, N 71.1%, Hb 116 g/L, PLT 442×10^9/L; ESR 65 mm/h, CRP 76.5 mg/L, ferritin 420 μg/L; coagulation function: PT 13.4 s, FIB 6.12 g/L, D-dimer <0.1 mg/L; blood culture: negative; autoantibodies are normal, liver and kidney functions are normal; urine routine is normal; T-SPOT.TB: negative; bone marrow cytology: no obvious evidence for malignant tumor; ultrasound: right inguinal lymph nodes enlarged with calcification (35 mm × 13 mm), no abnormal enlarged lymph nodes on the supraclavicular, left inguinal, armpit, neck, submandibular; No abnormalities in liver, gallbladder, pancreas, spleen, and kidney; Lung CT scan: small patchy ground-glass shadow in the posterior segment of the right upper lobe, and spot-like dense shadow under the pleura of the right middle lobe; ECG: sinus rhythm; left ventricular high voltage; Echocardiography: left ventricular enlargement. The inner diameter of the aorta is widened.

Patient is a middle-aged male. The main clinical manifestations are fever, arthralgia, visual impairment, and limited mandibular movement. Since physical examination revealed a large difference in blood pressure between the upper limbs on both sides. The possibility of arteritis should be considered first. Further examinations such as carotid artery ultrasound, coronary CTA, and thoracic artery MRA all indicated the presence of vascular lesions. Carotid ultrasound: bilateral carotid artery intima are rough and inner walls were thickened (8.3 mm on the right and 7.5 mm on the left); multiple plaques in the bilateral carotid arteries are up to 15 mm × 2 mm. Coronary CTA: mixed plaque formation in the proximal and middle segments of the right coronary artery, mild to moderate lumen stenosis; mixed plaque formation in the proximal left anterior descending branch, moderate lumen stenosis; soft plaque formation in the proximal left circumflex artery. The lumen is moderately or severely narrowed; the superficial myocardial bridge is formed in the distal right coronary artery (Fig. 4.10). Thoracic artery MRA: The bilateral subclavian arteries are slightly narrowed locally.

Although the patient's diagnosis is clear at this time, both physical examination and ultrasound showed that the patient had swollen lymph nodes in the right groin. Bone biopsy showed no evidence of malignant tumors; the tumor still needed to be excluded. Therefore, lymph node biopsy and PET/CT examinations were performed. Fortunately, lymph node biopsy revealed lymph epithelioid cyst.

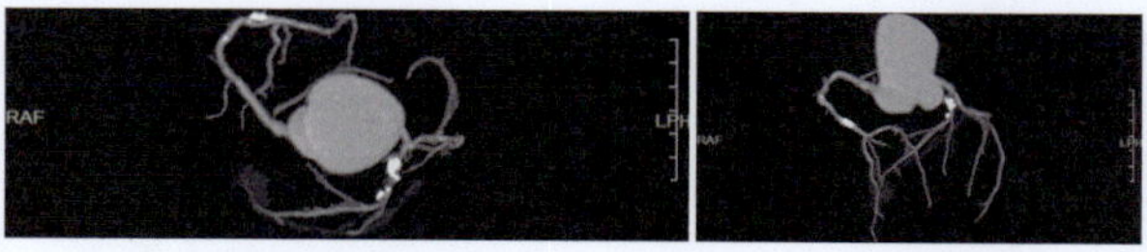

Fig. 4.10 The patient's coronary CTA. Mixed plaques can be seen in multiple vessels and the lumen is narrow

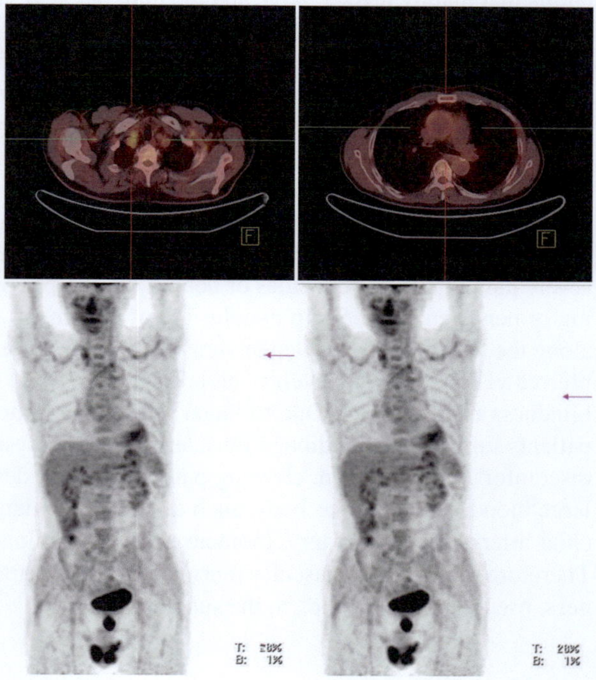

Fig. 4.11 PET/CT image of the patient. It can be seen that the FDG metabolism of the supraclavicular artery and aortic arch tube wall are increased

Interestingly, PET/CT found that the FDG metabolism in the walls of the bilateral supraclavicular artery and aortic arch were slightly and diffusely increased, with an SUV value of 2.8 (Fig. 4.11).

So far, combined with the characteristics of the patient's medical record and imaging and pathological examinations, the patient is likely to have giant cell arteritis. The patient refused to undergo further temporal artery biopsy. After consultation with the rheumatology department, the current diagnosis was confirmed. It is recommended to give patient oral methylprednisolone 40 mg/day combined with oral methotrexate 10 mg/week for anti-inflammatory. After consultation with cardiologists, the patient is advised to receive aspirin + talcom + atorvastatin for antiplatelet and plaque stabilization treatment. The patient's symptoms improved significantly after treatment. Later he was transferred to the rheumatology department for further follow-up and adjustment of the treatment.

4.7.3 Comments

Large vessel vasculitides (LVV) mainly include Takayasu's arteritis (TA) and Giant cell arteritis (GCA), both of which are chronic inflammatory granulation vasculitis mainly involving the large arteries and their branches. Small and medium blood vessels can also be involved. Takayasu arteritis (TA) and giant cell arteritis (GCA) are the two most common chronic inflammatory vascular diseases in systemic vasculitis that mainly involve large and medium blood vessels. Table 4.3 compares the clinical characteristics of TA and GCA.

The majority of GCA occurs over the age of 50, and the incidence in women is two to three times higher than in men. Prodromal symptoms include fatigue, anorexia, weight loss and low-grade fever. Fever is irregular, most of which are moderate (about 38 °C), and it can be as high as 39–40 °C in 15% of patients. The manifestations and severity of disease vary according to the location of the involved blood vessels and the length of the disease. Temporal and cranial arteries are most commonly involved. Headache is the most common symptom, manifesting as severe pain in one or both sides or behind the occiput, which are knife-cut or burning or persistent pain. Scalp nodules are of diagnostic value if they are distributed along the temporal artery. Ocular signs are also common, manifesting as amaurosis, blurred vision, drooping eyelids, and diplopia. In some severe cases, partial or total blindness can be found. Due to facial arteritis and poor local blood supply, some patients suffer from mandibular muscle spasm, manifesting as intermittent chewing discomfort, chewing pain, chewing pauses, and jaw deviation. GCA can affect the large blood vessels of the body, such as the subclavian artery, axillary artery, brachial artery, coronary artery, thoracic aorta, abdominal aorta, and femoral artery. Therefore, it can cause vascular murmur, weakened arterial pulsation or pulselessness, pseudoaneurysm, etc., in the subclavian artery.

Table 4.3 Comparison of clinical features between Takayasu's arteritis (TA) and giant cell arteritis (GCA)

Disease	Takayasu's arteritis (TA)	Giant cell arteritis (GCA)
Susceptible population	10–30 years old, common in women	Over 50 year old, common in women
Vessels involved	The aorta and its major branches	Most common in temporal artery
Manifestations	Systemic symptoms: fever, fatigue, joint pain, etc. Local symptoms: headache, intermittent dyskinesia of limbs	Temporal headache Intermittent mandibular movement disorder blindness
Signs	Brachial artery fluctuations weaken or disappear Systolic pressure difference between arms >10 mmHg Blood vessel murmur in the subclavian or abdominal aorta	Scalp tenderness Temporal artery dilation, weakened pulsation, tenderness Involved vascular signs

With high specificity, temporal artery biopsy is the gold standard for the diagnosis of GCA. Choosing the tender or nodular parts can increase the detection rate. Under local anesthesia, the temporal artery is cut out with a length of 1.5–3 cm for continuous pathological sections. The positive rate of biopsy is 40%–80%, and a negative test cannot rule out the possibility of GCA diagnosis.

In recent years, 18F-FDG PET/CT has been used for the diagnosis and treatment of various inflammatory and infectious diseases. Its value in auxiliary diagnosis of large vasculitis and follow-up of large vasculitis has been paid more attention. It also shows both high sensitivity and specificity for evaluating disease activity.

References

1. Rheumatology Branch of the Chinese Medical Association. Guidelines for the diagnosis and treatment of polymyalgia rheumatica and giant cell arteritis [J]. Chin J Rheumatol. 2011;15(5):348–50.
2. Rheumatology Branch of the Chinese Medical Association. Guidelines for the diagnosis and treatment of Takayasu arteritis [J]. Chin J Rheumatol. 2011;15(2):119–20.
3. Lindi J, Hejian Z. Primary vasculitis. In: Chen H, Lin G, Wang JY, editors. Practical internal medicine [M]. 14th ed. Beijing: People's Medical Publishing House; 2013. p. 2640–6.

4.8 ANCA-Associated Vasculitis with Hearing Loss

Jin Jialin

Patient, female, 49 years old, was admitted to the hospital on November 20, 2008 due to repeated fever for more than 7 months.

At the beginning of May 2008, the patient developed fever under no obvious predisposing cause, the maximum temperature reached 39 °C, mainly in the afternoon and evening, accompanied by chills, without cough and sputum, abdominal pain, diarrhea, frequent urination urgency. On May 14, she was hospitalized at a local hospital. CT revealed inflammatory changes in the lower and upper lobe of the left lung. Chronic inflammation and old tuberculosis lesions were visible in the lower lobe of the right lung. She was treated with cefepoxime for anti-infective treatment. Two weeks later, a CT scan showed that the pneumonia was significantly absorbed and she was discharged at the end of May. The patient developed fever again in mid-August and was hospitalized again. Details were not available. She was discharged at the end of August and still had fever when discharged. Later, the patient was hospitalized many times and was treated with ampicillin, sulbactam, metronidazole, azithromycin, etc., but the temperature did not drop significantly. On October 19, an MRI at another hospital showed mastoiditis, ethmoid sinusitis, and maxillary sinusitis. Oral mecobalamin and vinblastine treatment was given. On November 17, she came to our hospital, the blood test showed WBC 9.21 × 10^9/L, RBC 3.17 × 10^{12}/L, Hb 92 g/L, PLT 416 × 10^9/L, N 75.8%, ESR 120 mm/h. Abdominal ultrasound revealed enhanced echo of the cortical medulla of both kidneys and a cyst in the right kidney. For further diagnosis and treatment, she was admitted for FUO (Fever of Unknown Origin). The patient had been diagnosed with otitis media a year ago and then visited the local hospital many times. She suffered from hearing loss in the left ear for nearly a year, and the hearing loss in the right ear was significant, accompanied by tinnitus and otalgia. After onset of illness, the patient slept well and loses 3–5 kg in weight urination was normal.

4.8.1 Physical Examination on Admission

Temperature 37.5 °C, Bp 120/80 mmHg. conscious, in good spirits, no icteric subcutaneous no ecchymoses or petechias, no palpable swelling of superficial lymph nodes, soft neck, no thyroid enlargement, clear breath sounds in both sides of lung, no dry and moist rales. Rhythm was normal without murmurs. Liver and spleen were impalpable under the ribs. There was no edema in both lower limbs. Nervous system normal.

4.8.2 Diagnosis and Treatment

Relevant examinations had been complete after the patient was admitted to the hospital. Complete blood count: WBC 6.97 × 10^9/L, RBC 2.38 × 10^{12}/L, Hb 67 g/L, N 72.9%, PLT 370 × 10^9/L. Urine test: bacteria 2+, occult blood 3+, red blood cell 421/μL, white blood cell 393/μL. Liver function: ALT 17 U/L, AST 22 U/L, ALP 158 U/L, r-GGT: 112 U/L, albumin: 25 g/L, globulin: 38 g/L. Kidney function was normal. Reticulocytes: 1.6%. ESR: 120 mm/h, CRP: 111 mg/mL, anti-O and RF negative, ferritin 511 μg/L. Thyroid function was normal. RPR and HIV antibodies were negative. Hepatitis markers and tumor-related biomarkers (AFP, CEA, CA19-9, CA125, CY21-1, SCC, and NSE) were negative. Heart ultrasound: No obvious abnormality. Acid-fast staining of sputum smear (−), blood culture (−) × 3 times. ECG: mild T wave changes. Chest X-ray: slight inflammation of the lower right lung. Chest CT: the texture of both lungs increased, slight inflammation of lower right lung, and linear opacities in two lower lungs, changes after inflammation, and bilateral pleura was thickened. Bone marrow biopsy: The bone marrow was diluted by the peripheral blood.

After admission, patients still had fever and otalgia, infectious diseases were first considered: (1) ear infections and central nervous system infections caused by ear infection cannot be excluded, (2) urinary tract infections. Then, moxifloxacin, meropenem, meropenem + vancomycin and other anti-infective treatments were given successively. The mid-stream urine culture showed Escherichia coli >100,000 CFU/mL, producing ESBL, only sensitive to imipenem and cephalosporin sulbactam, resistant to all the others. Body temperature and symptoms did not improve significantly. Posterior cranial enhanced MR showed head dura mater of the right cerebral hemisphere, the tentorium cerebellum, and the falx were significantly enhanced, considering the possibility of meningeal infection. Bilateral mastoiditis, a few ischemic foci on both frontal lobes. In order to exclude central nervous system infection, cerebrospinal fluid examination was performed; pressure was 140 mmH_2O, colorless, clear, Pan's test 2+, WBC 8×10^6/L. Protein ↑ 1.415 g/L, sugar and chloride were normal.

Check autoantibody spectrum: ANA 1:320 (+) (granular type), pANCA (+), cANCA (−), PR3 is normal, MPO 79.4 RU/mL, ACA, ds-DNA, ENA, AMA negative, immunoglobulin and complement C3, C4 were normal. The abnormality rate of urinary red blood cells was 60% (most of them were spinous erythrocytes). Abdominal ultrasound showed the echo of both renal cortexes enhanced, and no abnormality in liver and spleen. The 24-h urine protein quantitatively increased by 1.35 g. Ultrasound-guided right kidney puncture was performed. Pathology reported 2 of 15 glomeruli had large cellular crescents, 3–4 capillaries have fibrinoid necrosis, and many mononuclear cell infiltrations in mesenchyme. One of the glomeruli had fibrinoid necrosis and many inflammatory cells packaged, forming granuloma-like structures. Immunoglobulins were all negative under the fluorescence microscope. Final conclusion indicated renal damage caused by vasculitis.

The patient is a middle-aged woman with repeated fever and the course of the disease is more than 7 months. Accompanied by tinnitus, otalgia and hearing loss. Laboratory tests showed anemia (Coomb's test positive, suggesting immune anemia), gross hematuria (high red blood cell abnormality rate, suggesting glomerular origin), proteinuria, suggesting kidney damage, ANA and pANCA positive, kidney biopsy confirmed vasculitis related kidney damage. Multiple blood cultures were negative. Although the mid-stream urine culture was positive, it could not explain the entire course of the disease. The effect of anti-infective treatment was not good, the effect of glucocorticoid treatment was good, and the tumor biomarkers (AFP, CEA, CA19-9, CA125, CY21-1, SCC, and NSE) were all negative, so malignant tumor can be excluded; thus, the diagnosis of ANCA-related vasculitis is clear.

Therefore, she was given intravenous methylprednisolone 40 mg bid, combined with amoxicillin and clavulanate. The patient's symptoms improved significantly, hearing improved, and body temperature gradually returned to normal. Blood and urine routine significantly improved, and she was allowed to be discharged, continuing glucocorticoid therapy outside the hospital, and follow-up regularly and timely.

4.8.3 Comments

ANCA-related vasculitis mainly refers to microscopic polyangiitis (MPA), granulomatous polyangiitis (Granulomatosis with polyangiitis, GPA) [formerly known as Wegener's granulomatosis (WG)] and Churg-Strauss syndrome (CSS). It is named since anti-neutrophil cytoplasmic antibodies (ANCA) can be detected in the serum of most patients. Among them, cytoplasmic ANCA (c-ANCA) is more common in GPA, and its target antigen is protease 3 (PR3). Pernuclear ANCA (p-ANCA) is mainly found in MPA, and its main target antigen is myeloperoxidase (MPO). In China, ANCA-related small vasculitis is dominated by MPA, which accounts for about 80% of all ANCA-related vasculitis, GPA accounts for about 20%, and CSS is relatively rare. Multi-organ involvement of the whole body is more common in patients with ANCA-related small vasculitis, and lung and kidney disease often prominent. GPA is more likely to invade the respiratory system, especially the upper respiratory tract and lungs, and destructive damage are easily formed. MPA usually manifests as lung-renal syndrome, focal segmental rapidly progressive glomerulonephritis (defined as renal function damage <50% and crescent formation >50% of glomeruli in several days or weeks) are characteristic changes. Patient of CSS mostly has a history of bronchial asthma and allergic diseases, and is characterized by hypereosinophilia. Histopathological changes and immunohistopathological examination are of great significance for the identifying of small vasculitis. MPA, GPA and CSS immunohistopathological examinations show no or only trace immunoglobulin deposits, which are oligoimmune small vasculitis, and Goodpasture syndrome has linear immune deposits. Other diseases that cause lung-renal syndrome include WG, Goodpasture syndrome and systemic lupus erythematosus, etc. However, Goodpasture syndrome has linear immune deposits, while systemic lupus erythematosus presents granular or massive immune deposits.

This patient's lung involvement is not obvious, and the prominent manifestations are kidney involvement and hearing loss. Generally speaking, ENT (ear, nose, and throat) lesions often suggest GPA, so this patient may be an overlap syndrome of MPA and GPA or an atypical manifestation of MPA. Considering that there is no evidence of granulomatous inflammation in the patient's pathology, the performance of renal biopsy is consistent with the performance of oligoimmune small vasculitis. Therefore, this patient should be considered MPA. At present, there are still differences in the understanding of MPA, and there is no internationally acknowledged diagnostic (classification) standard. At present, the diagnosis of MPA is mainly based on the overall judgment of five aspects: medical history, physical examination, serological examination, biopsy, and angiography; the first two aspects are the most important. Therefore, if such long-term fever cases are encountered in the clinic with multiple system involvements and the effect of anti-infection treatment is not good, the possibility of "connective tissue diseases" should be highly considered. In time immunological and histological examinations are helpful for diagnosis.

References

1. Mohan N, Kerr GS. ANCA-associated small vessel vasculitis: clinical and therapeutic advances. Curr Rheumatol Rep. 2010;12(6):406–13.
2. Baldini C, Talarico R, Della Rossa A, et al. Clinical manifestations and treatment of Churg-Strauss syndrome. Rheum Dis Clin N Am. 2010;36(3):527–43.

3. Tarabishy AB, Schulte M, Papaliodis GN, et al. Wegener's granulomatosis: clinical manifestations, differential diagnosis, and management of ocular and systemic disease. Surv Ophthalmol. 2010;55(5):429–44.
4. Qingjun W. Polyangiitis under the microscope. In: Rheumatism diagnosis and diagnosis review. Shanghai: Shanghai Science and Technology Press; 2004. p. 273–80.
5. Villiger PM, Guillevin L. Microscopic polyangiitis: clinical presentation. Autoimmun Rev. 2010;9(12):812–9.

4.9 A Case of Granulomatous Polyangiitis with Repeated Hemoptysis and Pulmonary Cavity

Liu YuanyuanQin Yanli, Zhang Shu and Chen Mingquan

The patient was a 23-year-old male from Jiangxi Province. He was admitted to our department on September 9, 2015 due to recurrent cough for 7 months, aggravation with fever and hemoptysis for 1 month.

The patient had dry cough without obvious trigger since February 2015. At that time, there was no fever, no expectoration, no hemoptysis, no chest tightness and chest pain. And the symptoms improved after treatment in the local hospital (details were not available). In July 2015, the patient developed severe paroxysmal dry cough without obvious causes, followed by a small amount of thick brown sputum without blood streaks, and no pharyngeal pain, rhinorrhea, fever, chest tightness, or shortness of breath. No medical management was given at that time.

On August 6, 2015, the patient developed fever with body temperature fluctuating between 38 and 39 °C, accompanied by drenching sweats and joint soreness. There was no significant difference between day and night. After the application of indomethacin suppository into the anus, the body temperature briefly dropped to normal, and the body temperature returned to normal after intravenous fluid rehydration treatment for 1 week (not specific). Afterwards, both eyes gradually became red and swollen, without obvious secretions, blurred vision and diplopia. On August 17, 2015, his routine scan at the local hospital showed mass shadows in the lower lobe of the right lung and the upper lobe of the left lung, with irregular cavity inside (Fig. 4.12). On August 19, 2015, the patient went to a local tertiary class A hospital and there were no significant abnormalities in blood routine, liver function and kidney function. The PPD and T-SPOT.TB were negative, and tumor markers such as CEA, NSE, CYFRA21, and other tumor markers were within normal range.

Bronchoscopy was performed on August 22, 2015, and inflammation in bronchial mucosa was seen in the left upper inherent lobe. Postoperative hemoptysis was observed, which was progressively worse, and chest sulking and shortness of breath was accompanied by severe cough. Due to 2.15×10^3 copies/mL of TB-DNA in alveolar lavage fluid, the patient was given HRZE diagnostic antituberculosis treatment. However, the patient developed scattered bright red petechiae in lower limbs on the day of medication initiation. When antituberculous drugs were discontinued,

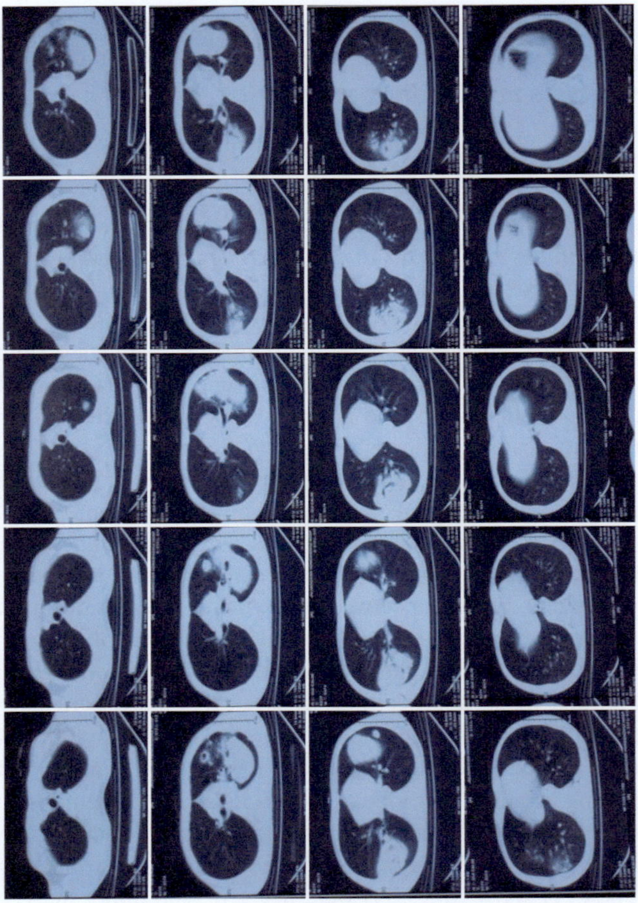

Fig. 4.12 Chest CT scan (August 17, 2015)

the skin rash of the patient's lower limbs gradually formed vesicles, and some of them became scabby after darkening, with occasional ulceration. The patient was discharged automatically.

On August 27, 2015, the patient transferred to another local hospital. Routine blood examination on admission showed that leukocytes were 8×10^9/L, neutrophils proportion 62.49%, eosinophils proportion 7%, hemoglobin 108 g/L. Liver and kidney function showed ALT 70 U/L; AST 66 U/L; ALB 26 g/L; LDH 261 U/L. Urine routine test showed protein +/−, occult blood +. ESR 54 mm/h, CRP 182.1 mg/L, D-dimer 1.86 mg/L. Blood cryptococcus latex agglutination test and T-SPOT. TB was all negative. Trichinella spiralis IgM (+), IgG (+), G test (−), GM test (−), weak positive for cANCA.

Anti-infective therapy was given with moxifloxacin, albendazole disinfestation (400 mg bid Po × 5 days), liver protection and hemostasis treatment, and the patient's body temperature did not drop. "Wegener granuloma" was not excluded, so dexamethasone was given 5 mg QD for 3 days, and the patient's temperature returned to normal. But the high temperature returned after 2 days, and had high fever again on September 8, 2015, with a temperature of 39 °C, accompanied by hemoptysis (about 15 mL). The patient was admitted to our hospital for further diagnosis and treatment.

4.9.1 General Physical Examination

Body temperature 37.6 °C, pulse 141 times/min, respiration 20 times/min, blood pressure 110/78 mmHg. Consciousness, mental retardation, normal development, medium nutrition, physical examination cooperation, conjunctive congestion in both eyes, anemia, scattered old vesicular rash on both lower limbs (Fig. 4.13), waist and both ear edges, partial ulceration, and partial scabby. Superficial lymph nodes were not palpable. The pharynx was not red, and the tonsils were not swollen. The respiratory sound in both lungs were coarse, and the respiratory sound in the upper left lung was low, and there were audible and palpable fine wet rales in left lung. The heart rhythm was uniform and no murmur was found in each valve area. Abdomen was soft, without any tenderness or rebound tenderness. Liver and spleen were not palpable under the costal region. Murphy's sign was negative. There was no tenderness at the Mullerian point or the ureteral point, and no pain on percussion in the bilateral kidney areas.

There was no edema in the lower extremities. Bilateral knee joints and ankles were tender. Muscle strength of both upper limbs was Grade 5, and muscle strength of both lower limbs was Grade 4. Muscle tension was normal, physiological reflexes were normal, and pathological reflexes were not elicited.

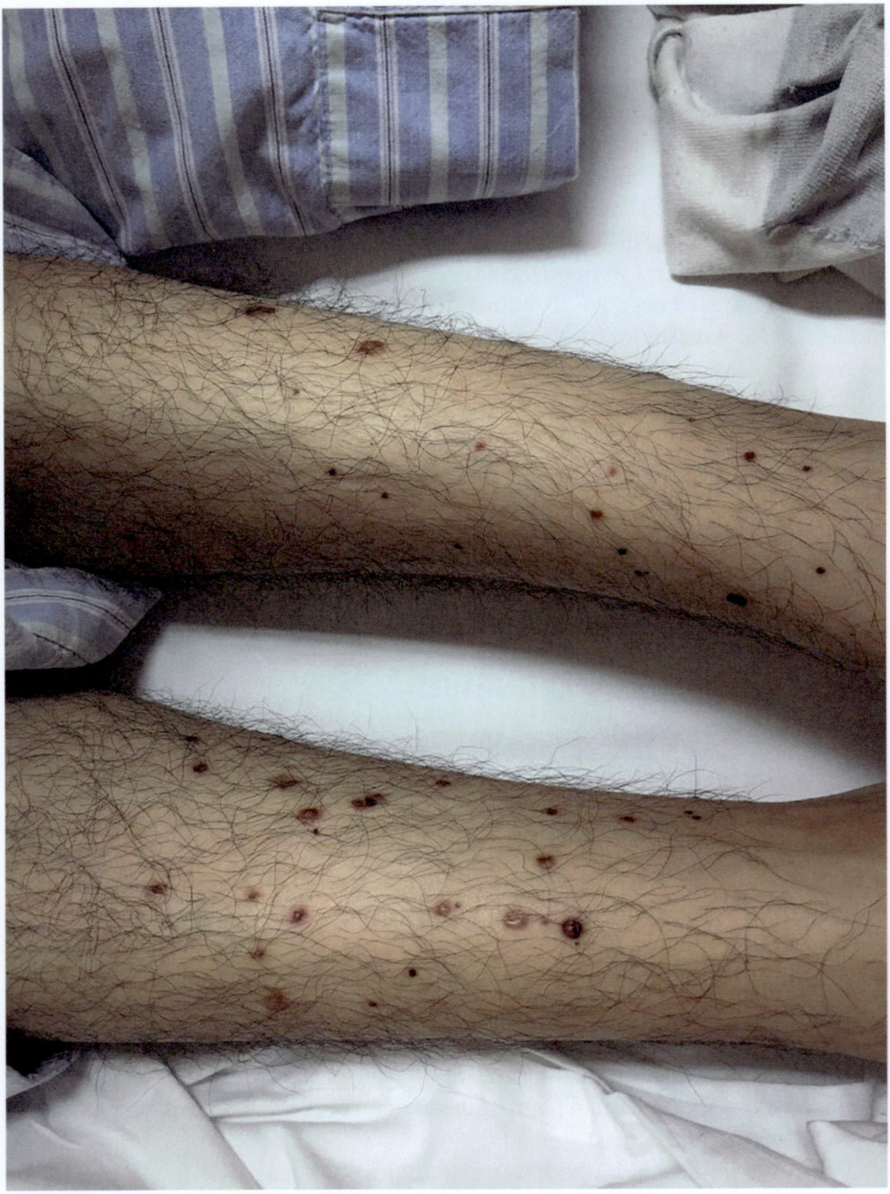

Fig. 4.13 Rash on lower limbs (September 9, 2015)

4.9.2 Diagnosis and Treatment

Clinical assessment was made after admission. Blood routine: leukocytes $12.69 \times 10^9/L$, neutrophils% 72.0%, monocytes% 6.1%, lymphocytes% 11.2%, eosinophils% 10.2%, hemoglobin 80 g/L, platelets $254 \times 10^9/L$, CRP was

133.40 mg/L, ESR 120 mm/h, PCT 0.64 ng/mL. Urine routine: trace protein, red blood cell 97.4/μL, white blood cell 5.4/μL. Liver function: ALT 46 U/L, AST 26 U/L, ALP 169 U/L, GGT 128 U/L, albumin 28.6 g/L, globulin 26.9 g/L, TBIL 19.7 μmol/L, DBIL 10.4 μmol/L. Renal function was normal. CPK and CK-MB were normal. LDH was 309 U/L. Blood glucose was 6.66 mmol/L and HbA1c was 5.2%.

HAV antibody, HBsAg and HCV antibody were all negative. Coagulation function showed PT 15.6 s, D-dimer 5.650 mg/L FEU, INR 1.30. Blood T-SPOT.TB was negative (A well: 0; B well: 1). Blood Cryptococcus latex agglutination test was negative. Serum parasite antibody was also negative (performed by Institute of Parasitology, Chinese Center for Disease Control and Prevention). Herpes simplex virus (HSV1 and HSV2) antibody IgG and IgM, Toxoplasma antibody IgG and IgM were all negative. CMV-IgG antibody was positive but CMV-IgM antibody was negative, and CMV-DNA was not detected. Rubella virus antibody IgG was positive and Rubella virus antibody IgM was suspected positive. EBV-DNA was not detected. Autoantibodies including ANA, ENA, ACA, ds-DNA, pANCA were negative, but cANCA was positive and PR3 elevated to 81.2 AU/mL, while MPO was 1.3 AU/mL. Immunoglobulins were in normal range except for total IgE of 249.00 IU/mL. Complement C3 was 0.92 g/L, while complement C4 reduced to 0.13 g/L. Rheumatoid factor elevated to 499.00 IU/mL. Blood and urine immunofixation electrophoresis was negative. Thyroid function: T3 0.64 ↓ nmol/L, T4 133.6 nmol/L, FT3 3.00 ↓ pmol/L, FT4 18.59 pmol/L, TSH 2.04 mIU/L. Tumor markers: CA125 38.93 ↑ U/mL, NSE 23.16 ↑ ng/mL, remaining negative. Chest CT scan: multiple lesions and multiple thick-walled cavities with liquid level in both lungs, possible inflammation (Fig. 4.14).

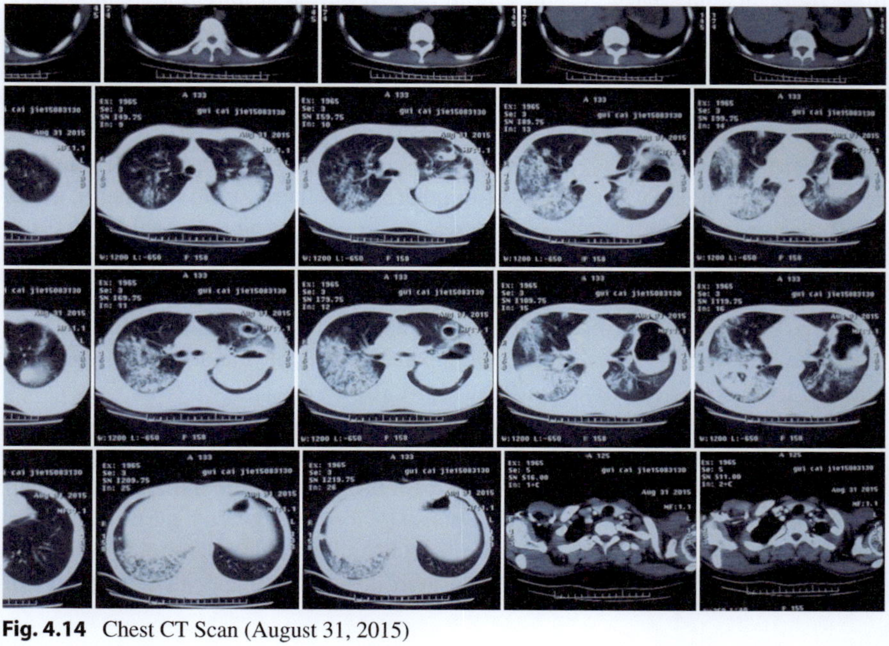

Fig. 4.14 Chest CT Scan (August 31, 2015)

The patient was a young male with fever, cough and hemoptysis. The first consideration was infection, and tuberculosis was most likely as with infection in this case. However, acid-fast bacilli were not found in the patient's sputum smear. Multiple PPD assays and blood T-SPOT.TB tests were negative, only TB-DNA in bronchial and alveolar lavage fluid was positive, and rash of both lower limbs emerged on the day of antituberculosis treatment (regimen: HREZ) initiation, so the diagnosis of tuberculosis still needed further etiological evidence. The patient had conjunctivitis, rash on both lower extremities, and weakly positive cANCA in the former hospital. The reexamination in our hospital showed positive autoantibody cANCA, increased PR3, negative pANCA, normal MPO, positive urine erythrocyte, vasculitis could not be excluded, and further pathological evidence was needed.

After admission, the patient still had hemoptysis twice, with 50 mL bright red blood for each time and was treated with snake venom hemagglutinin, pituitrin, and tranexamic acid for hemostasis. Considering that the patient still had fever and had a high possibility of infection and was in critical condition, he was given cefepime 1.0 q12h intravenous drip (later adjusted to meropenem 1.0 q8h intravenous drip), moxifloxacin 0.4 g qd intravenous drip, and linezolid 0.6 g q12h intravenous drip. Itraconazole was given at a dose of 250 mg qd intravenous drip (doubled on the first and second days) to cover probable fungal infection. Because the possibility of vasculitis (Wegener's granulomatosis) could not be ruled out, methylprednisolone 20 mg q12h was added intravenously, the patient's body temperature decreased, no more hemoptysis, lung rales decreased, and blood hemoglobin increased.

On September 11, 2015, the patient's sputum smear showed acid-fast bacilli (3+), and he was diagnosed with open tuberculosis (both lungs, sputum smear +++), but repeated sputum culture did not show *Mycobacterium tuberculosis*. He was given isoniazid, clarithromycin, ethambutol, and moxifloxacin for diagnostic treatment (pyrazinamide wasn't used for drug fever occurred at initiation), and methylprednisolone 30 mg was given to suppress the inflammatory response.

The patient was hospitalized in our hospital again on October 8, 2015. Combined with previous medical history, the patient had multiple systemic lesions, positive cANCA, and elevated PR3, so the possibility of vasculitis was still considered. Consequently, the patient was given methylprednisolone 60 mg qd intravenous drip combined with the above-mentioned antituberculosis therapy. On October 9, 2015, skin biopsy of the right lower limb rash was taken, and the pathological results suggested focal epidermal necrosis and massive inflammatory necrosis in the surrounding epidermal stratum corneum. On October 14, 2015, the reexamination of chest CT scan (Fig. 4.15) suggested multiple lesions in both lungs, multiple thick-walled cavities with liquid level and surrounding patches, which were absorbed compared with the images on September 9, 2015 (Fig. 4.16).

Subsequently, the patient was consulted in the rheumatology department. Combined with the patient's age, lung lesions and rash, and necrotizing lesions revealed in skin biopsy, 0.34 g protein in 24-h urine protein quantitative test, positive cANCA and elevated PR3, good response to hormone therapy, the clinical diagnosis of granulomatosis with polyangiitis (GPA) was made. The patient has no history of cocaine consumption and hyperthyroidism; a rash appeared on the day of

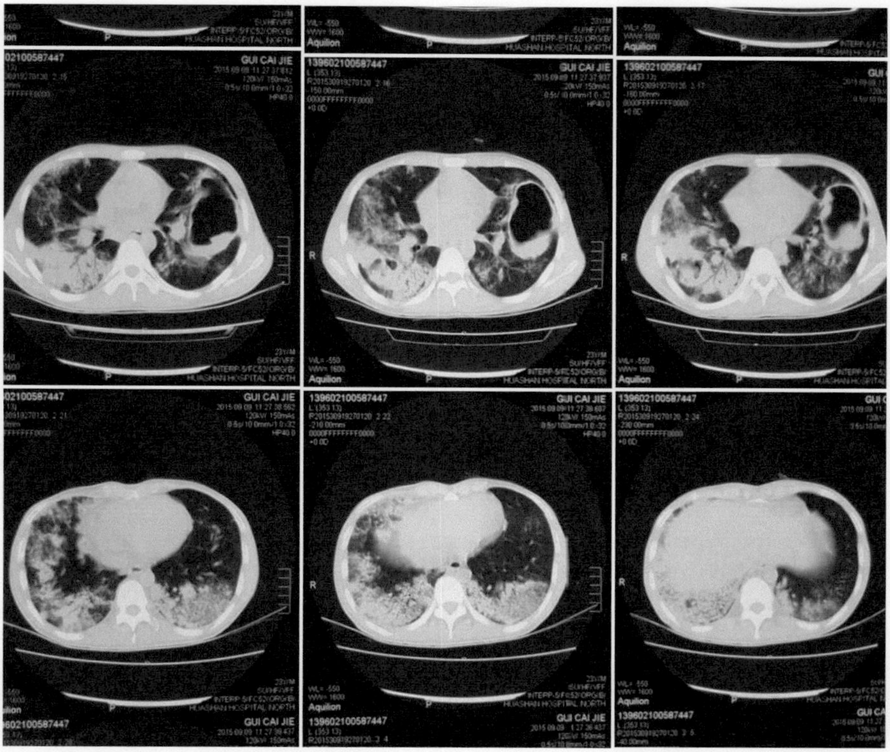

Fig. 4.15 Chest CT scan (October 14, 2015)

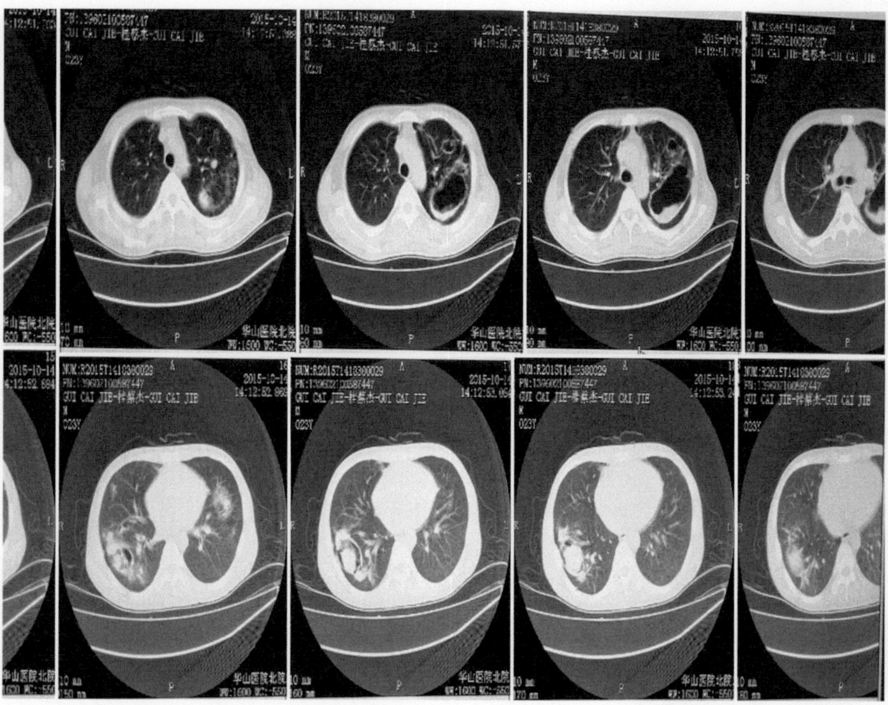

Fig. 4.16 Chest CT scan (September 9, 2015)

antituberculosis initiation. There was no evidence for drug-induced ANCA-related small vasculitis. Therefore, the patient was diagnosed with primary GPA and could be treated with glucocorticoid combined with cyclophosphamide (CTX). The treatment was adjusted to methylprednisolone 40 mg qd po. Since acid-fast bacilli was found in the sputum, isoniazid was retained and other anti-infective drugs were discontinued. Later, the patient was transferred to the rheumatology department for further treatment, and received methylprednisolone combined with CTX. In the follow-up of rheumatology department outpatient, chest CT scans showed improvement.

4.9.3 Comments

Granulomatosis with polyangiitis (GPA), formerly called Wegener's granulomatosis (WG), is a type of ANCA-associated vasculitis. At the beginning of 2011, the American Society of Rheumatology, the American Society of Nephrology and the European Society of Rheumatology proposed to update the name of the disease from "WG" to "GPA" together. GPA is a kind of necrotizing granulomatous vasculitis, an autoimmune disease.

This disease involves small arteries, small veins and capillaries, and occasionally large arteries. The pathology is characterized by inflammation of blood vessel walls, mainly affecting the upper and lower respiratory tracts and kidneys, usually initiating with focal granulomatous inflammation of nasal mucosa and lung tissue, and progressing to diffuse necrotizing granulomatous inflammation of blood vessels. The clinical manifestations include nasal and paranasal sinusitis, pulmonary degeneration and progressive renal failure. It can also affect joints, eyes, skin, heart, nervous system and ears.

The diagnostic criteria of GPA was made by the American College of Rheumatology (ACR) in 1990: (1) nasal or oral inflammatory reactions: painful or painless oral ulcers, purulent or bloody nasal secretions; (2) chest X-ray examination: nodules, fixed infiltrating lesions or cavities; (3) abnormal urinary sediment: microscopic hematuria (erythrocyte >5/high-power field) or red blood cell casts; (4) pathological granulomatous inflammatory changes: arterial wall or around the artery, or neutrophil infiltration in the outer area of blood vessels (artery or arteriole) to form granulomatous inflammatory lesions. GPA can be diagnosed when two or more items of the criteria were met, and the sensitivity and specificity of the criteria for diagnosis were 88.2% and 92.0%, respectively.

In this case, the patient was a young male with cough, fever, hemoptysis, cavities in the lungs, and one positive acid-fast staining of sputum smear. The patient was easily diagnosed as tuberculosis at first, but the antituberculosis effect was poor. Repeated reexamination of sputum acid-fast staining was negative, accompanied by multi-system changes, and the diagnosis was primary GPA combined with the final pathological biopsy. GPA is often misdiagnosed in clinical practice. In order to make an early diagnosis, repeated biopsies should be performed for patients with the following conditions: fever of unknown cause with respiratory symptoms;

chronic rhinitis and paranasal sinusitis, mucosal erosion or granulation tissue proliferation after examination; ulceration, necrosis, or granuloma of eyes and oral mucosa; variable nodular shadows or cavities in the lungs; purpura, nodules, necrosis and ulceration of skin.

References

1. Jennette JC, Falk RJ, Bacon PA, et al. 2012 revised international Chapel Hill consensus conference nomenclature of vasculitides. Arthritis Rheum. 2013;65:1–11.
2. Rheumatology Branch of the Chinese Medical Association. Guidelines for the diagnosis and treatment of microscopic polyangiitis. Chin J Rheumatol. 2011;5:259–61.
3. Chen M, Cui Z, Zhao MH. ANCA-associated vasculitis and anti-GBM disease: the experience in China. Nephrol Dial Transplant. 2010;25(7):2062–5.
4. Chen M, Yu F, Zhang Y, et al. The clinical and pathological characteristics of Chinese patients with anti-neutrophil cytoplasmic autoantibodies associated systemic vasculitide: a study of 426 patients from a single center. Postgrad Med J. 2005;81:723–7.
5. Chen M, Yu F, Zhang Y, et al. Clinical and pathological characteristics of Chinese patients with antineutrophil cytoplasmic autoantibody associated systemic vasculitides: a study of 426 patients from a single Centre. Postgrad Med. 2005;81:723–7.

4.10 Polyarteritis Nodosa Presenting as Fever and Hematuria

Jin Jialin

The patient is a 45-year-old male, admitted to the hospital on April 27, 2000 with repeated fever for more than half a year and gross hematuria for 5 months.

The patient had a sudden rapidly decreased visual acuity in left eye and left eyeball pain while watching TV on September16 last year. Seeing a doctor at a local hospital, he was diagnosed with left posterior optic neuritis. After treatment with dexamethasone for more than 1 month, the pain in the left eye was significantly relieved, and the vision partly restored (nearsighted 6.0 diopters before the illness, now 13 diopters). On October 21, the patient developed fever without obvious cause, and the body temperature was as high as 38.8 °C. Routine blood test revealed the following: leukocyte count, 13.4×10^9/L, percentage of neutrophils, 80.9%, hemoglobin, 147 g/L. Body temperature was low in the morning and gradually rose in the afternoon, accompanied by flushing, night sweats, fatigue, etc., without chills. Ultrasonography of the abdomen showed "hepatosplenomegaly, no ascites". After that, the dexamethasone was gradually stopped, and the body temperature fluctuated. In November, the patient developed backache on the right side, tawny urine, frequent and inexhaustible urination, and was diagnosed as acute pyelonephritis, epididymitis, and prostatitis. After treatment with imipenem and cilastatin, the body temperature gradually dropped to normal. And no abnormality was found in the urine routine. In mid-February of this year, the patient had fever again with shivering and chills without obvious predisposing cause. The body temperature was as high as 40 °C. After self-administration of cefradine and paracetamol, the fever continued for about 2 weeks and then subsided without seeing the doctor. At the end of February, the patient again felt sore back on the right side, which was worse than before, accompanied by soy sauce-colored urine, and the patient had a burning sensation when urinating. At the same time, the patient had persistent low fever, with a body temperature of 37.5–38.5 °C. The rate of red blood cell abnormality in the urine indicated "renal hematuria", the intravenous pyelography was negative, and the renal biopsy at another hospital showed mild focal segmental hyperplastic nephritis, and the patient was given symptomatic hemostasis treatment. Condition was unrelieved. On February 25, the patient was re-admitted to the hospital for a renal biopsy, which still showed mild focal segmental proliferative nephritis. After taking cisapride, the patient developed symptoms of increased stool frequency in mid-March, and stools were not formed, like jam. The patient had colic in the left lower abdomen before going to the toilet, and the abdominal pain was relieved after going to the toilet, and the symptoms were relieved after treatment with *clostridium butyricum* tablets. On April 25, colonoscopy showed "nothing unusual on the ascending colonoscopy," and clean midstream urine culture showed "*Staphylococcus epidermidis* growth, colony count 6000/mL." After taking cefuroxime anti-infection treatment, the patient did not relieve, and still had fever, which was as high as 38 °C. The urine routine showed more than 100 red blood cells/HP. The patient was admitted due to fever of unknown. The patient had poor appetite and night sweats. His weight increased by 20 kg after using dexamethasone.

Past Medical History: The patient has a history of duodenum ulcer for more than 20 years. Confirmed by gastroscopy, he had a history of upper gastrointestinal bleeding 4–5 times, and his condition was stable recently. Surgical resection was performed for acute appendicitis more than 20 years ago. In 1987, the patient suffered "cervical dislocation and fracture of the upper end of the left femur" due to a fall from a great height, and healed after head traction therapy.

4.10.1 Physical Examination on Admission

His body temperature was 38 °C, blood pressure was 120/85 mmHg. His consciousness was clear, his left eye vision was almost completely lost, and his left ear hearing decreased. There was a 1 cm-sized pigmented patch on the right upper abdomen, the surface was not smooth, the middle was sunken, the edges were still clear, and there was no hair. Multiple lymph nodes were touched below the posterior edge of the patient's bilateral mastoid muscles, ranging from mung bean to peanut size, which were medium quality, smooth surface, obvious tenderness, and moderate mobility. Breath sounds in both lungs were clear, heart rate was 84 beats/min, and the rhythm was uniform. No pathological murmur was heard. The abdomen was distended. There was moderate tenderness in the upper left abdomen, upper right abdomen, and lower right abdomen. The lower edge of the liver was two fingers below the ribs. There was percussion pain in the liver area. The lower edge of the spleen was three fingers below the ribs. And the spleen's texture was soft and there was tenderness in the spleen. Bowel sounds were reduced. There was percussion pain in the left kidney area. Somatic sensation on the right is less than that on the left. The muscle tone of the limbs is normal. The muscle strength of the left limb was grade V, and the muscle strength of the right limb was grade IV. There was no edema in both lower limbs.

4.10.2 Medical History

Relevant examinations were completed after admission, leukocyte count, 6.16–11.89 × 10^9/L, hemoglobin, 148–156 g/L, platelet count, 201–280 × 10^9/L. Urine routine test showed erythrocyte count 80–120/HP, leukocyte count 10–12/HP. The three-cup urine test showed hematuria throughout the course. His liver and kidney function, electrolytes, blood sugar, immunoglobulin, and rheumatoid factor were all normal. The hepatitis B marker showed HBsAb (+). ASO was slightly elevated, 129 IU/mL. The proportion of reticulocytes was 1.8%. The abnormality rate of urine red blood cells was 82%. Urine Bence-Jones protein test was negative. ANA, ENA, ANCA were negative (repeated twice). Ham's test, sugar water test, Coomb's test, and snake venom factor hemolysis test were all negative. Antibodies to EBV, CMV, HSV, and Coxsackie virus were all negative. Tumor biomarkers (AFP, CEA, CA19-9, CA125, CA153, CA50, CA72-4, PSA, FPSA, and PAP) were all negative. Blood cultures were negative, a couple of times. Nothing was unusual in the full chest radiograph. Ultrasonography of the abdomen showed fatty liver and no swelling of retroperitoneal lymph nodes. Two separate bone marrow punctures showed "underactive bone marrow proliferation". Gastroscope showed antral inflammation (congestion and exudative type, moderate to severe), inflammation of the duodenal bulb. Intravenous pyelography showed two patches of high-density shadows were seen in the pelvic cavity. Urinary system B-ultrasound showed chronic inflammation of the prostate, no abnormality in the kidneys, ureters, and bladder. Head MRI showed inflammation of the right frontal sinus.

After admission, the patient continued to have a fever, with a body temperature between 37 and 38 °C, feeling backache, frequent urination, and had a burning sensation when urinating. On April 28, the urine culture reported the growth of *Staphylococcus epidermidis*, the colony count was 10,000 cfu/mL, and the combination of norvancomycin combined with fosfomycin was given for nearly 3 weeks. The treatment effect was not obvious, and there were still fever and urinary tract irritation. Consider vasculitis very likely probably and tuberculosis cannot be ruled out, the HRE triple antituberculosis treatment was used from May 12. After antituberculosis treatment, the patient still had fever, and from May 18, he developed dull mid-upper abdominal pain with vomiting of coffee-like substances, fecal occult blood (+++). On the 19th, he passed black stools three times, which were tarry;

subsequently, the black stools changed from formed to unformed. He got better after acid suppression and symptomatic treatment. Antituberculosis treatment was discontinued after 4 weeks due to no obvious improvement. In late May, because of heavy hypertension, benazepril, amlodipine, metoprolol, and other antihypertensive treatments were added. Due to decreased vision in the left eye, visual field examination revealed that the visual field of the left eye was reduced, the central visual acuity decreased, and the blind spot was pathologically enlarged. Because the ophthalmologist considered the diagnosis of retrobulbar optic neuritis, he started to receive dexamethasone 15 mg/day intravenously from June 7. The patient's fever and abdominal distension improved, but as the dexamethasone was gradually reduced to 5 mg/day, the fever reappeared. The dexamethasone was increased to 10 mg/day, and the body temperature still fluctuated at 37–39 °C. Abdominal distension was even more obvious, the abdominal circumference increased progressively, and causes such as hypokalemia and ascites were all ruled out. Small bowel MRI and celiac arteriography (DSA) showed no obvious abnormalities in the intestine, no stenosis of the intestine cavity, no vascular abnormality was identified in the celiac axis and superior and inferior mesenteric artery. Follow-up urine routine, the result showed mainly hematuria, occasionally proteinuria. The patient had a refractory hypertension (treated with the quadruple antihypertensive agents, benazepril + amlodipine + metoprolol + indapamide), the blood pressure reached 160/110 mmHg maximum. The fecal occult blood gradually attenuated and turned negative in mid-July, but blood in the stool and bloody stools appeared again on July 22. As for medical history, the patient had a history of testicular pain.

The patient was a middle-aged male, started with retrobulbar optic neuritis and multiple system organs involvement, prominent clinical manifestation including persistent high fever, impaired vision, repeated hematuria, and gastrointestinal bleeding, unexplained abdominal distension, resistant hypertension, and nervous system damage. He had testicular pain, epididymitis, and had evidence of hepatitis B virus infection (positive surface antibody). The patient had fever with percussion pain in the left kidney area, and a positive mid-section urine culture. As the colony count was negative and anti-infective therapy ineffective, infectious diseases could be excluded. Head MRI, chest radiograph, abdominal ultrasound, bone marrow examination, and serum tumor biomarkers were negative and no evidence of tumor was found. According to the American Rheumatism Association's classification criteria for polyarteritis nodosa (1990), the patient meets 4 out of 10 criteria (testicular pain + polyneuropathy + hypertension + hepatitis B virus infection) and can be diagnosed as nodular polyarteritis.

The treatment plan was changed as follows: (1) CTX was added to glucocorticoid application, first, 200 mg intravenously every other day, and after 1 month, it was changed to 800 mg intravenously every 2 weeks. (2) Switched to methylprednisolone, 120 mg/day for intravenous infusion, and then tapered to 80 mg/day for long-term treatment. After adding CTX, blood pressure was well controlled, however, body temperature and hematuria were still not restored to normal, and abdominal distension was obvious. Adhere to 80 mg methylprednisolone treatment, supplemented with treatments such as urinary tract infection control (netilmicin, etc.), gastric acid suppression, and Chinese medicine. After 2 months, the patient's symptoms improved, his body temperature was normal, and the urine color was clear, and the abdomen was soft, and the glucocorticoid was gradually reduced. After being discharged from the hospital, he was changed to oral glucocorticoid and asked to go to the clinic for follow-up.

4.10.3 Reviews

Polyarteritis nodosa (PAN), also known as periarteritis nodosa or polyarteritis, is a necrotizing arteritis that mainly affects the medium and small arteries. The disease can invade the blood vessels of the whole body, or it can be limited to the blood vessels of a certain organ or tissue, such as kidney, skin, muscle and peripheral nerves. The clinical manifestations vary greatly among individuals, depending on the location and extent of damaged blood vessels. The disease can occur at any age, the ratio of male to female is 2:1, and the average age of onset is 40–60 years old. The cause of this disease is unknown. About 30% of patients are related to hepatitis B virus infection. Other causes include human immunodeficiency virus infection, cytomegalovirus infection, and paravirus B19 infection. Currently, PAN is considered to be a disease mediated by immune complexes.

At present, clinical diagnosis of PAN mainly refers to two standards: the classification standard of PAN by the American Rheumatism Association in 1990 and the definition standard of PAN in the 1994 Chapel Hill International Vasculitis Conference. The American Rheumatism Association's classification standards for PAN (1990) include the following: (1) otherwise unexplained weight loss ≥4 kg (weight loss ≥4 kg at the beginning of the disease, except for dieting or other factors), (2) livedo reticularis (extremities or trunk showing spots and nets Plaque), (3) testicular pain or tenderness (excluding infection, trauma or other factors), (4) myalgia, weakness or lower limb tenderness (diffuse myalgia (except shoulder girdle and pelvic girdle) and muscle weakness or lower limb muscle pain), (5) mononeuropathy and polyneuropathy (single neuropathy, polyneuropathy, and polyneuropathy), (6) Diastolic blood pressure ≥ 90 mmHg (hypertension), (7) elevated levels of serum blood urea nitrogen (≥14.3 mmol/L (40 mg/dL) or creatinine ≥132.7 μmol/L (1.5 mg/dL), excluding dehydration or obstruction), (8) evidence of hepatitis B virus infection via serum antibody or antigen serology, (9) characteristic arteriographic abnormalities not resulting for noninflammatory disease processes (arteriography shows aneurysm or obstruction in the visceral arteries, excluding for arteriosclerosis, muscle dysplasia or other non-inflammatory factors), and (10) A biopsy of small- or medium-sized artery containing polymorphonuclear cells (defective tissue shows granules and monocytes infiltration in the arterial wall). The presence of at least three of these criteria can be diagnosed as PAN. In 1994, the Chapel Hill International Vasculitis Conference defined PAN as necrotizing inflammation of medium-sized and small arteries, without glomerulonephritis, or vasculitis in arterioles, capillaries or venules. Although this patient's intestinal DSA examination did not find abnormal changes, the diagnosis of "polyarteritis nodosa" was clear based on the numerous clinical manifestations and therapeutic effect. The prognosis of this disease without treatment is poor, and glucocorticoid is the drug of first choice. If the condition of the patient is severe, hormone therapy is not effective for more than 1 month or for those with visceral damage, cytotoxic drugs should be included, such as cyclophosphamide, azathioprine, or methotrexate. Although the patient was diagnosed one year after the onset of illness, fortunately, the patient has been under follow-up by the doctor. Therefore, when there is clinically unexplained fever, weight loss, skin damage, abdominal pain, kidney damage, high blood pressure, nervous system damage and other multi-system damage, the diagnosis of polyarteritis nodosa should be considered. Angiography and tissue biopsy are helpful for diagnosis.

References

1. Pettigrew HD, Teuber SS, Gershwin ME. Polyarteritis nodosa. Compr Ther. 2007;33(3):144–9.
2. Baig S, Alamgir M. The extrahepatic manifestations of hepatitis B virus. J Coll Physicians Surg Pak. 2008;18(7):451–7.
3. Lightfoot RW Jr, Michel BA, Bloch DA, et al. The American College of Rheumatology 1990 criteria for the classification of polyarteritis nodosa. Arthritis Rheum. 1990;33(8):1088–93.

4.11 Recurrent Pulmonary Infection with Atelectasis with the Background of Relapsing Polychondritis

Wang Xinyu

A 46-year-old woman from Shanghai was admitted to our hospital with a 2-month history of repeated fever, cough and fatigue.

Two months ago, the patient developed fever without obvious inducement, accompanied by cough, expectoration, chest pain, fatigue and anorexia. She presented to the local hospital for treatment. Blood routine examination: WBC: 10.59 8%, hemoglobin: 84 g/L, neutrophil: 87.4%, lymphocyte: 6, CRP: 129.3 mg/L. Sputum culture showed normal flora growth. Chest CT: atelectasis of right middle lobe, bronchoscopy is recommended. Echocardiography showed normal size of atrioventricular cavity, normal left ventricular systolic function, CDFI showed mild mitral, tricuspid and aortic regurgitation, mild pulmonary hypertension. EF = 78%. Considering the acute exacerbation of COPD, levofloxacin and etimicin were given for the treatment of infection. Three days later, the symptoms of fever, cough, and expectoration relieved and the patient was discharged. Fifteen days after discharge, the patient had fever, cough, and expectoration symptoms again. Bronchitis was considered in the outpatient department of another hospital, and the effect of levofloxacin was not effective. Two weeks later, he was admitted again. WBC: 8.33 3%, lymphocyte: 17.4%, hemoglobin: 89 g/L, CRP: 99.54 mg/L. Sputum culture showed normal flora growth. Chest CT Reexamination showed that there was a little chronic inflammation near the heart margin of the middle lobe of the right lung, which was roughly similar to the front film; considering pneumonia, moxifloxacin, and clindamycin were given for infection treatment, and the patient still had fever. Levofloxacin, dexamethasone, and methylprednisolone were given. In order to identify the cause of fever, the patient presented to our hospital for further diagnosis and treatment.

The patient has a history of asthma for more than 10 years and is currently taking salbutamol sulfate; the patient has Guillain-Barre syndrome for 5 years and is currently taking furan thiamine; the patient also has a history of primary adrenocortical dysfunction for 3 years and is taking cortisone acetate tablets long term for supplementary treatment.

4.11.1 Physical Examination

Mentally clear, general spirit, anemia appearance, no abnormal skin and mucosa, no liver palms, no swelling of superficial lymph nodes. No subcutaneous bleeding point or rash was found. No head deformity, normal eyelids, no abnormal eyelid conjunctiva, no yellow sclera. Bilateral pupils were equal in size and circle, sensitive to light reflex, tragus structure collapsed, no abnormal secretion in external auditory canal, no mastoid tenderness. Nasal bridge collapse (Fig. 4.17), good nasal

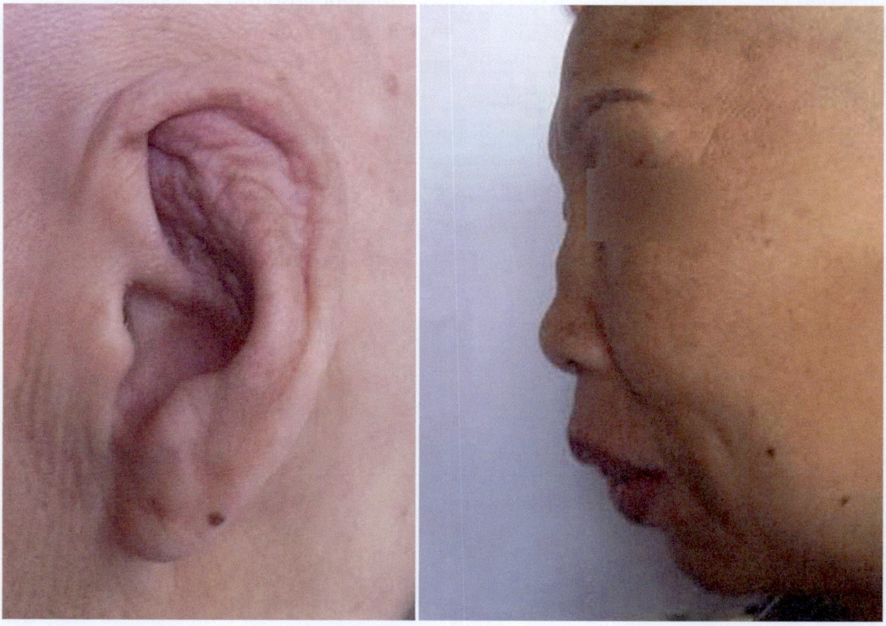

Fig. 4.17 The appearance of patients with ear cartilage damage and collapse of the nose, hair loss the patient showed the appearance of ear cartilage damage, the collapse of nasal bridge and loss of hair

ventilation, no deviation of nasal septum, no flapping of nasal wings, no tenderness in bilateral paranasal sinuses, no cyanosis in lips. There was no enlargement of bilateral parotid gland, soft neck, no resistance, no distention of jugular vein, middle trachea, and no enlargement of thyroid gland. The chest was symmetrical without deformity, the sternum without tenderness, the breath sounds of both lungs were clear, and dry and wet rales were not heard. The heart rate was 82 beats/min, regular; the abdomen was flat, the abdominal wall was soft, the whole abdomen had no tenderness, muscle tension and rebound pain, the liver and spleen were not touched under the ribs, the liver and kidney had no percussion pain, and the bowel sounds were 5 beats/min. No abnormality of anus and genitalia, no deformity of spine and limbs, no swelling of joints, no clubbing fingers (toes), no edema of lower limbs. Normal muscle strength, normal muscle tension, normal physiological reflex, no pathological neural reflex.

4.11.2 Diagnosis and Treatment Process

Laboratory examination after admission. Blood routine: white blood cell count: 7.35 × 10^9/L, lymphocyte%: 13.60% ↓, neutrophil%: 81.40% ↑, hemoglobin: 106 G/L ↓, erythrocyte sedimentation rate: 27 ↑, reticulocyte: 5.10% ↑. Lymphocyte subsets (2014-08-01): Total NK: 3% ↓, T + B + NK: 91% ↓; ANA: positive, titer: 1:100, ENA antibody spectrum, anti-centrocyte cytoplasmic antibody, double stranded DNA antibody were negative, blood immunoglobulin E: 2308.80 ng/mL ↑, blood immunoglobulin M: 3G/L ↑; thyroid function: free triiodothyronine: 2.90 pmol/L ↓, free thyroxine: 23.97 pmol/L ↑, thyroid stimulating hormone: 2.90 pmol/L ↑ T-SPOT TB: (negative), antigen A (ESAT-6) well: 0, antigen B (CFP-10) well: 0, positive control well: (normal), negative control well: 0, procalcitonin: 0.04.

Enhanced Lung CT: right middle lobe bronchial obstructive pneumonia with atelectasis, right middle lobe bronchial proximal wall was not smooth with suspicious small nodules shadow (Fig. 4.18). Echocardiography: structural

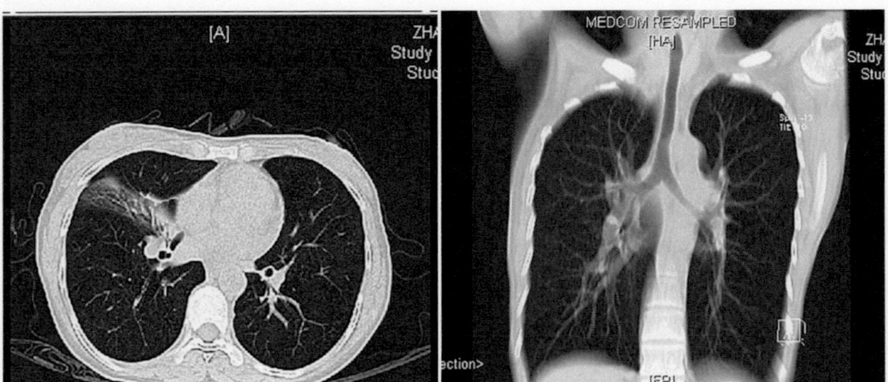

Fig. 4.18 CT scan showed bronchial obstructive pneumonia with atelectasis in the right middle lobe, and the proximal wall of right middle lobe bronchial was not smooth with suspicious nodules

echocardiography: mild to moderate mitral regurgitation. Ultrasound showed a small nodule in the isthmus of the thyroid, which may be benign. Bilateral supraclavicular lymph nodes were enlarged, bilateral cervical lymph nodes showed no obvious abnormal enlargement, bilateral parathyroid glands were not shown, multiple cholesterol crystals were found in gallbladder. No obvious abnormality was found in liver, pancreas, spleen, kidneys, ureters and bladder. PET-CT: (1) The metabolism of FDG in the irregular shadow of right hilar was slightly increased, and the metabolism of FDG in mediastinal and bilateral hilar lymph nodes was slightly increased. PET imaging of the rest of the body (including brain) showed no abnormal increase of FDG metabolism. (2) Laryngitis. (3) Right middle lung atelectasis. Small nodule shadow of right lower lung, no increased FDG metabolism, considered as benign, recommended follow-up. Bilateral axillary lymph node hyperplasia. Bullae in both lungs. (4) Hemorrhoids. Colitis. (5) Low density shadow of left adnexal area, no increase of FDG metabolism, considered benign, gynecological follow-up is recommended. (6) Low density shadow of left femoral head, slightly increased FDG metabolism, considered as benign, recommended follow-up, cervical hyperosteogeny.

The patient is a middle-aged female with recurrent fever for 2 months. She has a history of asthma, Guillain-Barre syndrome and primary adrenocortical hypofunction. However, her condition is under stable control, and there is no diagnosis that can be explained by recurrent fever and cough. The patient has recurrent pulmonary infection, accompanied by atelectasis of the right middle lobe, and repeated sputum culture, and no pathogen growth. Repeated pulmonary infection with atelectasis should be considered as bronchial obstruction caused by abnormal pulmonary bronchial structure, which leads to atelectasis. The right middle lobe is especially prone to chronic or recurrent infection and atelectasis, which is called middle lobe syndrome. The causes include bronchial lung cancer (20%–40%), benign tumor, other types of bronchial stenosis (including bronchial stones), exogenous compression, bronchiectasis, chronic infection, etc. The most common cause is nonspecific infection, and this kind of atelectasis is mostly non obstructive.

CT scan of this case showed that the right middle lobe bronchial obstructive pneumonia with atelectasis occurred repeatedly, which was consistent with the description of middle lobe syndrome. The diagnosis should consider bronchial lung cancer, benign tumor, other types of bronchial stenosis (including bronchial stones), exogenous compression, bronchiectasis, chronic infection, etc. But the patient's appearance has characteristic changes, including external ear relaxation, collapse, deformity, and nasal cartilage local collapse. Combined with the patient's atelectasis, mitral regurgitation, and other clinical manifestations, it can be explained by recurrent chondritis (RP). After consultation with a rheumatologist, the patient was diagnosed with the disease and began to be treated with methylprednisolone and methotrexate. The patient's symptoms were relieved and discharged from the hospital after the temperature was normal. Two weeks after discharge, sputum mycobacterium culture: positive, molecular identification: M. tuberculosis. So, the antituberculosis treatment was performed. The patient's fever did not recur, and the sputum mycobacterium culture turned negative after 3 months.

4.11.3 Comment

Relapsing polychondritis (RP) is a rare disease involving multiple systems of the whole body. It has progressive inflammatory and destructive lesions with repeated attacks and remission, involving cartilage and other connective tissues of the whole body, including ear, nose, eye, joint, respiratory tract and cardiovascular system. The clinical manifestations were chondritis of ear, nose and respiratory tract, accompanied by the involvement of eyes, ear vestibule and other organs. Polyarthritis and vascular involvement are also common. The disease can occur in all age groups, and the peak incidence age is 40–50 years old. Both men and women were involved, but the respiratory tract was more involved in women.

The clinical process of this disease is various, and most cases have been involved in multiple systems when diagnosed. There can be a sudden attack, a sudden aggravation of the disease, or fulminant attack, with respiratory failure. Cartilage is distributed in all kinds of tissues and organs of the whole body. Usually, the manifestations of chondritis are multiple organ damaged and vary with the involved organs, and also due to the combined connective tissue disease or vasculitis. Auricular cartilaginitis is the most common symptom. It is characterized by sudden pain, swelling, redness and scalding of the outer ear. The inflammation can subside by itself or by treatment. The common symptom is symmetry, and unilateral is rare. The manifestation of nasal chondritis, such as repeated attacks, can cause local collapse of nasal cartilage, forming saddle-nose deformity. Most of the patients with tracheobronchial and bronchial tree ossifying cartilage lesions complained of chronic cough and expectoration, followed by shortness of breath. They were often diagnosed as chronic bronchitis, which lasted for 6 months to decades. Eventually, they had dyspnea, repeated respiratory tract infection and wheezing. Sometimes, they had tenderness, hoarseness, or aphasia in front of trachea and thyroid gland cartilage.

The diagnosis of relapsing polychondritis is usually based on clinical features, not necessarily biopsy. McAdam et al. proposed the following diagnostic criteria: symmetrical otochondritis, non-destructive, seronegative polyarthritis, rhinochondritis, ophthalmitis, respiratory tract chondritis, and cochlear or vestibular dysfunction. By meeting at least three of the diagnostic criteria, the diagnosis can be established. If the clinical manifestations are uncertain, chondritis caused by other causes must be excluded, especially infectious diseases. Biopsies and cultures or other necessary tests are required to exclude syphilis, leprosy, fungal or other bacterial infections.

Repeated pulmonary infection with atelectasis is not uncommon in clinic, but the root causes of atelectasis are different. There are obstructive and nonobstructive type in the aspect of mechanism, and tumor and nontumor type in the aspect of etiology. Clinicians tend to explain the manifestation of the disease by monism, but it is not uncommon that tumor accompanied with infection or connective tissue disease accompanied with infection. Through the programmed clinical thinking mode, we can avoid finding a possible surface reason and missing the hidden reason, which is worthy of reference for clinicians. In this case, recurrent fever with cough for more than 2 months, the appearance of auricle and abnormal nasal cartilage are important indications for the diagnosis of rare recurrent polychondritis.

In addition, the incidence of secondary infection of autoimmune diseases, especially after systemic hormone therapy, is higher than that of the general population, and the abnormality of airway structure is also one of the high-risk factors of tuberculosis. Intermittent use of respiratory quinolones in this case may temporarily cover up the symptoms of tuberculosis, and glucocorticoid treatment may also affect the determination of T-SPOT TB examination results. Therefore, even if the diagnosis of connective tissue disease is relatively clear, we should pay more attention to the presence of other infections at the same time.

References

1. Belot A, Collardeau-Frachon S, Bellil D, Descours G, Gillet Y. It sounds like a relapsing polychondritis. Lancet Infect Dis. 2013;13(7):638.
2. Xuhua S, Jinmei S, Zhike C, et al. Clinical analysis of 56 cases of relapsing polychondritis. Chin J Gen Pract. 2006;5(10):607–9.
3. Haili H. Pulmonary tuberculosis and connective tissue diseases. Chin J Clin Dr. 2004;32(8):10–2.
4. Xuhua S, Jinmei S, Zhike C, et al. Clinical analysis of 56 cases of relapsing polychondritis. Chin J Gen Pract. 2006;5(10):607–9.
5. Haili H. Chinese clinician of tuberculosis and connective tissue diseases. Chin Clin. 2004;32(8):10–2.

4.12 Polymyalgia Rheumatica

Hu Yuekai

A 61-year-old woman was admitted to the hospital with a 1-month history of fever.

A month ago, she caught a fever without obvious cause (temperature, 37.5–38 °C). The temperature usually started to rise in the morning and reached the highest at night fall, accompanied by general fatigue, musculoskeletal aches, night sweats, occasional cough with no sputum. She showed no obvious sign of intolerance of cold and chills. Then she went to a local hospital. Chest CT scan did not find anything obviously abnormal. Cephalosporin antibiotics and hormones were given orally (specific details not available) but the effect was not good. Her body temperature fluctuated between 38.5 and 38.9 °C. The results of routine blood check are as follows: leukocytes, 9.6×10^9/L; neutrophil ratio, 77.5%; lymphocytes, 13.1%; hematocrit, 98 mm/h; hsCRP, 10 mg/dL. The thyroid function, tumor index, and immune index were normal while the results of sputum bacterial culture, fungal culture and antacid bacilli searching were all negative. No abnormality was shown during the ultrasound of upper abdomen, ultrasound of uterine adnexa, cardiac ultrasound, and chest CT scan. Bone marrow aspiration found nothing. For further diagnosis and treatment, the patient was transferred to our hospital with the diagnosis of fever of unknown origin. During the course of the disease, she had no nausea, no vomiting, no bellyache, no diarrhea, no urinary frequency nor urgency, no urodynia, no headache, no vomiting of blood, no black stool, no arthralgia, no rash, no hair loss, and no photosensitization.

Since the illness, the patient was mentally well, with normal appetite and sleep, normal urination and defecation, and no obvious weight loss.

4.12.1 Admission Checkup

T:37.9 °C	P:80 bpm	R:20 bpm	BP:122/70 mmHg

The patient was sane and in good mental condition. She was well nourished with normal development. She walked into the ward in an autonomous position. And she was able to cooperate in physical examination and answer questions relevantly. The skin and sclera were not yellowish, and the superficial supraclavicular lymph nodes were not enlarged. The head had no deformity and the features are regular. The neck was soft, the trachea was centered and the thyroid was not enlarged. The respiratory motion was normal and symmetrical on both sides. The breath sounds of both lungs were clear and no obviously dry or wet rales were heard. HR: 80 bpm. The heart beat with regular rates and no pathological murmurs were heard in each valve area. The abdomen was soft, no pressure pain, no rebound pain, and no detection of the liver and spleen. The joints were movable and not deformed. There was no edema in both lower limbs and the knee reflex was normal. The pulsation of the temporal artery and dorsalis pedis artery were also normal, without tortuosity or stiffness. Neuropathological signs were not elicited.

4.12.2 Diagnosis and Treatment

The patient was admitted to the hospital and the relevant tests were completed. Blood routine examination: white blood cells, 10.03×10^9/L; red blood cells, 3.46×10^{12}/L; hemoglobin, 95 g/L; neutrophils, 83.2%; lymphocytes, 8.9%; platelets, 515×10^9/L.

The results of urinary and fecal routine are normal. Liver function (2011-09-28): ALT, 107 ↑ U/L; AST, 98 U/L; ALP, 186 ↑ U/L; GGT, 133 ↑ U/L. Lymphocyte subsets: CD3 Total T, 60%; CD4 T cell, 50%; CD8 T cell, 9%; CD19 Total B, 8%; Total NK, 26%; CD4+/CD8+, 5.56. CD19 Total B, 8%; Total NK, 26%; CD4+/CD8+, 5.56; hematocrit, 78 mm/h; RF (−), blood culture, negative; T-SPOT.TB, negative. Serum immunofixation electrophoresis: monoclonal immunoglobulins were not found.

Thyroid ultrasound: no significant abnormalities were seen. Sacroiliac CT: degeneration of the sacroiliac joint on both sides. PETCT: (1) PET imaging of the whole body (including the brain) did not show any significant abnormal foci of increased FDG metabolism. (2) Uneven density of the thyroid gland with hypodense foci, which was considered to be benign lesions since no abnormal foci of increased FDG metabolism are found. Ultrasound is recommended. (3) Scattered small nodules in both lungs with no abnormal increase in FDG metabolism, considered to be benign lesions. (4) Gastritis; cholecystitis. (5) Arthritis of shoulder joint, hip joint and knee joint on both sides. Mild osteophytes in cervical, thoracic and lumbar vertebrae.

The patient complained of persistent muscle soreness, especially around the neck and pelvis, which was obvious in the morning. Combining the patient's symptoms, physical signs and laboratory results, she was considered to have rheumatic polymyalgia. And she was given prednisone 8 mg tid. with omeprazole, calcium D and potassium chloride extended-release tablets as symptomatic supportive treatment. The patient's fever and muscle aches resolved rapidly. The patient was followed up after discharge and was in stable condition.

4.12.3 Comments

Rheumatic polymyalgia has a group of syndromes characterized by pain and stiffness in the proximal muscles of the scapularis, pelvic girdle and cervical muscles, with a significant increase in blood sedimentation and nonspecific systemic symptoms. The etiology of the disease is unknown. It is generally a benign process and closely related to age, positively. Few people suffer from the disease before the age of 50. In addition, there are 2–3 times more women than men and there are family clusters. HLA-DR4 haplotype is an important genetic phenotype of the disease.

The various diagnostic criteria for rheumatic polymyalgia are similar, while the Chinese ones are: age of onset ≥50; muscle stiffness with morning stiffness in the neck, scapula and pelvis, at least two sites, lasting 4 weeks or more; elevated blood sedimentation of more than 50 mm/h (Weil's method); antinuclear antibodies and rheumatoid factor, both negative; good response to low-dose glucocorticoid therapy; secondary polymyalgia excluded. 70%–95% of patients have stiffness in shoulder muscles, with slightly less involvement of the neck and buttocks (50%–70%). Some may involve the tendon attachments of the limb girdle muscles. There may also be pain and edema in the wrist and interphalangeal joints, and a small amount of synovial fluid in the joints of shoulders, knees or hip. Less than one-third of patients with rheumatic polymyalgia may present with anemia and abnormal liver function. Blood sedimentation is usually elevated, with 10.8% of the patients less than 50 mm/h, while only 5.4% have a sedimentation of less than 40 mm/h.

In this case, it was an elderly female starting with a low to moderate fever and pain in the muscles and joints of shoulders and pelvic. Blood sedimentation was elevated while the antinuclear antibodies and rheumatoid factor were negative. The results of electromyography were normal. Results of repeated blood cultures and other pathogenic tests were all negative. No significant abnormalities on PET-CT. So, the diagnosis was considered to be rheumatic polymyalgia, which was further supported by the effectiveness of low-dose glucocorticoid therapy. This case suggests us that after excluding infections, tumors and other rheumatic diseases, rheumatic polymyalgia needs to be considered when elderly people have unexplained fever with increased blood sedimentation, unexplained mild to moderate anemia, muscle aches and pains with difficulties in raising arms, dressing, squatting and standing up. And it is important to note that rheumatic polymyalgia is often combined with giant cell arteritis. Thus, in this group of patients, extra attention should be paid to headache, abnormal temporal artery pulsation, *jaw claudication*, visual impairment and arm *claudication*. Necessarily, a biopsy can be performed to confirm the diagnosis.

References

1. Salvarani C. Polymyalgia rheumatica and giant-cell arteritis. N Engl J Med. 2002;347:261–71.
2. Salvarani C. Polymyalgia rheumatica and giant-cell arteritis. Lancet. 2008;372(9634):234–45.
3. Watts A. Systemic vasculitis: an epidemiological perspective. Curr Immunol Rev. 2011;4(7):388–93.
4. Diagnosis and treatment guideline on polymyalgia rheumatica (draft). Chin J Rheumatol. 2004;8(8):506–7.

4.13 The Mysterious Driving Force Behind Repeated Fever for 6 Years—Familial Mediterranean Fever

Zhang Yanliang, Ruan Qiaoling, Wu Jing, and Zhang Wenhong

A student, 19 years old, from Nanjing, Jiangsu, was referred to our hospital on March 14, 2018 with a 6-year history of fever. In July 2012, the patient was hospitalized in a children's hospital due to fever, and was diagnosed with juvenile idiopathic arthritis. After treatment, he improved and was discharged. After that, he took long-term oral methylprednisolone and methotrexate drugs treatment for follow-up observation. During the withdrawal process, he developed fever in November 2012 and was readmitted to the hospital. At that time, the routine blood test showed: Hb 137 g/L, WBC 9.54×10^9/L, N% 86.4%, L% 8.8%, PLT 99×10^9/L, CRP 62 mg/L; Abdominal CT showed "bilateral pleural effusion, plump spleen", suspected diagnosis with upper respiratory tract infection. After using prednisone and naproxen and other drugs, symptoms improved. He continued prednisone and methotrexate therapy. Since then, there was a similar attack in February 2013, which improved after similar treatment. Taking prednisone, methotrexate, and naproxen and other drugs for 1 year, drugs were gradually reduced and then stopped. There was no fever in the next 2 years. In June 2017, the patient had fever again without obvious cause, and the body temperature reached 38.4 °C. The laboratory test results showed ESR 41 mm/h, CRP 71.7 mg/L, ferritin (−); ANA antibody profile (−), neutrophil antibody (−), rheumatoid factor (−), AKA (−), CCP (−); liver and kidney function, autoimmune antibodies, thyroid function, tumor indicators, immunoglobulin were all negative; the other tests showed mycoplasma pneumoniae IgM was positive and respiratory syncytial virus, influenza virus, adenovirus were negative. The chest CT scan revealed local thickening of oblique fissure on the right side; a small amount of fluid in the right pleural cavity; splenomegaly. The local hospital gave azithromycin intravenous infusion and oral administration of oseltamivir. Four days later, the patient's temperature was still high, reaching 39.5 °C. He came to our hospital for treatment and was admitted to the rheumatology department. He was diagnosed as connective tissue disease and was given prednisone 20 mg/day, methotrexate 10 mg/week. After 2 weeks treatment, the patient was improved and discharged, and went to the outpatient clinic regularly. The prednisone dose was gradually tapered. In September 2017, it was changed to methylprednisolone 6 mg/day. Due to the increased bilirubin in the liver function after review, the methotrexate was discontinued and started liver protection treatment to improve liver function. At 23:00 on the evening of March 13, 2018, the patient had a fever again without obvious cause, and his temperature reached 38.9 °C. There was no chill, no headache and vomiting, no sore and itching throat, no cough and sputum. In the emergency department of our hospital, he was given cefuroxime for anti-infection. The temperature was measured at 37.2 °C on the morning of the March 14. For further diagnosis and treatment, he was admitted to the hospital with a fever of unknown origin. During the course of the disease, the patient had poor appetite and sleep, and his bowel movements were basically normal.

The patient was physically fit. A history of allergy to penicillin drugs. No family genetic history has been found yet.

4.13.1 Physical Examination

T 37.1 °C, P 87/min, R 19/min, BP 120/70 mmHg, height 176 cm, weight 60 kg. Consciousness, fair spirit, normal development, and good nutrition. The skin and mucous membranes of the whole body were not yellowish or rash, and the superficial lymph nodes were not palpable and enlarged. There was no swelling of the bilateral tonsils. Percussion on both lungs was clear, and breath sounds in both lungs were slightly lower, and rales were not heard. There is no expansion of the heart dullness boundary, the heart rate is 87 beats/min, the rhythm is uniform, and no pathological murmur is heard in the auscultation area of each valve. The abdomen was soft, no tenderness and rebound pain in the abdomen, no masses or lumps in the abdomen, no palpable under the liver and spleen ribs, negative Murphy's sign, negative mobile dullness, and no obvious percussive pain in the kidney area. The muscle strength and muscle tension of the limbs are normal, and the physiological reflex is present, but the pathological reflex is not elicited.

4.13.2 Diagnosis and Treatment Process

The relevant examinations were complete after the patient was admitted to the hospital. Blood routine: WBC 5.9 × 10^9/L, N% 68.8%, L% 16.5% (↓), Hb 128 g/L, PLT 86 × 10^9/L (↓), ESR 14 mm/h. There were no obvious abnormalities in liver and kidney function, thyroid function, and coagulation function. Routine urine and feces: no obvious abnormalities. Autoantibodies and tumor markers were negative; hepatitis B surface antibodies were positive; hepatitis C, HIV, and syphilis were all negative. Pathogenic microorganisms: *Mycoplasma pneumoniae* IgM, Chlamydia IgM, Legionella pneumophila IgM, Influenza A IgM, Influenza B IgM, Parainfluenza IgM, Respiratory syncytial virus IgM, Q fever Rickettsia IgM, Adenovirus IgM were all negative.

Cardiac color Doppler ultrasound: a small amount of pericardial effusion, mild mitral regurgitation, and mild tricuspid regurgitation. Chest CT: increased texture of both lungs, bronchial disease (Fig. 4.19). Full abdominal MR: The spleen is slightly larger; there is a small amount of fluid in the abdominal cavity and pericardium (Fig. 4.20).

After admission, the patient was treated with methylprednisolone 8 mg/day orally and cefuroxime intravenously for anti-infection treatment. In the afternoon of March 15, the patient's body temperature rose to 38.5 °C. Considering that the original immune system disease may not be controlled, the oral methylprednisolone was stopped and dexamethasone 5 mg/day was used instead. Cefuroxime was stopped on the 16th and changed to azithromycin to against infection, and continuous application of dexamethasone 5 mg/day intravenously, the patient's body temperature was around 37.5 °C during the treatment, but the patient's body temperature rose to 38.5 °C again on March 20.

The patient had been diagnosed with juvenile idiopathic arthritis, and the course of the disease was as long as 6 years. During this period, he had never had joint symptoms, which seemed to be inconsistent. Therefore, we doubted the original diagnosis. Combined with the clinical performance of the patient, we consider whether there is the possibility of autoinflammatory disease. Auto-Inflammatory

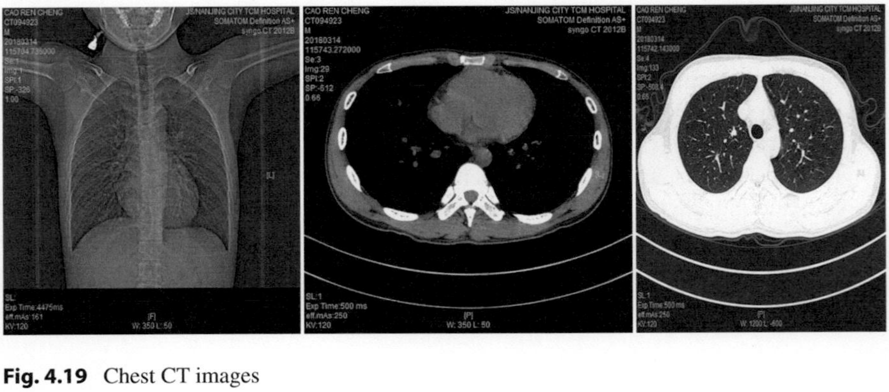

Fig. 4.19 Chest CT images

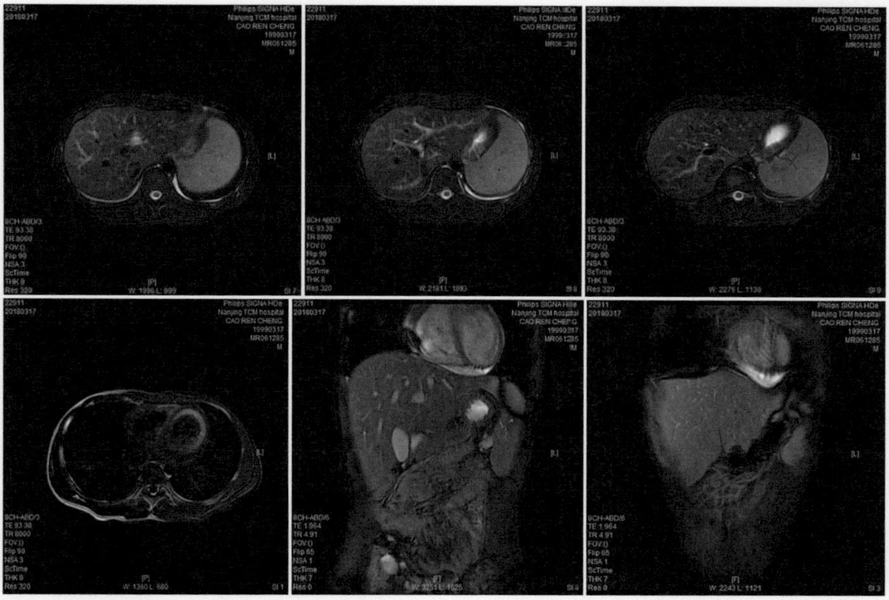

Fig. 4.20 Abdominal MR images

Disease (AID) is a hereditary, periodic, noninvasive inflammatory disease. The age of onset is early, and the clinical manifestations are mainly recurrent systemic inflammatory reactions such as fever, rash, arthritis, serositis, etc. During the onset of the disease, acute inflammatory reaction substances (increased C-reactive protein, increased erythrocyte sedimentation rate, increased neutrophils). Therefore, blood samples of the family were collected for genetic testing. Intravenous infusion of methylprednisolone 40 mg/day and methotrexate 10 mg/week were added. Afterwards, the patient's body temperature gradually returned to normal. He was discharged from the hospital on April 2 with gradual glucocorticoid reduction, and the condition was stable. On May 10, sequencing of 535 genetic immunodeficiency-related genes in the patient's family showed that the patient's MEFV (Familial Mediterranean Fever-related gene) had E148Q compound heterozygous mutations, and both mutation sites had been reported to cause related disease, the patient was diagnosed with familial Mediterranean fever (Table 4.4, Fig. 4.21).

4.13.3 Reviews

Auto-Inflammatory Disease (AID) is a hereditary, periodic, noninvasive inflammatory disease. The onset age is early, and the clinical manifestations are mainly recurrent systemic inflammatory reactions such as fever, rash, arthritis, and serositis. Familial Mediterranean Fever (FMF) is a kind of hereditary periodic fever syndrome, which is a single-gene inherited autoinflammatory disease, which can be divided into type 1 and type 2. FMF is mainly caused by mutations in the MEFV

Table 4.4 Changes in blood routine and inflammatory markers

Date classification	Hb (g/L)	WBC (10^9/L)	RBC (10^{12}/L)	N%	PLT (10^9/L)	ESR (mm/h)	CRP (mg/L)	High sensitive CRP (mg/L)
3.15	128	5.8	4.11	66.9	86	14	26.9	
3.16	137	7.0	4.29	68.8	107	10		36
3.19	132	7.1	4.24	76	118		14.7	
3.20	135	8.1	4.47	85.71	134			30
3.21	128	6.81	4.27	93.8	128			38
3.26	136	8.4	4.32	79.6	153		5.19	
3.31	140	10.0	4.53	82.2	128	10	<3.13	

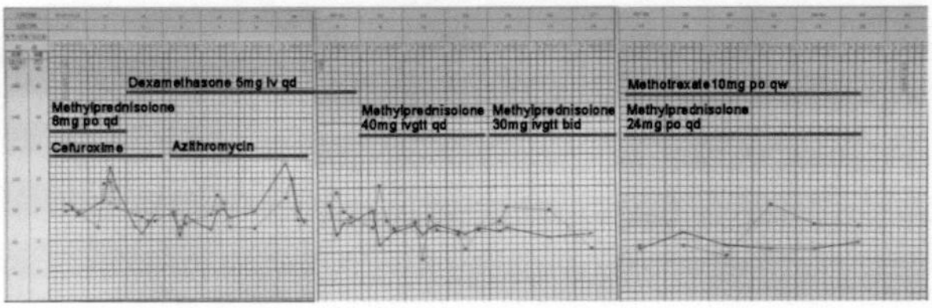

Fig. 4.21 Main anti-infection treatment and changes in body temperature

gene. MEFV is located on chromosome 16p13.3. The pyrin protein encoded by this gene is closely related to the innate immune system. Mutations in MEFV lead to a decrease in the number of pyrin or changes in function, resulting in excessive activation of the NALP3 inflammatory complex and causing inflammation reaction. FMF is traditionally considered as autosomal recessive inheritance, but recently more and more studies have found that only one mutation, a heterozygous mutation, has been detected in FMF patients, and it is believed that heterozygous mutations may be more common than homozygous mutations. Its exact pathogenesis needs to be further studied.

FMF is mostly seen in people along the Mediterranean coast (such as Jews, Armenians, Turks, and Arabs in Spain and Portugal), with a prevalence of 1/1000 to 1/200. Usually, the age of onset is 5–15 years old. About 20% of the children have the first attack before 2 years old; 67% have the onset before 10 years old; and 90% have the onset before 20 years old. The clinical manifestations of FMF are greatly affected by environmental factors. Common clinical manifestations include repeated fever, abdominal pain, and joint damage. In a few cases, fever is the only symptom. The specific symptoms are as follows: (1) Repeated fever (99%–100%): sudden stop, fever lasts for 1–3 days, and the fever interval ranges from 1 week to several years; (2) Abdominal pain (70%–95%): It can develop from local abdominal pain to total abdominal pain, and may have symptoms of peritoneal irritation or paralytic intestinal obstruction; (3) Chest pain (40%–45%): It is related to aseptic pleurisy and pericarditis, which can be self-limitingly improved within a few days; (4) Arthralgia (45%–75%): more large joints are involved, but fewer joints are involved, and the symptoms peak within 24–48 h, and then often resolve spontaneously without leaving joint damage; (5) erysipelas-like rash (7%–40%): No antibiotic treatment is needed, and it can resolve spontaneously; (6) AA amyloidosis: It is common in untreated FMF patients, manifested by persistent large amounts of proteinuria, reaching the level of nephrotic syndrome, and gradually progressing to end-stage renal disease. In some patients, renal amyloid becomes its only clinical manifestation, called type 2 FMF.

The diagnosis of FMF is mainly based on family history, typical attack characteristics, response to colchicine, and other causes that can cause similar manifestations need to be excluded. At present, the most commonly used standard for adults is still the Tel Hashomer standard, see Table 4.5.

The patient's fever characteristics are in line with the typical onset of FMF, arthralgia, WBC and CRP increase, and a good response to colchicine. The onset can be resolved spontaneously. There is a period of asymptomatic remission. What's more, the genetic testing found E148Q heterozygous mutation of MEFV gene. In short, the patient has a diagnosis of FMF. When diagnosing and differentially diagnosing patients with long-term fever, it is necessary to be alert to the possibility of auto-inflammatory diseases. If necessary, select relevant genetic testing to reduce misdiagnosis and missed diagnosis.

Table 4.5 FMF clinical diagnostic criteria

Primary standard	Secondary standard	Supplementary standard
Have a typical episode of peritonitis (diffuse)	Incomplete paroxysmal chest pain	FMF family history
Have a typical episode of pleurisy (unilateral) or pericarditis	Incomplete paroxysmal abdominal pain	FMF susceptible population
Have typical episodes of monoarthritic (hip, knee, ankle)	Incomplete paroxysmal mono-arthralgia	Onset <20 years old
Only typical onset of fever symptoms	Exertional lower limb pain	Symptoms are severe at the time of attack, requiring bed rest
	Good response to colchicine treatment	Onset symptoms resolve spontaneously
		Asymptomatic between onsets
		Evidence of transient inflammatory response at the onset, such as white blood cell, erythrocyte sedimentation rate, serum amyloid, fibrinogen increase, etc.
		Intermittent proteinuria/hematuria
		Laparoscopy is negative or normal appendix is removed
		Parents marry close relatives

Clinical diagnosis needs to meet ≥1 primary criterion or ≥2 secondary criteria. Incomplete seizures refer to pain and recurrent symptoms but fail to meet the typical attack criteria

References

1. Ozen S, Demirkaya E, Erer B, et al. EULAR recommendations for the management of familial Mediterranean fever. Ann Rheum Dis. 2016;75(4):644–51.
2. Hentgen V, Grateau G, Kone-Paut I, et al. Evidence-based recommendations for the practical management of famiilial Mediterranean fever. Semin Arthritis Rheum. 2013;43(3):387–91.
3. Özen S, Bilginer Y, Ayaz NA, et al. Anti-interleukin 1 treatment for patients with familial Mediterranean fever resistant to colchicine. J Rheumatol. 2011;38(3):516.
4. Bilgen SA, Kilic L, Akdogan A, et al. Effects of anti-tumornecrosis factor agents for familial Mediterranean fever patients with chronic arthritis and/or sacroiliitis who were resistant to colchicine treatment. J Clin Rheumatol. 2011;17(7):358–62.

Fever of Unknown Origin Other Disease

5

Chen Chen, Chen Shu, Yu Shenglei, Zhu Chong, Li Ning, Zhang Jiming, Zhu Haoxiang, Sun Feng, Wang Ting, Yang Feifie, Huang Yuxian, and Liu Qihui

5.1 Miscellaneous Disorders

The miscellaneous disorders account for approximately 10% of the spectrum of FUO, including drug fever, granulomatous disease, thrombophlebitis, hemolytic attacks, occult hematoma, periodic fever, and factitious fever, among others. Many of the uncommon causes of FUO will be systematically described in this chapter. Apart from drug-induced fever, none of the miscellaneous causes of fever are found very frequently in patients with FUO.

The miscellaneous disorders include several disparate groups of diseases; therefore, no similar characteristics or generally applicable laboratory tests could be summarized. Here is a list of several miscellaneous disorders specifically.

1. Drug-induced ever:

   Drug-induced fever may result from allergic or idiosyncratic reactions, or from alterations in thermoregulatory mechanisms. Although eosinophilia and rash are present in only approximately 25% of cases, their absence should not deter clinicians from considering a potential drug etiology. The most common drugs that cause fever include: antimicrobials (sulfonamides, penicillin, nitrofurantoin, vancomycin, and antimalarials), H1- and H2-blocking antihistamines, antiepileptic drugs (barbiturates and phenytoin), iodides, nonsteroidal anti-inflammatory drugs (including salicylates), antihypertensive drugs (hydralazine, methyldopa), antiarrhythmic drugs (quinidine, procainamide), antithyroid drugs, contaminants such as quinine that accompany injected cocaine or heroin, etc.

C. Chen · C. Shu · Y. Shenglei · Z. Chong · L. Ning · Z. Jiming · Z. Haoxiang · S. Feng · Y. Feifie · H. Yuxian · L. Qihui (✉)
Department of Infectious Diseases, Huashan Hospital, Fudan University, Shanghai, China

W. Ting
Department of Infectious Diseases, Jing'an District Central Hospital of Shanghai, Shanghai, China

W. Zhang, X. Weng (eds.), *Fever of Unknown Origin*,
https://doi.org/10.1007/978-981-95-1401-4_5

Drug-induced fever can manifest soon after the initiation of medication; however, delayed onset—ranging from several weeks to months or even years—has also been reported. Diagnosis is typically established through a therapeutic trial involving stopping the suspected agent. In most instances, defervescence occurs within 72 h following drug withdrawal, although some may be prolonged in certain cases. Reintroduction of drugs within the same class is not recommended during diagnostic evaluation.

2. Factitious fever:

   Factitious fever typically reflects an underlying psychiatric disorder and is more commonly observed among women and healthcare professionals. Affected individuals deliberately feign illness to achieve secondary gain. Falsification of fever is often accomplished by manipulating thermometers, resulting in exaggerated temperature readings that may exceed 41 °C. These artificially elevated temperatures are frequently inconsistent with typical physiological responses; characteristic signs such as chills, cool or warm extremities, sweats, and tachycardia may be absent or incongruent with the recorded fever pattern.

3. Venous thrombosis and thromboembolism:

   Although the more common presentations include dyspnea, pleuritic pain, cough, and hemoptysis, a small number of patients with thrombosis present with fever. D-dimer test and enhanced CT scans could be useful for differential diagnosis.

4. Hyperthyroidism and subacute thyroiditis:

   These conditions are most frequently diagnosed clinically. However, when the patient's medical history, physical signs, and laboratory tests are not typical, it may be misdiagnosed as another disease, and the diagnosis of subacute thyroiditis will be difficult.

5. Familial Mediterranean fever (FMF) and cyclic fever:

   Familial Mediterranean fever manifests as an intermittent fever of unknown cause. It usually starts in childhood. In addition to fever, there may be peritoneal and pleural serous inflammation and characteristic skin lesions (painful erythema). Occasionally, FMF presents symptoms such as joint pain and headache. Spontaneous remission and recurrence often alternate. White blood cells increase and erythrocyte sedimentation rate increases during the attack, and return to normal in remission. The disease is more common in Jews, Armenians, and Arabs, but it also occurs in other ethnic groups such as Western Europeans. Without special treatment, it may progress or cause specific complications.

The miscellaneous category contains both varied and individually rare causes of classic FUO. During the diagnosis and treatment of these miscellaneous disorders, some cases are easily diagnosed, while others have a complicated and process. What needs to be emphasized again is that the evaluation of a patient with FUO typically includes a comprehensive history, verification that the patient actually has fever, consideration of the fever pattern, repeated physical examinations, a host of laboratory investigations, key imaging studies, and invasive diagnostic procedures.

5.2 Subacute Thyroiditis with Fever, Neck Pain and Sore Throat

Chen Chen and Chen Shu

A 55-year-old female with a fever for 21 days was admitted to the hospital.

Since March 14, 2004, she has developed chills and fever without obvious inducements with herbody temperature going up to 38.4 °C. She felt pain while swallowing approximately 5 days before fever, with pain in the left neck for more than 1 month and without a runny nose, cough, fear of fever, hand shaking, and palpitation. After self-administration of compound chlorphenamine and cefradine, her body temperature was still high, and she went to the other hospital. The routine blood check was as follows: WBC 13.3 × 10^9/L, N 70.3%, CRP 54 mg/L. Although she was given cefuroxime and other treatments, it was ineffective. The body temperature was as high as 39.5 °C. The treatment plan was switched to ceftriaxone and ciprofloxacin for anti-infective treatment. Her body temperature still fluctuated at around 38 °C. Before admission, the routine blood test was WBC 9.7 × 10^9/L and N 60.9%. The appetite was fair, and there was no significant change in weight, so she was transferred to this hospital for further diagnosis and treatment.

5.2.1 Admission Check

Her body condition was fine, with a temperature of 36.7 °C. She had no ecchymosis on the skin and mucous membranes of the whole body, with unpasted and enlarged superficial lymph nodes and a soft neck. There was tenderness of the left thyroid, with no enlarged thyroid on both sides. Clear breath sounds was present in both lungs, and the heart rate was 70 beats/min with regular rhythm and no murmur. Her abdomen was soft, nontender, and nondistended. Liver, spleen, and ribs were not reached. Neither of the lower limbs were swollen. Hands trembling was negative, and pathological signs were not elicited.

5.2.2 Diagnosis and Treatment

After admission, routine blood test was as follows: WBC 6.99 × 10^9/L, N 65.3%, RBC 4.09 × 10^{12}/L, HB 111 g/L, PLT 315 × 10^9/L; liver function A/G was 33/35, the rest was normal. Thyroid function was as follows: TSH 0.01 mIU/L, TT4 201 nmol/L, TT3 2.92 nmol/L, FT4 40.3 pmol/L, FT3 11.7 pmol/L, thyroglobulin antibody (TGA) 24.1%, thyroid microsomal antibody (MCA) 19.4%, and TPO-Ab 57.65 IU/ml. Thyroid iodine uptake rate was 2.78% for 3 h and 0.96% for 24 h, both significantly lower than the normal level; ESR 30 mm/h, ANA 1:100, with Extractable Nuclear Antigen (ENA), dsDNA, and Anti-Neutrophil Cytoplasmic Antibody (ANCA) negative. Urine routine, stool routine, renal function, electrolytes, coagulation function, blood glucose, immunoglobulin, complement, CRP, anti-“O”, tumor markers (Alpha-Fetoprotein (AFP), CEA, CA153, CA199, CA125, CA50, and CA724) were all within the normal range. B-ultrasound: thyroid gland with diffuse lesion, consistent with inflammation. There was no obvious enlargement of the superficial lymph nodes throughout the body, and no obvious abnormalities in the liver, gallbladder, pancreas, spleen, or kidney. The 24-h dynamic ECG showed occasional ventricular premature beats, occasionally with double rhythm and two bursts. Echocardiogram was normal. The gastroscope indicated gastritis (congestion and exudation, moderate). After admission, with her history of left neck pain, iodine uptake rate was significantly decreased, and T4 increased, and thyroid B-ultrasound showed diffuse changes, so she was diagnosed with subacute thyroiditis. She then received methylprednisolone 10 mg tid po. After her condition was stabilized, she was discharged.

5.2.3 Reviews

Subacute thyroiditis, also known as de-Quervain thyroiditis, granulomatous thyroiditis, and giant cell thyroiditis, is a self-limited, inflammatory disease of the thyroid that is manifested by pain. The diagnosis of subacute thyroiditis is mainly based on clinical manifestations and laboratory examinations: acute onset, often accompanied by symptoms and signs of upper respiratory tract infection; goiter with single or multiple nodules, hard and obvious tenderness; pain in the thyroid area with radiation to the submandibular, locations behind the ears, and neck. The pain can be transferred to the opposite side; the early erythrocyte sedimentation rate increases significantly, often greater than 50 mm/h; the thyroid iodine uptake rate is low, and the two-way separation phenomenon of transient serum thyroid hormone concentration increases. Thyroid antibody is negative or slightly elevated; thyroid puncture or biopsy has multinucleated giant cells or granuloma changes.

The diagnosis of subacute thyroiditis is relatively easy to determine; it is a rare cause of fever. However, when the patient’s medical history, physical signs, and laboratory examinations are not typical, it may be misdiagnosed as other diseases, and the diagnosis of subacute thyroiditis will be difficult. This patient started with fever and had neck pain with no palpitations, hand tremors, hyperhidrosis, and increased white blood cells. Anti-infective treatment was given until the thyroid function report was clear, which delayed the diagnosis and treatment. Therefore, patients with pharyngeal soreness during the course of the disease should be alert to the possibility of subacute thyroiditis. It is necessary to carefully ask about the medical history and check the neck signs, especially the tenderness in the thyroid area, so as to avoid misdiagnosis.

References

1. Chinese Medical Association Endocrinology Branch. Guidelines for diagnosis and treatment of thyroid diseases in China-thyroiditis. Chin J Intern Med. 2008;9:784–8.

2. Karachalios GN, Amantos K, Kanakis KV, et al. Subacute thyroiditis presenting as fever of unknown. Int J Clin Pract. 2010;64(1):97–8.
3. Yi W. Diagnosis and treatment of subacute thyroiditis. Chin J Pract Surg. 2004;24(1):25–6.
4. Ying G, Yanming G. Subacute thyroiditis. Int J Endocrinol Metab. 2009;29(5):358–360.
5. Lin C, Yue C, Weiwei Z, et al. Ultrasound diagnosis of subacute thyroiditis. Chin J Med Imaging Technol. 2010;26(9):1678–81.

5.3 A Case of Central Hyperthermia

Yu Shenglei and Chen Shu

A 20-year-old man presented to our institution with a 10-day history of fever and epigastric discomfort.

Ten days before presentation, the patient with no notable inducement, noted the onset of fever and epigastric discomfort with nausea, fatigue, and slight myalgia in both lower extremities. During this time, he had temperatures as high as 38.9 °C and dined chills, rigors， vomiting, rashes, joint pain or swelling, cough, sputum, diarrhea, urinary frequency or urgency, and painful urination. Passage of flatus and feces was normal. Laboratory evaluation from outside hospital revealed that the white blood cell (WBC) count was 11.6×10^9/L and the percentage of neutrophils was 66.7%. The patient was treated with cefuroxime for antimicrobial treatment, but the symptoms did not improve. Three days later, he was admitted to the emergency department, and the blood test showed that WBC count was 10.97×10^9/L and the percentage of neutrophils was 57.2%. Both renal and liver function tests were normal. Ultrasound imaging displayed solid nodules on the right lobe of the liver, which seemed to be angiomas. The computed tomography (CT) of the abdomen was unremarkable. He was treated with levofloxacin for antimicrobial therapy, but his temperature remained unimproved. He was then transferred to our institution. Since the onset of the disease, the patient was alert, and he had normal mentation. There was no notable change in his weight, defecation, or urination. The patient's medical history was remarkable for urticaria, which occurs once a year.

5.3.1 Physical Examination

T: 38.6 °C, P: 90 bpm, R: 16 bpm, BP: 110/70 mmHg. The patient's general physical condition was relatively normal. Cardiopulmonary examination results were unremarkable. His abdomen was flat and soft, while tenderness was noted below the xiphoid and above the umbilicus, without rebound tenderness, and there was no tenderness in the other part of the abdomen. Murphy's sign was negative. The liver and spleen did not reached below the costal margin. The patient had pain with percussion in the hepatic area but not in the costovertebral angle. The bowel sounds were about 7 times/min. The patient had no shifting dullness or lower extremities edema. The physical examination revealed mild tenderness in the gastrocnemius, while muscular tension was normal.

5.3.2 The Process of Diagnosis and Treatment

On presentation, the patient underwent a blood test, which showed that the WBC count was 11.34×10^9/L and the percentage of neutrophils was 60.2%. Since the duration of the fever was only 2 weeks, the diagnosis was drawn to acute fever. Infectious diseases were considered in combination with gastrointestinal symptoms. Levofloxacin was added for anti-infective treatment. But the patient complained about upper abdominal skin pruritus with extensive skin redness in the chest and abdomen. Drug eruption and drug fever were considered, and all the drugs were discontinued. However, there was no improvement in the fever type. Then doxycycline was used for replacement, but it was ineffective.

The blood peripheral smear was performed, and the results revealed the following: the percentage of neutrophilic multinucleated cells was 58%; lymphocytes, 33%; large mononuclear cells, 4%; eosinophils, 0%; atypical lymphocytes, 5%. The patient was considered to be infected with the Epstein-Barr virus. He was treated with methylprednisolone(40 mg) and acyclovir for antiviral therapy, but the fever did not improve.

Ultrasound revealed left supraclavicular lymphadenopathy. No remarkable abnormality in morphology and structure was identified in the bilateral cervical and axillary lymph nodes. Bone marrow biopsy displayed proliferative bone marrow, and there was a mature obstacle in the granulocytes series with some of them degenerated. Plasma cells were easy to see, while reticular macrophages with a few hemophagocytic cells and atypical lymphocytes could be seen, too. The results of gastroscopy were unremarkable.

The patient kept febrile for 3 weeks after admission, and the temperature ranged from 39 to 40 °C. Though treated with multi-antibiotics, including levofloxacin, doxycycline, imipenem, fosfomycin, and amikacin, the fever did not improve. Fever could not be attenuated or moderated by steroids (such as methylprednisolone and dexamethasone), amidopyrine compound, and nonsteroidal anti-inflammatory drugs (NSAIDs), as well as physical cooling therapy.

The detailed medical examination was performed again and revealed the following: The patient had a clear level of consciousness. He was obese, and his appetite was normal. The right limb was more sensitive than the left. Notable medical history was added that the patient had a history of hypohidrosis and diaphoresis only presented on the back. He drank water frequently as he needed to drink every hour in the daytime, 3–4 times in the nighttime. The patient also drank a large amount of water with a daily intake and output of more than 4000 mL. Combined with the fact that multiple antipyretic drugs were ineffective, the diagnosis was drawn to hypothalamic syndrome, and brain magnetic resonance imaging (MRI) was necessary.

Brain-enhanced MRI findings were normal.

Pituitary MRI scan demonstrated swelling of the pituitary with low-signal intensity.

Pituitary Enhanced MRI Reports: coronal views of the T1W1 scan showed that the pituitary was uneven, the upper edge of the pituitary was swollen, the pituitary stalk was thickened, and the position was in the middle. The saddle bottom was slightly collapsed, and the sella was slightly enlarged. After enhancement, the pituitary gland and the anterior pituitary stalk were enhanced, and the left basal ganglia area saw filiform and uneven enhancement. Conclusion: There was an abnormal enhancement in both the sellar area and left basal ganglia. Combining the clinical considerations of inflammatory lesions, the possibility of histiocytosis X needed to be excluded.

Brain Magnetic Resonance Spectroscopy(MRS) Reports: The N-Acetylaspartate (NAA) peak and Cholesterol (CHO) peak in part of the left basal ganglia decreased, while the NAA/CHO ratio increased slightly. The cerebellar sulcus widened.

Radiology consultation recommended: Tumors in the basal ganglia should be considered, and germ cell tumors should be considered in combination with the patient's age and the location of the lesion. Lumbar puncture was performed, and the results of the cerebrospinal fluid routine examination, as well as the biochemical test, were unremarkable. Tumor cells were not found in the cerebrospinal fluid, but cysticercosis antibody showed a weak positive. A blood hormone test was performed, including sex hormones, growth hormone, adrenal cortex hormones, and thyroid function, and the results were normal. β-HCG and AFP did not increase. The water deprivation and pressurization experiment was difficult to complete because the patient was extremely thirsty and could not tolerate long-term deprivation of water.

Diagnostic treatment with bromocryptine was performed. Then the body temperature decreased slightly, and the peak was maintained below 38 °C. The family refused to treat with chlorpromazine. The neurosurgery consultation recommended that diagnostic puncture of intracranial lesions should be performed through the nose to clarify the nature of the disease, but the family considered the risk and refused the operation.

The patient was followed up regularly in the outpatient department of our hospital after discharge. His temperature returned to normal, though he still suffered from frequent polydipsia and polyuria. Considering the results of brain MRI reexamination, which displayed enlarged sellar lesions, the final diagnosis was drawn to sellar germ cell tumors. After radiotherapy in the neurosurgery department of our hospital, the lesions were reduced, and the symptoms of polydipsia and polyuria were improved (Figs. 5.1, 5.2, and 5.3).

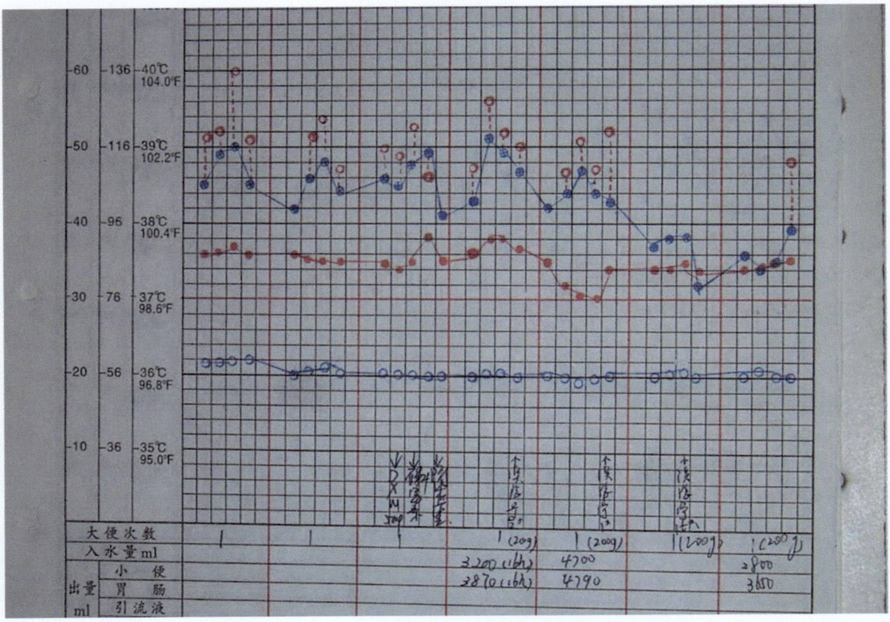

Fig. 5.1 The patient's body temperature decreased after treatment with bromocriptine

Fig. 5.2 The pituitary stalk was thickened at the arrow point

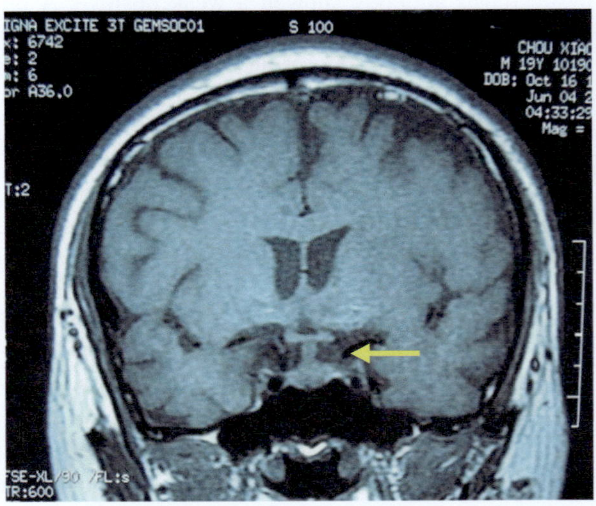

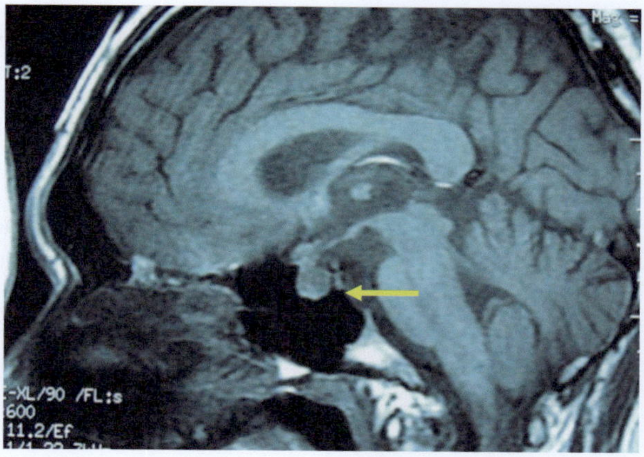

Fig. 5.3 The pituitary gland was irregularly enhanced at the arrow point

5.3.3 Discussions

Hypothalamic syndrome refers to hypothalamic diseases caused by many reasons. Endocrine and metabolic disorders are the main clinical manifestations of hypothalamic syndrome, which may combine with autonomic dysfunction such as regulation disorders of body temperature, diet, and sleep. The clinical manifestations are diverse, and the symptoms appear in a different order, thus making it sometimes difficult to draw a clinical diagnosis. It is easy to be clinically misdiagnosed for some people who suffer from autonomic dysfunction (including hypohidrosis, anhidrosis, heat intolerance, polydipsia, etc.) and lack of endocrine changes in the early stage of the disease. Therefore, attention should be paid to some special manifestations in the medical history, especially the medical history of central dysregulation of hormones and autonomic disorders. Physical examination and laboratory examinations can help confirm the diagnosis. Additionally, the results of physical examination and laboratory tests will also be helpful for the correct diagnosis.

Central hyperthermia is uncommon. When the patient has the following manifestations, clinicians should be highly alert to central hyperthermia, and it is recommended to perform pituitary MR and lumbar puncture for further confirmation.

1. Burst hyperthermia: The body temperature rises linearly and it can reach up to 40–41 °C. Hyperthermia can last for hours to days, eventually leading to the death of the patient. However, sometimes the body temperature can suddenly drop to normal.
2. The temperature of the trunk is high, followed by the temperature of the limbs. The body temperature can be asymmetric, and the difference sometimes exceeds 0.5 °C.
3. Although the patient is febrile, the toxemic symptoms are unremarkable, and there can be no history of chills.
4. No flushing of facial or body skin can be seen. On the contrary, the body skin can be generally dry, with hypohidrosis and cold limbs.
5. Generally, no increase in pulse and breathing accompanies the increased body temperature.

6. There is no evidence of infection. And the number of WBC usually keeps within the normal range. Or the amount of WBC increases while the ratio of different types of WBC remains the same.
7. Due to the dysfunction of thermoregulation, the patient's body temperature fluctuates with the changes in external temperature.
8. Antibiotics and antipyretic drugs (such as acetylsalicylic acid, etc.) are generally ineffective during hyperthermia. Due to the impairment of central thermoregulation, antipyretics are ineffective for decreasing –body temperature. However, chlorpromazine and cold therapy may work.

References

1. Wenxin S, Fengsheng C. Diagnosis and treatment of hypothalamic syndrome [J]. Chin J Pract Pediatr. 2006;21(11):806–8.
2. Chunlian W, Linyi H, Suting L. A case of hypothalamic syndrome caused by intracranial tumor [J]. Chin J Pediatr. 2004;42(12):958.
3. Qinghua G, Li Z, Yiming M, et al. The value of cerebrospinal fluid human chorionic gonadotropin measurement in the diagnosis and treatment of intracranial germinomas [J]. Chin J Intern Med. 2010;49(10):851–4.
4. Ogawa K, Shikama N, Toits T, et al. Long-term results of radiotherapy for intracranial germinoma. Int J Radiat Oncol Biol Phys. 2004;158:705–13.
5. Xin L, Fuquan Z, Ke H, et al. Analysis of the therapeutic efficacy of radiotherapy in 74 cases of intracranial germinomas [J]. Chin J Radiat Oncol. 2009;18(3):173–5.
6. Bloom H. Primary intracranial germ cell tumors. Clin Oncol. 1983;2:233–57.
7. Liang L, Korogi Y, Sugahara T, et al. MRI of intracranial germcell tumors. Neuroradiology. 2002;44(5):382–8.

5.4 Pseudo-fever

Chen Shu

A 17-year-old female was admitted to the hospital because of a persistent fever for more than 2 months.

The patient started with a cough and a sore throat 2 months ago. There was a gradual increase in body temperature up to 40 °C, accompanied by fear of cold and irregular fever, no chills. During the course of the disease, the patient had pain in the left shoulder and left knee, occasional headache and dizziness, no rash, no abdominal pain, no diarrhea, no urinary urgency, no urinary frequency, or other concomitant symptoms. She was considered to have a cold and given antipyretic and anti-infective treatment in the community hospital, which did not work. And then she consulted the local hospital. All the results were negative, including blood culture, sputum culture, chest X-ray, bone marrow aspiration, chest CT, ENA/ANA/anti-ds-DNA/ESR, and Widal test. She was treated with penicillin, cephalosporin, levofloxacin, and other antibiotics at the hospital, but did not achieve the expected effect. Now she was admitted to our hospital for further diagnosis and treatment.

5.4.1 Admission Checkup

The general condition was well, and no significant abnormalities were observed.

5.4.2 Diagnosis and Treatment

After checking her three routines, blood culture, sputum to find antacid bacillus, serology, and autoimmunology indicators, we got nothing but negative results. Nor did we find anything positive in chest X-ray, B-ultrasound, heart ultrasound, electrocardiogram, or other imaging tests. Anti-infection treatment was ineffective. We considered the possibility of connective tissue disease and then applied hormone therapy, but no significant effects occurred. Over the course of the treatment, the nurse coincidentally found her hand temperature normal when touching her hand to give an injection, while the patient's self-reported body temperature was 38.5 °C. After that, the nurse personally measured the patient's axillary temperature to be 36.7 °C and rectal temperature 37.3 °C. She immediately reported it to the doctors in charge and drew their attention. After discussion, the possibility of pseudo-fever was taken into consideration. All treatment was soon stopped and the nurse was asked to test the patient's temperature in person. The nurse took her temperature several times afterwards, and the outcomes were all normal. The doctor let the family out and communicated with the patient directly. At this time, the patient confessed that she was facing the college entrance examination and was too burdened. She did not perform well in her study and therefore felt stressed out about going on to higher education. So, she tried to use her illness to escape from her studies. After psychological counseling, the patient was discharged, and the family was instructed to provide psychological support. No fever was reported in the follow-up phone call (Fig. 5.4).

5.4.3 Comments

The onset of pseudo-fever is mostly in young and middle-aged people, especially among those stressed ones who are close to graduation or examinations. The clinical manifestations are good appetite, good spirits, no fever at night; all auxiliary tests are normal, and antibiotic treatment is ineffective. The diagnosis is usually confirmed after a strict observation of body temperature and exclusion of other diseases.

Pseudo-fever is involved in many cases of fevers of unknown origin and accounts for 1%–3% in total. Although the proportion is not high, it should not be neglected to avoid misdiagnosis and mistreatment. In fact, it is not difficult to identify pseudo-fever; usually, the fact that the skin temperature does not correspond to the fever is an important clue to the suspicion of pseudo-fever, the same with heart rate not increasing accordingly with fever and the absence of sweating during fever reduction. In addition, the body temperature of these patients does not change at different times of the day. And the patient lacks the common manifestations of fever, such as

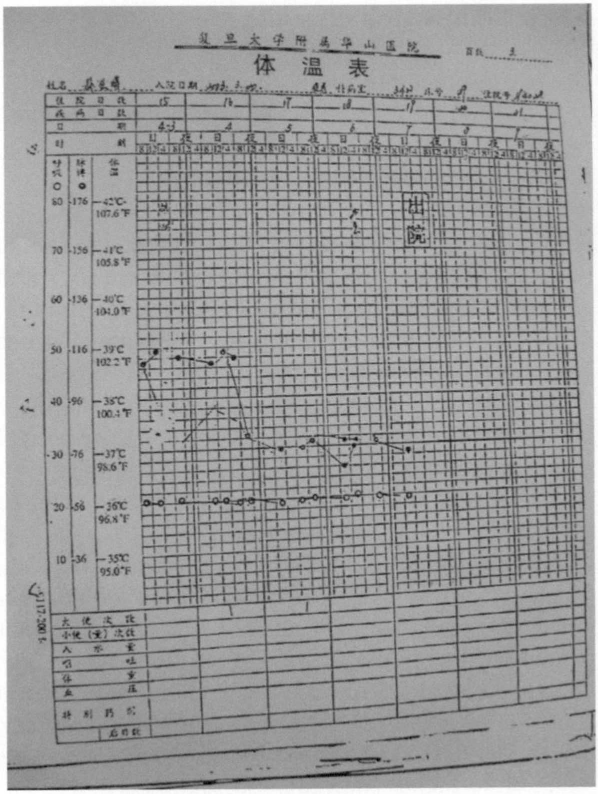

Fig. 5.4 The thermometer shows that the fever pattern of the patient was continuously high and maintained at about 39 degrees with little fluctuation. The body temperature was completely normal after monitoring her temperature measurement

chills, skin flushing, etc. In this case, we should watch out for the possibility of false body temperature reports. The medical staff can make a diagnosis based on the points above, and reveal the true cause by monitoring the body temperature.

5.5 Entered with Fever and Symptoms of Encephalitis, Suspected as Viral Encephalitis Initially, and Diagnosis Confirmed with MELAS (Mitochondrial Encephalomyopathy, Lactic Acidosis and Stroke-Like Episodes) at Last

Zhu Chong, Li Ning, and Zhang Jiming

On January 6, 2016, a 20-year-old woman presented to our institution with recurrent headache, fever, and altered mental status for 1 month.

On the night of December 7, 2015, the patient developed a bilateral tension headache without an obvious cause, accompanied by nausea and vomiting, which was non-ejection. At 8 am the next day, she had mental and behavioral disorders in school, such as speech disorder, failure to recognize people, accompanied by fever (up to 37.8 °C), severe headache, nausea, and vomiting. The patient was then sent to the neurology department of the local hospital for hospitalization. She was treated with foscarnet sodium, acyclovir (dose details were unknown), and methylprednisolone 0.5 g for 3 days. The patient's condition did not improve and was further aggravated. During hospitalization, the patient had epileptic seizures twice, manifested as sudden right gaze of both eyes, accompanied by disturbance of consciousness, lasting for about 1–3 min, and was given oral oxcarbazepine and levetiracetam (dose details were unknown) to control the symptoms. As her symptoms continued, further diagnosis and treatment needed to be implemented in our department. The patient's medical history showed hearing loss in both ears in May 2015, diagnosis of moderate nerve deafness by audiometry. The patient's mother had been short and had hearing loss for several years.

5.5.1 Physical Exam

On examination, the patient was alert. Her temperature was 37 °C; heart rate was 98 beats/min; breath frequency was 20 times/min; blood pressure was 124/79 mmHg, with the height of 156 cm and the weight of 35 kg. She had maldevelopment, poor nutrition, malaise, irrelevant answers, indifferent reaction, passive contact and communication, free movement, and lack of cooperation during the physical exam. There were no abnormal findings in the physical examination of the chest and abdomen. The muscle strength of the limbs was grade 4, and the muscle tension was decreased. The physiological reflexes were normal, and the pathologic reflexes were not elicited. She found it difficult to stand with eyes closed; the finger-to-nose test and heel-to-shin test could not be completed. There was no abnormality in deep and superficial sensation.

5.5.2 Assessment and Treatment Plan

Blood test: white blood cell: 13.31 × 10^9/L, neutrophil: 78.9%, red blood cell: 3.77 × 10^{12}/L, platelet: 278 × 10^9/L. Liver function: ALT 94 μ/L, AST 52 μ/L, creatine kinase 65 μ/L, LDH 362 μ/L; blood lipids: cholesterol 7.49 mmol/L, triglyceride 2.09 mmol/L, HDL 1.85 mmol/L, LDL 5.25 mmol/L. fasting blood lactic acid: 2.99 mmol/L, fasting blood glucose: 3.9 mmol/L, HbA!c 6.1%; OGTT: fasting glucose: 4.10 mmol/L, half-hour glucose: 5.60 mmol/L, 1 h glucose: 8 mmol/L, 2 h glucose: 9.20 mmol/L, 3 h glucose: 9.10 mmol/L. Thyroid function: TSH: 1.31 mIU/L, TT3: 1.02 mmol/L, TT4: 108.1 mmol/L, FT3: 3.77 mmol/L, FT4: 11.5 mmol/L; EBV-IgM (−), EBV-IgG (+), EBV-IgA (−). ANA: 1:100, other autoimmune indexes were normal. Cerebrospinal fluid biochemistry: glucose 2.90 mmol/L, chlorine 116 mmol/L, protein 394 mg/L. Cerebrospinal fluid routine: colorless, clear, Pan's test ±, RBC 146 × 106/L, WBC 8 × 106/L. T-SPOT: negative. The levels of Parathyroid Hormone (PTH) and prolactin were 3.9 ng/L and 42.01 ng/mL, respectively.

Electroencephalogram (December 8, 2015): abnormal electroencephalogram, a large number of wide-range б waves, slow spike-waves were seen in both hemispheres, which were periodic, and the left temporal and occipital parts was obvious.

Head MRI (December 11, 2015): high T2 signal and high Diffusion-Weighted Imaging (DWI) signal in the left temporal occipital lobe; Magnetic Resonance Angiography (MRA) was normal.

Head MRI (December 31, 2015): swelling of the left temporal occipital lobe and right temporal cortex, high T2W signal, high DWI signal; no obvious abnormality was found in MRA. There was progress compared with the MRI on December 11.

Head CT (December 31, 2015): low-density lesions in the left occipitotemporal lobe and right temporal lobe, bilateral basal ganglia calcification (Fig. 5.5).

ECG (January 9, 2016): sinus arrhythmia, T wave change.

Echocardiography (January 14, 2016): normal.

Electromyography (January 11, 2016): myogenic damage was found in some muscles of upper limbs.

The characteristics of the patient's medical history: (1) 20-year-old female; (2) an acute onset, with "fever + encephalopathy" as the core symptom; (3) short stature, family history of nerve deafness; (4) transcranial lesions mainly involving the cortex on MRI, bilateral basal ganglia calcification on CT; (5) suspected maternal inherited disease. In conclusion, we clinically diagnosed mitochondrial encephalomyopathy, lactic acidosis, and stroke-like episodes (MELAS). In order to further confirm the diagnosis, we will send blood samples of this patient and her mother for gene testing. The results of gene detection showed that both the patient and her mother had a heterozygous mutation of mitochondrial gene m.3243A > G (Fig. 5.6), and the patient was finally diagnosed as MELAS.

Meanwhile, after the clinical diagnosis of MELAS, we began to give this patient intravenous arginine 1 g qd, levocarnitine 3 g qd, butylphthalide 25 mg bid, lipoic acid 0.6 g qd, oral coenzyme Q10 20 mg tid, levetiracetam 500 mg qd, oxcarbazepine 150 mg qd, quetiapine 25 mg qn, and rosuvastatin 20 mg QD. After that, the patient's symptoms gradually improved steadily. By the time of discharge on January 27, 2016, the patient had no headache, speech confusion, or convulsions, but still had a weak reaction and less active speech. The patient was followed up in the outpatient department of our hospital on April 5, 2016, and the symptoms basically disappeared: no headache, vomiting, epileptic seizure, or abnormal mental behavior but had memory loss compared with that before the disease onset. Physical exam: clear mind, alert, fluent answers, quick response, automatic posture, physical exam cooperation. The muscle strength of the limbs was grade 4 and had normal muscle tension as well as normal physiological reflexes. She was difficult to stand with eyes closed and had no pathological reflex, with negative finger-to-nose test and negative heel-to-shin test. There was no abnormality in deep and superficial sensation. Head MRI (April 5, 2016) showed old lesions in the left temporal occipital lobe, high T2WI signal, and no obvious abnormality on DWI. Now the patient is being treated with oral L-carnitine, coenzyme Q10, vitamin B2, and levetiracetam.

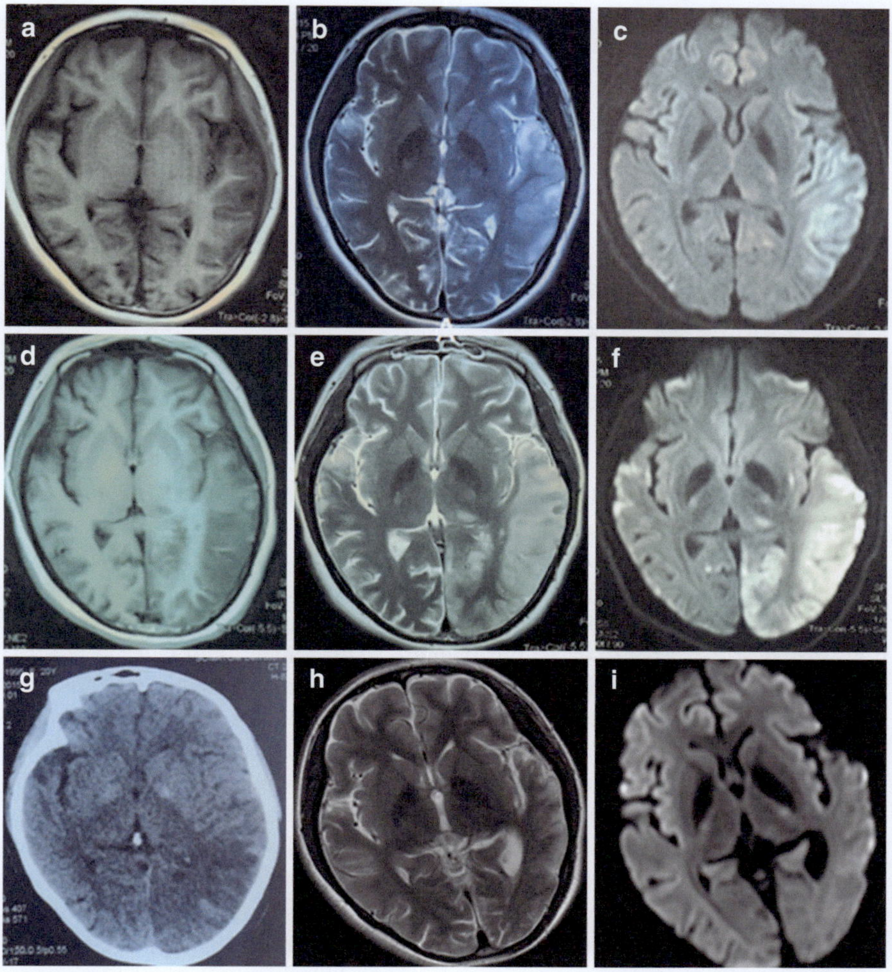

Fig. 5.5 Head MRI. (**a**) (2015-12-11): Abnormal signal is seen in the left temporal occipital lobe, showing low signal on T1WI; (**b**) (2015-12-11): Corresponding to the lesion in Image a, the left temporal occipital lobe presents high signal on T2WI; (**c**) (2015-12-11): The aforementioned left temporal occipital lobe lesion shows high signal on DWI; (**d**) (2015-12-31): Swelling is observed in the left occipitotemporal lobe and right temporal lobe cortex, with low signal on T1WI; (**e**) (2015-12-31): Corresponding to the swollen lesions in Image d, high signal is noted on T2WI; (**f**) (2015-12-31): The swollen lesions in Images d-e show high signal on DWI; these findings are deteriorated compared with the lesions in Images a-c (2015-12-11); (**g**) (2015-12-31): Low signal foci are seen in the left occipitotemporal lobe and right temporal lobe cortex; calcification is present in the bilateral basal ganglia (arrow); (**h**): Old lesions are present in the left temporal occipital lobe, manifesting as high signal intensity on T2WI. (**i**) (2016-04-05): No obvious abnormal signal is detected on DWI corresponding to the old lesions in Image h

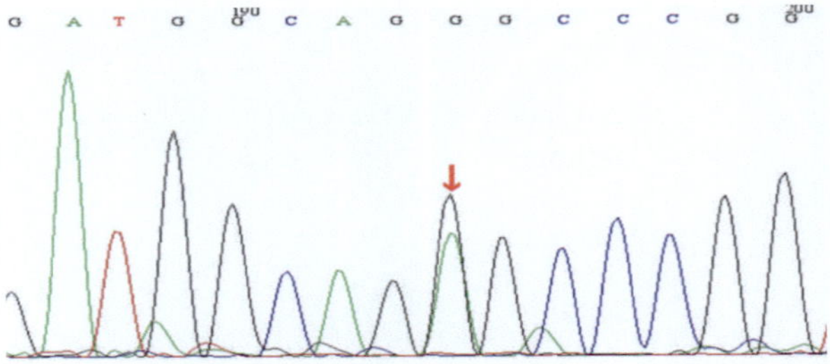

Fig. 5.6 Gene test results. The red arrow indicates the m.3243A > G mutation

5.5.3 Comments

MELAS is one of the most common types of mitochondrial diseases, which often occurs in youth before 20 years old, and sometimes occurs in middle-aged and older people. Stroke is the typical manifestation, which has the characteristics of maternal inheritance, and has typical neuroimaging and muscle biopsy. 80% of MELAS is considered to be caused by m.3243A > G.

The clinical manifestations of mitochondrial encephalomyopathy are different, so it is difficult to make an early diagnosis. Due to the lack of understanding or limited examination by doctors, especially doctors from the department of infectious diseases, it is easy to cause misdiagnosis. This patient with fever, headache, and vomiting as the initial symptoms was misdiagnosed as viral encephalitis. The reasons may be as follows: (1) same clinical manifestations as viral encephalitis (fever, headache, vomiting, convulsions, and mental disorders); (2) abnormal EEG; and (3) similar lesions (temporal lobe and temporal occipital lobe). However, the cerebrospinal fluid examination of this patient was basically normal, and antiviral therapy as well as large-dose hormone therapy did not have any effect. It is important that the patient had the characteristics of bilateral moderate nerve deafness and short stature, which were similar to her mother and suspected of maternal inheritance. On head MRI, the lesions mainly involved the cortex and appeared repeatedly. On head CT, the calcification of bilateral basal ganglia was proven, which was unique to MELAS, but viral encephalitis rarely occurred. Although there were recurrent encephalitis-like manifestations, we should be highly alert to the possibility of MELAS. We should detect the blood lactate level, arterial blood gas analysis, and perform a head MRI scan. When we find that there are multiple abnormal signal foci in the brain with nonparallel vascular distribution, combined with muscle biopsy and mitochondrial gene detection, we can make a clear diagnosis. The prognosis of patients with MELAS varies greatly. Patients often suffer from limb paralysis, progressive mental retardation, and even dementia due to the superimposed effect of recurrent seizures or stroke mimics seizures. Therefore, early diagnosis and timely as well as long-term maintenance treatment are very important to improve the prognosis of patients.

References

1. El-Hattab AW, Adesina AM, Jones J, et al. MELAS syndrome: clinical manifestations, pathogenesis, and treatment options[J]. Mol Genet Metab. 2015,116(1–2):4–12.
2. Lorenzoni PJ, Werneck L C, Kay CSK, et al. When should MELAS (Mitochondrial myopathy, Encephalopathy, Lactic Acidosis, and Stroke-like episodes) be the diagnosis?[J]. Arq Neuro-Psiquiatr. 2015;73(11):959–67.
3. Parikh S, Goldstein A, Koenig MK, et al. Diagnosis and management of mitochondrial disease: a consensus statement from the Mitochondrial Medicine Society[J]. Genet Med. 2015;17(9):689–701.
4. Nesbitt V, Pitceathly RDS, Turnbull DM, et al. The UK MRC Mitochondrial Disease Patient Cohort Study: clinical phenotypes associated with the m.3243A>G mutation—implications for diagnosis and management[J]. J Neurol Neurosurg Psychiatry. 2013;84(8):936–8.
5. Yatsuga S, Povalko N, Nishioka J, et al. MELAS: a nationwide prospective cohort study of 96 patients in Japan[J]. Biochim Biophys Acta (BBA) – Gen Subj. 2012;1820(5):619–24.

5.6 Acute Disseminated Encephalomyelitis Easily Misdiagnosed as Viral Meningoencephalitis

Li Ning and Zhang Jiming

A 29-year-old man was admitted to the hospital on December 11, 2014, with fever and head discomfort for half a month. The patient felt uncomfortable after catching a cold on the morning of November 27, 2014, and felt "cold" without attention or treatment. He played football in the rain on the afternoon of November 30, then chills and fever appeared at night with a peak of 39 °C. The patient sweated a lot and his body temperature dropped after taking analgin, but presented with projectile vomiting twice without warning. The stomach contents were vomited about 300 mL; no abnormality of blood color or coffee color was observed. Sore throat and runny nose appeared then. The next day (December 1), he went to a local hospital. The blood routine test showed that white blood cells: 6.56×10^9/L, neutrophil ratio: 66%, monocyte ratio: 11.1%, platelets: 237×10^9/L, Hemoglobin (HB): 142 g/L. Chest X-ray: no obvious substantial lesions were seen. Considering infectious diseases, oral cefdinir was prescribed by doctors, but chills and fever still existed with a peak value of 39.7 °C; from December 2nd, he was given intravenous cefoxitin intravenous therapy, but there was no improvement; On December 3, the peak temperature was 38.9 °C, and the fever could be reduced by the administration of indomethacin. On December 4, the patient's peak temperature rose again to 40.2 °C, and new symptoms such as difficulty in passing urine and stool, mild abdominal distension, and mild weakness of the lower limbs appeared. He went to the central hospital of the district and rechecked the blood routine: white blood cell:

8.06×10^9/L, the ratio of neutrophils: 69.9%, the ratio of monocytes: 14%, a lumbar puncture on cerebrospinal fluid (CSF) pressure (December 8): 295 cmH $_2$O, CSF routine: 80% red blood cells, 40% white blood cells, and 86% lymphocytes. CSF biochemical examinations: protein 2615 mg/L, glucose 2.0 mmol/L (synchronous blood glucose 6.5), chlorine 110 mol/L. Cranial MRI plain scan showed scattered ischemia in the bilateral deep frontal and parietal lobes and abnormal signals in the left posterior frontal lobe. On the evening of December 8, the patient was clear, but he was more excited and talked a lot; after falling asleep, he gradually started talking nonsense and other situations, and returned to normal the next morning. Considering central nervous system infections, doctors administered anti-microbial agents including intravenous penicillin, ceftriaxone, and moxifloxacin; antiviral agents including acyclovir, ribavirin, and dexamethasone (specific usage and dosage are unknown). During the treatment, the body temperature would temporarily decrease, but the patient still had chills and fever every day, the peak temperature was slightly lower than before, mostly within 38.5 °C. Also, the patient still had a headache, poor mental state, difficulty in defecation, abdominal distension, no improvement of lower limb weakness, and developed chest distress and tachypnea. Then he came to our hospital's emergency department on December 10, and the blood test: white blood cells: 8.25×10^9/L, neutrophil ratio: 89%, monocyte ratio: 11.9%, platelets 326×10^9/L, HB 141 g/L, CT scan of the lower abdomen: the abdominal intestines are obviously dilated (Fig. 5.7). Blood gas analysis (oxygen inhalation 2 L/min): PH 7.512, carbon dioxide partial pressure 4.46 kPa, oxygen partial pressure 16.68 kPa, oxygen saturation 99%. For further diagnosis and treatment, he was admitted to our ward on December 11. Since the illness, the patient's mental state is normal, the appetite is good, but the sleep is not good with insomnia.

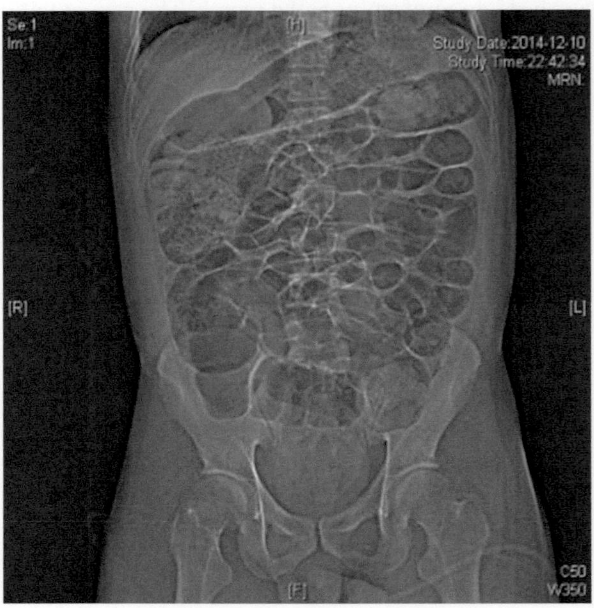

Fig. 5.7 Obvious dilatation of part of the intestine

From December 4, the patient gradually developed abdominal distension and difficulty in urination and defecation. He was given an indwelling urinary catheter, glycerin enema, and an oral administration of lactulose, and then a small amount of stool was discharged. There has been no significant change in weight recently.

History: physical fitness, regular exercise, and a denied history of major and recent trauma. Suffered from nephritis when young (about 6 or 7 years old), and was cured without recurrence.

5.6.1 Physical Examinations

General condition: On examination, the patient was conscious, responsive to questions, and well-oriented; she/he had normal calculation ability, normal development, and good nutritional status. The patient was admitted to the ward with a passive posture and was able to cooperate in examinations. Chest, heart, and lungs: normal. Abdomen: abdominal distension, percussion drum sounds, abdomen soft, deep abdominal pressure pain of full abdomen, no rebound tenderness, Murphy's sign was negative, bowel sounds: 2 times/min. Extremities: no edema in both lower limbs. The muscle strength of both upper limbs was basically normal, and the muscle strength of both lower limbs was decreased (grade III), with normal muscle tone. Nervous system: normal physiological reflexes, pathological reflexes were not elicited.

5.6.2 Case History

Routine blood examination after admission was as follows: HB: 145 g/L, white blood cell count: 10.82×10^9/L, neutrophil %: 81.20%, platelet count: 334×10^9/L. ESR: 7 mm/h. Liver function: alanine transaminase: 84 U/L, lactate dehydrogenase: 327 U/L, γ-glutamyl transferase: 84 U/L, α-hydroxybutyrate dehydrogenase: 256 U/L, total bile acid: 11 μmol/L, bilirubin, muscle anhydride normal. Electrolytes: potassium: 4.60 mmol/L, sodium: 133 mmol/L, chloride: 95 mmol/L. The coagulation function is basically normal. CSF pressure: 170 mmH2O, CSF biochemistry examinations: chlorine: 111 mmol/L, CSF sugar: 1.80 mmol/L (synchronous blood sugar: 6.6 mmol/L), CSF protein: 3747 mg/L; CSF routine: monocytes: 85%, coenocytes: 15%, Pan's test: (3+), red blood cells: 4×10^6/L, white blood cells: 189×10^6/L.

In regard to treatment, purulent meningitis could not be excluded temporarily, so we administered antiviral treatment, dexamethasone (5 mg q12h) for anti-inflammation, and meropenem plus vancomycin for antimicrobial treatment. Also, we used dehydration to reduce cranial pressure, replenished energy and electrolytes, promoted gastrointestinal peristalsis and relieved defecation, and provided other symptomatic treatment.

However, the patient's condition progressed rapidly. He complained of abdominal distension and lower limb weakness on the next day (12.12), accompanied by fever and shortness of breath, with 95% terminal oxygen (3 L/min oxygen inhalation), heart rate 100 beats/min, regular rhythm, and neck rigidity is slightly less than before, and there is still resistance. Cardiopulmonary examination is the same as before, but abdominal distension and tension have increased. Slight depression and edema of both lower limbs were observed. Proximal muscle strength of both upper limbs Grade II, grip strength Grade II, both upper limbs tendon reflex (+++), Hoffman sign on the left (+), right (−); abdomen reflex (−), muscle strength of both lower limbs Grade III, tendon reflexes (±), pathological signs (−), and deep and shallow sensations below four-4 on both sides disappear or decrease. We urgently call a neurology consultation and consider spinal cord disease: Acute Disseminated Encephalomyelitis (ADEM)? It is recommended to perform an MRI of the thoracic spine centered on the T4 and reexamine the head MRI and high-dose glucocorticoids therapy after controlling the infection. We then completed the relevant examinations urgently, the head MRI showed: Some pia mater were enhanced with abnormal signal shadow in the bilateral basal ganglia region. The local mucosa of the bilateral maxillary sinus was thickened (Fig. 5.8). An MRI of the thoracic vertebra indicated that there were multiple abnormal signals in the thoracic medulla at the level of scan field T1–7. The inflammation could not rule out the uniformity of the signals in the lumbar medulla, and no obvious abnormal enhancement was observed after enhancement (Fig. 5.9). At this time, we considered that ADEM was

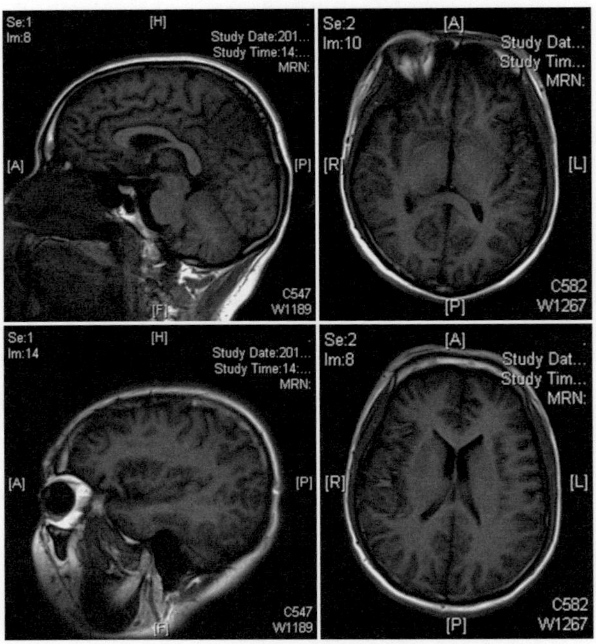

Fig. 5.8 Cranial MRI enhancement (December 12, 2014): speckled abnormal signal shadow was seen in bilateral basal ganglia, FLAIR cerebral sulcus in the posterior occipital region was blurred, no obvious abnormal signal shadow was seen in the parenchyma of the remainder brain, no obvious abnormal signal shadow was seen in the size and shape of the ventricle system, and no displacement was observed in the midline structure. After enhancement, the partial pia meninges were enhanced with linear enhancement of local mucosal thickening in the bilateral maxillary sinus

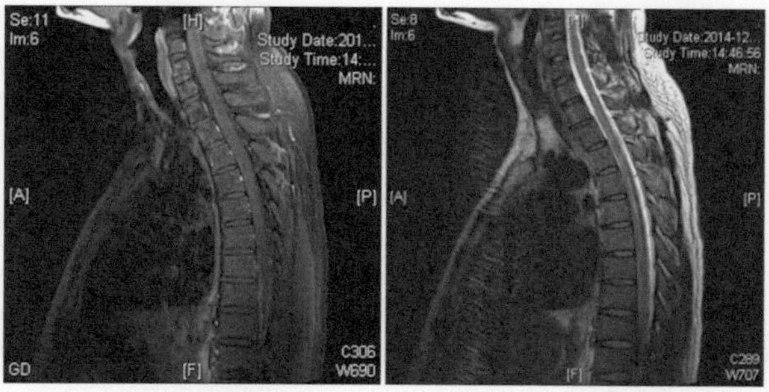

Fig. 5.9 MRI enhancement of thoracic vertebrae centered on thoracic 4 (December 12, 2014): there was physiological curvature of thoracic vertebrae, and no obvious bone hyperplasia was observed at the vertebral body margin; at the level of scanning field T1–7, there seemed to be small patches of abnormal signal shadow in the thoracic medulla, and there were no signs of bulging herniation in the thoracic intervertebral disc after enhancement

highly possible. On the third day of admission (12.13), based on the effective antimicrobial therapy, large amounts of glucocorticoids (methylprednisolone 1 g qd) were given for 3 days, and gamma globulin for 5 days (30 g/d), combined with life support therapy. On the same day, the patient's peak body temperature began to drop to 38 °C, and the general condition improved, and there was no obvious swelling of the lower limbs. Abdominal distension had relieved, and he had more anal exhaust, a small amount of paste-like stools in normal color. The muscle strength and tension of the limbs were the same as before, the depth of sensation below T4 on both sides of the chest disappeared or decreased, and the sensory level did not change significantly. From the third day of glucocorticoid therapy (December 15), the patient began to feel better, and his mental state improved. The peak body temperature was controlled at about 38 °C, and vital signs, such as blood pressure, heart rate, and breathing, became stable. Abdominal distension is further relieved, and the anus has more exhaust and defecation, the stools were unformed, paste-like in normal color. The muscle strength of both upper limbs is basically normal, and the muscle strength of both lower limbs is slightly improved compared with the previous one, belonging to grade I, tendon reflex (±), pathological signs (−), sensory disturbance level begins to drop (1–2 cm lower than before). On December 16, the patient's body temperature fluctuated with a peak value of 38.5 °C. Due to the patient being on high-dose glucocorticoids for many days, and the current ADEM-related symptoms and signs becoming better, the patient's body temperature rebounded. Blood routine test reexaminations: white blood cell count: 21.97×10^9/L, Neutrophils%: 91.50%, platelet count: 244×10^9/L, hemoglobin: 135 g/L, combined with the patient's lung lesions and tachypnea, were highly correlated with lung bacterial infections or fungal infections. Therefore, on the basis of the current anti-infection treatment plan, itraconazole for antifungal therapy is added. On physical examination, the level of sensory disturbance was lowered by 2 cm again. Combined with the recommendations of the neurology consultation, the glucocorticoids were gradually reduced: 500 mg/d × 5d, 240 mg/d × 5d, 120 mg/d × 5d. After that, the patient's sensory disturbance level decreased daily at a rate of 1–2 cm/d. Although fever was still present, the peak body temperature started to reduce (37.5–38 °C), and the blood routine test, heart rate, and respiratory rate gradually fell to the normal range. Abdominal distension and difficulty in defecation were almost relieved. Upper limb muscle strength recovered well, but lower extremity muscle strength was still poor (only Class I). The sensory disturbance level had dropped below the symphysis surface when discharged on December 26. After the patient was discharged from the hospital, the glucocorticoids were reduced, and the patient continued exercising. As of the latest follow-up (April 2015), the patient's lower limbs had returned to normal, and the muscle strength of both lower limbs had returned to grade IV.

5.6.3 Discussion

Acute disseminated encephalomyelitis (ADEM) is an acute inflammatory demyelinating disease that extensively affects the white matter of the central nervous system, mediated by cellular immunity. ADEM is an autoimmune disease targeting the myelin protein of the central nervous system. The disease usually occurs after infection (such as mycoplasma pneumonia, Epstein-Barr virus, or cytomegalovirus infection etc.), rash (measles, chickenpox, smallpox, and rubella), or vaccination (rabies vaccine, smallpox vaccine). It is a kind of activated immune disorder syndrome.

This patient was featured with a sudden onset of fever, headache, and transient mental disorders. At the beginning, the symptoms were very similar to viral encephalitis, but then the disease progressed with difficulty in defecation, progressive decline in muscle strength, sensory disturbances, and even paraplegia, which were not consistent with viral encephalitis, and the final diagnosis was ADEM. The patient should have had the experience of viral infection at the beginning of the disease, and then, within 1–2 weeks, he developed sensory disturbance below T4, significant decrease in muscle strength of the limbs, and difficulty in urination and defecation, which belong to transverse myelitis. Transverse myelitis might be associated with recent viral or bacterial infection and could be secondary to immune injury. The viruses involved in the pathogenesis of transverse myelitis include coxsackie virus, ECHO, cytomegalovirus, herpes zoster virus, measles virus, enterovirus and so on. For bacteria, it includes *Mycobacterium, Pneumococcus,* and *Legionella.* Moreover, ADEM could be accompanied by encephalitis, causing encephalomyelitis in patients. In order to clarify the correlation between viral infection and viral infection-related immune encephalitis or encephalomyelitis, it is urgent to establish virological examinations.

References

1. Menge T, Hemmer B, Nessler S, et al. Acute disseminated encephalomyelitis: an update Arch Neurol. 2005;62(11):1673–80.

2. Rossi A. Imaging of acute disseminated encephalomyelitis. Neuroimaging Clin N Am. 2008;18(1):149–61.
3. Qiang D. Analysis of clinical features of 86 cases of acute disseminated encephalomyelitis [J]. J Chongqing Med Univ. 2007;(08):874–6.
4. Caigui G, Xiaoyi W, Limeng D, et al. MRI differentiation between viral encephalitis and acute disseminated encephalomyelitis[J]. J Clin Radiol. 2005;(02):112–5.
5. Chuanzhen L. Neurology. Fudan University.

5.7 IgG4-Related Disease Onset with Fever Accompanied by Multiple Lymph Node Enlargement

Zhu Haoxiang, Sun Feng, and Zhang Jiming

A 59-year-old male was admitted to our hospital on November 22, 2016, due to "fever for more than 2 months."

The patient reported no obvious cause of fever since September 20, 2016, with the highest temperature of 38.2 °C, which was obvious in the afternoon. He took medicine by himself and began to develop a systemic wheal-like rash that afternoon without special treatment. He went to the local hospital on September 26, and the blood routine test showed a white blood cell count level of 13.11×10^9/L, a hemoglobin level of 118 g/L, a platelet level of 373×10^9/L, a C-reactive protein (CRP) level of greater than 5 mg/L, an erythrocyte sedimentation rate(ESR) level of 56 mm/h. His chest CT showed diffuse miliary shadow in both lungs. The local physician did not give him specific treatment, and the condition did not improve. On October 4, 2016, he went to another hospital, and his laboratory examination showed an albumin level of 28.7 g/L, a globulin level of 42.4 g/L, a rheumatoid factor level of 242 IU/mL, and a CRP level of 36.5 mg/L. His blood culture was negative four times. On October 8, reexamination of chest CT showed multiple small nodules in the left lung, implying multiple inflammatory proliferative foci, with little pleural effusion on both sides. The patient was treated with dexamethasone and loratadine for antiallergic treatment. The patient was discharged from the hospital when his symptoms were relieved with normal body temperature and subsiding rash. The patient was readmitted to the hospital because of recurring fever and rash in November 2016. Chest CT (November 7) showed enlarged multiple lymph nodes with peripheral exudation changes in the mesenteric root and retroperitoneum region; enlargement of the prostate with calcification; infection in the lower lobe of both lungs, and a little pleural effusion on both sides. Bone marrow smear (November 8) showed nucleated cells proliferated actively with obvious granulocytic proliferation, and the proportion of erythroid and lymphatic cells was low. Heteromorphic lymphocytes (2%), plasma cells (4%), and occasional hemophagocytes were seen on the bone marrow smear. The patient was prescribed with low-dose of methylprednisolone (dose unknown), but he still had a fever with rash. The physician stopped glucocorticoid use 2 days later due to positive fecal occult blood. His IGRA was higher than 400 pg/mL, so the local physicians considered that tuberculosis and lymphoma could not be excluded temporarily and arranged for his discharge. Then, triple antituberculosis therapy (INH + RFP + EMB) was initiated on November 8. Because of worsened rash, antituberculosis drugs were stopped after 3-day treatment. He was admitted to our hospital to clarify the diagnosis. Since the onset of the disease, the patient suffered from poor appetite and weight loss (5 kg).

5.7.1 Physical Examination

The temperature was 38.8 °C, the blood pressure 126/78 mmHg, the heart rate 88 beats per minute, and the respiratory rate 21 breaths per minute. The patient was conscious, with a slightly dispirited spirit. He had a general nutritional status, with slightly pale conjunctivae and no jaundice. Multiple lymph nodes were palpable in the whole body, especially the cervical and inguinal regions, with good mobility, normal texture, and no obvious tenderness. The remainder of the examination was normal.

5.7.2 Presentation of Cases

He was admitted to our hospital for further examination on November 23:

Blood routine: White blood cell 8.21×10^9/L; Neutrophil percentage 61%, Lymphocyte percentage 22%; Eosinophil percentage 15%; Hemoglobin: 96 g/L; Platelet 133×10^9/L. Urine routine: protein +. The remainder was normal.

Liver function: glutamic-pyruvic transaminase 13 U/L, glutamic-oxalacetic transaminase 12 U/L, total bilirubin <12.0 μmol/L, alkaline phosphatase 231 U/L, gamma-glutamyl transpeptidase 101 U/L, total protein 69 g/L, albumin 23 g/L, globulin 46 g/L, prealbumin 91 mg/L. Renal function, blood amylase, autoimmune antibodies were all normal. Tumor markers were all normal except for CA125 at 79.38 U/mL.

Erythrocyte sedimentation rate 109 mm/h, procalcitonin 0.09 ng/mL, C-reactive protein 10.6 mg/L, ferritin 603 ng/mL, RF-IgG: 77.5 U/mL.

Antibodies to nine respiratory pathogens, three sets of blood culture, urine culture, urine sediment for acid-fast bacilli; G test, latex agglutination test, HIV, RPR, and hepatitis markers were all negative.

T-SPOT.TB: positive (antigen A > 200, antigen B > 20).

EBV-DNA: 2.70×10^4 copies/mL.

Urinary series protein: urinary transferrin: 2.91 mg/L, urinary α-1 microglobulin: 109 mg/L, urinary immunoglobulin G: 39.4 mg/L, urinary albumin: 21.6 mg/L.

Immunoglobulin: IgG: 37 g/L, IgA: 1.47 g/L, IgM: 1.88 g/L, IgG4: 72.1 g/L.

Blood light chain: κ-light chain: 7.24 g/L, λ-light chain: 4.12 g/L, KAP/LAM: 1.76.

Urine light chain: urine-κ-light chain: 909 mg/L, urine-λ-light chain: 317 mg/L, urine KAP/LAM: 2.87.

Serum Immunofixation electrophoresis: positive for monoclonal Immunoglobulin IgG-lambda.

Urine immunofixation electrophoresis: No Bence-Jones protein was found.

Blood gas analysis was normal.

Chest CT scan: multiple inflammations in left upper lobe and bilateral lower lobe, with bilateral pleural effusion. Coronary artery calcification.

B-ultrasonography of lymph nodes and thyroid: follicular nodules of the right thyroid lobe, TI-RADS type 2. Multiple enlarged lymph node in right cervical (maximum 20 × 6 mm), bilateral supraclavicular (maximum 15 × 6 mm on the right, maximum 29 × 14 mm on the left), left axillary (maximum 16 × 10 mm), bilateral inguinal (maximum 49 × 9 mm on the right, maximum 47 × 9 mm on the left) region, especially obvious in the supraclavicular region, irregular in shape.

Bone marrow morphology: bone marrow hyperplasia, myeloid hyperplasia, and increased proportion of eosinophils and granulocytes were seen, mostly mature and a few naive, partially mature neutrophils with degeneration. Neutrophil Alkaline Phosphatase (NAP) points are high. The erythroid part has insufficient hemoglobin filling, and iron staining shows iron utilization disorders. A few abnormal lymphocytes and macrophages can be seen on the film. Plasma cells accounted for 3%.

Bone marrow biopsy: bone marrow biopsy shows 7–8 medullary cavities. Hematopoietic cells account for about 60%. Megakaryocytes can be seen, and there are no obvious abnormalities in hematopoietic cells of various lines. Reticular staining was negative.

Bone marrow flow cytometry was normal.

PET-CT: (1) Multiple patchy nodules of the lungs, multiple systemic lymph nodes, prostate, and seminal vesicle glands increased Fluorodeoxyglucose (FDG) metabolism, considering the possibility of inflammatory proliferative lesions. Lymph node biopsy is suggested to exclude neoplastic lesions, and the rest of the body (including the brain, lower extremities, etc.) PET-CT imaging showed no abnormal increase in FDG metabolism. (2) Left upper pulmonary branch dilatation, left lower lung bullae, bilateral pleural effusion, pelvic effusion; (3) Fatty liver, liver cyst, and cholecystitis; (4) Bone marrow and spleen FDG metabolism increased, considering the reactive hyperplasia; (5) Hyperosteogeny of cervical, thoracic, and lumbar vertebrae.

The biopsy of the left inguinal lymph node was performed on November 30. The lymph node pathology showed that the structure of the lymph node was still present, and the T cell in the paracortical area was highly proliferated with plasma cell infiltration. It was first considered Castleman's disease according to the histology and was recommended to exclude T-cell lymphoma by the T Cell Receptor (TCR) gene test. The TCR gene rearrangement was negative on December 16. On December 27, the pathology consultation by Shanghai Cancer Hospital reported lymphoid tissue hyperplasia, with immunohistochemistry of CD20 part+, CD3 part+, CD4 part+, CD8 minority+, CD10 focal+, PD -1 Minority+, CXCL13−, CD15−, CD30 scattered+, cyclin D1−, plasma cell IgG minority+, IgG4 part+, kappa part+, lambda part+; follicular dendritic cell CD21+; Ki-67+ (about 30%). There was no clonal rearrangement of TCRG, TCRB, and TCRD genes in the duplicate gene test.

Combined with morphology and immunophenotype, they tended to consider the patient as proliferative lymphoid tissues and focal dysplasia.

Because of the progressively increased level of IgG4 and bile enzyme during the patients' hospitalization, with the highest Alkaline Phosphatase (ALP) of 815 U/L and γ-GT of 3801 U/L, Magnetic Resonance Cholangiopancreatography (MRCP) was performed to rule out IgG4-related cholangitis. The MRCP result only showed the gallbladder body folds. At the same time, liver puncture was performed, whose pathology showed mild edema of liver cells and scattered spot necrosis, which was consistent with acute hepatitis. In addition, we found inflammatory injury of small bile ducts in portal tract, without inflammatory fibrosis changes. Hepatocytes had a small amount of vesicle lipidosis and eosinophil infiltration, and fibrinoid necrosis was suspected. The pathologist reminded us to differentiate the drug-induced liver damage. In addition, lymphoproliferative diseases (IgG4-related diseases) may also be considered. After communication with hematology and pathologists and reconsideration of the film (see Fig. 5.10 for details), the patient was finally diagnosed with an IgG4-related disease based on the patient's clinical manifestations and laboratory examinations.

We gave the patient methylprednisolone 40 mg per day since December 13 after the diagnosis of IgG4-related disease. The patient's temperature returned to normal on the next day, and the blood eosinophil ratio and count returned to normal after 3 days of treatment. The dose of methylprednisolone 40 mg per day was maintained for 2 weeks. Since the body temperature continued to be normal, and the indicators

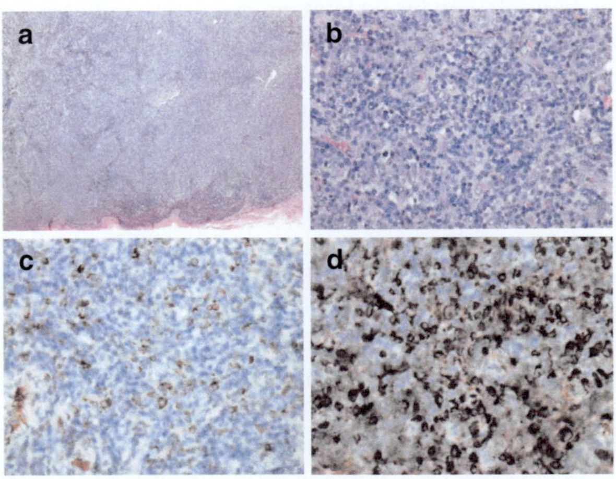

Fig. 5.10 The pathological and immunohistochemical results of the patient's inguinal lymph node biopsy. (**a**) The low-power microscope showed partial destruction of the lymph node structure, diffuse lesions in the paracortical area, reduced follicles, and no obvious fibrosis and sclerosis. (**b**) The lesions under high magnification are mainly immature plasma cells, accompanied by a large number of immunoblasts, histiocytes, and lymphocytes. Small blood vessels proliferate, but no hyaline degeneration, cell abnormalities are not obvious, and mitotic phases are few. (**c**) Immunohistochemical staining of IgG4, IgG4-positive cells are scattered in the field of high-power microscope, >10/HPF. (**d**) Immunohistochemical IgG staining, diffuse IgG-positive cell distribution under high-power microscope, but IgG4/IgG ratio <30%

improved, we gradually reduced his methylprednisolone. On January 16, 2017, we did the reexamination after 1 month of methylprednisolone treatment. The lymph node B-ultrasound showed that multiple lymphadenopathies in the cervical, supraclavicular, axillary, and inguinal region had disappeared, and the chest CT scan showed that the inflammation lesions and pleural effusion had been absorbed compared to that of 1 month ago. Blood routine test showed a white blood cell level of 14.75×10^9/L, eosinophil ratio of 0.2%, an erythrocyte sedimentation rate level of 34 mm/h, and his liver function returned to normal. The IgG4 level is 13.6 g/L, which is obviously lower than before. Blood immunofixation electrophoresis was negative. The steroid was reduced by one tablet per week, and one tablet every 2 weeks in the later period until the drug withdrawal.

5.7.3 Pathological Discussion

The clinical manifestation of IgG4-related diseases (IgG4-RD) is the enlargement of multiple organs or hyperplasia of nodules, which are caused by infiltration of IgG4-positive lymphoplasma cells, accompanied by fibrosis. IgG4-RD can involve multiple organs, most often in the pancreas (which can cause autoimmune pancreatitis (AIP)), biliary tract, salivary glands, lacrimal glands, retroperitoneal tissues, and lymph nodes. It can also involve organs and tissues such as the kidney, thyroid, and pituitary. It is usually a chronic inflammatory disease. Multiple organs are simultaneously or successively affected in most patients, but in some patients, only a single organ is affected. The clinical manifestations also vary greatly depending on the involved organs. Some will have serious complications, such as organ enlargement caused by compression and dysfunction caused by cell infiltration or fibrosis. Steroid treatment is often effective.

The patient started the disease with fever and multiple lymphadenopathies, accompanied by obvious wasting symptoms (anemia, hypoalbuminemia, etc.). After admission, it was found that eosinophil ratio and globulin IgG increased significantly, and the IgG4 level reached more than 30 times the normal value. Although there are many positive clues, the diagnosis is still very difficult. It is hard to be diagnosed even if we did various pathological examinations such as bone marrow biopsy, lymph node biopsy, and liver biopsy during hospitalization. Differentiating the IgG4-related diseases from Castleman disease is the hardest part. The final diagnosis of IgG4-related diseases is the comprehensive consideration of consultation with a hematologist and pathologist, and the effectiveness of glucocorticoid therapy. We have a certain understanding of IgG4-related diseases through this case report.

References

1. Stone JH, Zen Y, Deshpande V. Igg4-related disease. N Engl J Med. 2012;366(6):539–51.
2. Caruthers MN, Khosroshahi A, Augustin T, et al. The diagnostic utility of serum igg4 concentrations in igg4-related disease. Ann Rheum Dis. 2015;74(1):14–8.

3. Izumi Y, Takeshita H, Moriwaki Y, et al. Multicentric castleman disease mimicking igg4-related disease: a case report. Mod Rheumatol. 2017;27(1):174–7.
4. Uehara T, Hamano H, Kawakami M, et al. Autoimmune pancreatitis-associated prostatitis: distinct clinicopathological entity. Pathol Int. 2008;58(2):118–25.
5. Khosroshahi A, Wallace ZS, Crowe JL, et al. Intemational consensus guidance treatement on the management and treatment of igg4-related disease. Arthritis Rheumatol. 2015;67(7):1688–99.
6. Zen Y, Nakanuma Y. lgg4-related disease: a cross-sectional study of 114 cases. Am J Surg Pathol. 2010;34(12):1812–9.

5.8 Hepatitis B Cirrhosis Complicated with Superior Mesenteric Vein Thrombosis with Fever, Abdominal Pain and Ascites Resembling Bacterial Peritonitis

Wang Ting, Yang Feifie, and Huang Yuxian

A 46-year-old female was admitted to the hospital for a 3-week fever with abdominal pain on October 8, 2016.

On September 15, 2010, the patient developed persistent epigastric pain with no obvious inducement, accompanied by paroxysmal colic, nausea, and vomiting of gastric contents 3–4 times a day, diarrhea 5–6 times a day, with yellow and watery stool. She had a fever with body temperature of 39 °C, accompanied by chills and no shivering, anorexia, and fatigue. The patient was diagnosed with "acute gastroenteritis" as a local hospital outpatient, and was given symptomatic treatment such as anti-infection, antispasmodic, and analgesic therapies. The symptoms of abdominal pain and abdominal distension did not improve; still feverish, the abdominal pain presented as total abdominal pain, and the abdominal distension aggravated progressively. On September 23, 2010, she was admitted to the local hospital. Physical examination showed abdominal tenderness, mild muscle guarding, rebound pain (+), shifting dullness (+). Abdominal B-ultrasound showed a large amount of ascites, cirrhosis, and splenomegaly. Abdominal paracentesis was performed and ascites routine examination showed that: Micro mixed, nucleated cell count 1180 × 106/L, lobulated nucleus 45%, lymphocyte 55%, ascites biochemical test showed that: total protein 19.3 g/L, albumin 12.7 g/L, lactic dehydrogenase 165 U/L, glucose 11.6 mmol/L, adenosine deaminase 11 U/L. Ascites bacterial culture (−), then the local hospital considered the diagnosis of "decompensated cirrhosis, spontaneous bacterial peritonitis", successively given ceftriaxone, ceftazidime and other anti-infection treatment, the abdominal pain of the patient was slightly relieved, body temperature returned to normal. But 5 days later, she developed fever again with body temperature above 38 °C, without obvious shivering, but abdominal pain and abdominal distension aggravated again. So, on October 8, 2010, she was admitted into our department for further diagnosis and treatment. Since the onset of the disease, the patient has had no obvious night sweats, no obvious weight loss, stool two times per day, into a paste, and no bloody stool. The patient had a history of "e antigen positive chronic hepatitis B" for 9 years. One year ago, he was diagnosed with compensated liver cirrhosis and received lamivudine antiviral therapy. During the treatment, HBV DNA decreased, but did not fall to the detection limit, and transaminase remained normal. He had a history of bilateral ovarian cyst resection more than 10 years ago, and had venous thrombosis in the lower and upper limbs after the operation. She had a history of mitral valve repair 9 years ago.

5.8.1 Physical Examination at Admission

Conscious, weary spirit, skin and sclera without obvious yellow staining, facial telangiectasia, suspicious liver palm. Low breath sounds in both lungs, and there were no obvious dry and wet rales. The heart rate was 100 beats per minute, and the rhythm was regular. No obvious pathological murmur was found in each valve auscultation area. Abdominal distention, abdominal wall veins exposed, tenderness positive in the right middle and lower abdomen, especially in the right lower abdomen, rebound pain positive, no muscle tension, Murphys (±), unsatisfied with liver and spleen palpation, whole abdominal percussion showed voiced sound, no hyperactivity of bowel sounds, no pitting edema in both lower limbs, and negative neuropathological signs.

Blood routine examination after admission: WBC $5.52 \times 10^9/L$, RBC $3.45 \times 10^{12}/L$, Hb 98 g/L, neutrophils 75.2%, monocytes 13.2%, platelets $88 \times 10^9/L$. Liver function test: ALT 19 μ/L, TBIL 22.8 μmol/L, ALB 29 g/L. Coagulation function test: prothrombin time 15.7 s, international standard ratio 1.48; ascites routine examination: yellow, turbid, Rivalta test 1 +, RBC 4320×10^6 L, nucleated cells count $440 \times 10^6/L$, 20% lymphocytes and 80% neutrophils; ascites biochemical examination: total protein 25 g/L, ascites adenosine deaminase negative, ascites exfoliated cells negative, ascites bacterial smear and culture negative, acid-fast stain of ascites smear and tuberculosis culture of ascites was negative. T-SPOT.TB test was negative. Antinuclear antibody and soluble nuclear antigen were negative. HBsAg positive. HBeAg positive, anti-HBC positive, HBV DNA 7.11×10^6 IU/mL, YMDD mutation positive. Abdominal B- ultrasound: cirrhosis, ascites, gallbladder wall rough thickening, splenomegaly. Chest X-ray, CT: chest postoperative changes, pneumonia in both lower lungs, left pleural effusion. The anti-infection therapy was adjusted to imipenem and cilastatin sodium, amikacin, metronidazole, vancomycin, and other anti-infection treatments, and diuretic and supportive therapy were strengthened. The patients continued to have high fever, persistent fever, persistent abdominal pain, and a large amount of ascites. X-ray abdominal plain film: see bowel gas and a small fluid level, no obvious obstruction or perforation sign. Abdominal CT: liver cirrhosis, massive ascites, splenomegaly, no mass. Abdominal CT venography- abdominal Computed Tomography Venography (CTV) (Figs. 5.11 and 5.12) found superior mesenteric vein thrombosis, tortuous dilation of the portal vein and its tributaries. The patient was diagnosed with "superior mesenteric vein thrombosis". After fasting, low molecular weight heparin anticoagulation, promoting blood circulation and removing blood stasis, and other comprehensive treatment, the symptoms of this patient were gradually relieved, and a good curative effect was achieved.

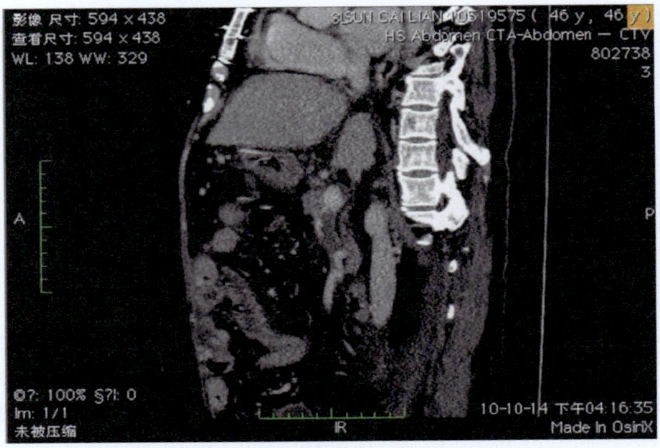

Fig. 5.11 Abdominal CTV showed a long filling defect in superior mesenteric vein

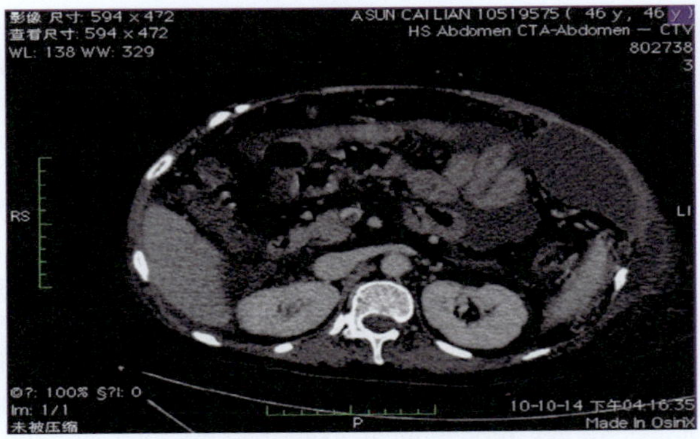

Fig. 5.12 Abdominal CTV showed a wedge-shaped filling defect in the section of the superior mesenteric vein

5.8.2 Comment

The clinical manifestations of mesenteric venous thrombosis (MVT) were not specific. The main clinical manifestations of mesenteric venous thrombosis are abdominal pain, abdominal distention, peritoneal irritation sign, bloody ascites, vomiting, fever, abdominal X-ray findings of intestinal gas, and liquid levels as well. The most common complications were intestinal infarction and peritonitis. MVT is easy to miss and misdiagnosed due to a lack of specific clinical manifestations. Enhanced CT can be used as a common diagnostic method, and its value is to reduce the potential risk of delayed treatment. Early diagnosis, timely anticoagulation and thrombolytic therapy are the keys to improving the prognosis, which can avoid further intestinal ischemia and necrosis and recover.

According to the results of etiological examination and therapeutic effect after admission, it is difficult to explain this case with "spontaneous bacterial peritonitis", whether there are other causes of fever, abdominal pain and ascites, such as focal abscess, intestinal obstruction or perforation, vascular disease, etc., especially the patient had "e antigen positive chronic hepatitis B, decompensated cirrhosis after hepatitis", Ascites, a hallmark of decompensated liver cirrhosis, is mildly bloody and composed mainly of nucleated cells. Considering that the patient had a history of venous thrombosis in the upper and lower limbs, and the patient had persistent fever, abdominal pain, and refractory ascites, this time we should be highly aware of the possibility of mesenteric venous thrombosis. Therefore, X-ray abdominal plain film, abdominal enhanced CT, and abdominal CTV are particularly important for the diagnosis. The diagnosis of this patient was finally confirmed by the above examination, and has achieved a good therapeutic effect.

References

1. Wiest R, Krag A, Gerbes A. Spontaneous bacterial peritonitis: recent guidelines and beyond. Gut. 2012;61:297–310.
2. Runyon BA. Management of adult patients with ascites due to cirrhosis: update 2012. Hepatology. 2013.
3. European Association for the Study of the Liver. EASL clinical practice guidelines on the management of ascites, spontaneous bacterial peritonitis, and hepatorenal syndrome in cirrhosis. J Hepatol. 2010;53:397–417.
4. Hotoleanu C, Andercou O, Andercou A. Mesenteric venous thrombosis: clinical and therapeutical approach. Int Angiol. 2008;27:462–5.
5. Niu YL, Zhang ST, Yu ZL, et al. Clinical characteristics of mesenteric venous thrombosis. Zhongguo Shiyong Neike Zazhi. 2007;27:603–5. (in Chinese).
6. Niu Yinglin, Zhang Shutian, Yu Zhonglin. Clinical characteristics of mesenteric venous thrombosis. Chin J Pract Internal Med. 2007;27:603–5.
7. Hedayati N, Riha GM, Kougias P, et al. Prognostic factors and treatment outcome in mesenteric vein thrombosis. Vasc Endovascular Surg. 2008;42:217–24.
8. Harnik IG, Brandt LJ. Mesenteric venous thrombosis. Vasc Med. 2010;15:407–18.
9. Zhang XC, Chen Zl, Ding XM, et al. The treatment of superior mensenteric venous thrombosis. Zhongguo Putong Waike Zazhi. 2010;19:655–8. (in Chinese).
10. Xicheng Z, Zhaolei C, Xiangmin D, et al. Treatment of superior mesenteric vein thrombosis. Chin J Gen Surg. 2010;19:655–8.

MIX
Papier aus verantwortungsvollen Quellen
Paper from responsible sources
FSC® C105338
FSC
www.fsc.org

If you have any concerns about our products,
you can contact us on
ProductSafety@springernature.com

In case Publisher is established outside the EU,
the EU authorized representative is:
Springer Nature Customer Service Center GmbH
Europaplatz 3, 69115 Heidelberg, Germany

Printed by Libri Plureos GmbH
in Hamburg, Germany